STRESS AND HEALTH

BIOBEHAVIOURAL PERSPECTIVES ON HEALTH AND DISEASE PREVENTION

From the perspective of behavioral science, the series examines current research, including clinical and policy implications, on health, illness prevention, and biomedical issues. The series is international in scope, and aims to address the culturally specifc, as well as the universally applicable.

Series Editor: Lydia R. Temoshok, PhD., Institute of Human Virology, Division of Clinical Research, University of Maryland Biotechnology Center, 725 West Lombard Street, Room N548, Baltimore, Maryland 21201, USA

Volume 1
Stress and Health: Research and Clinical Applications
*edited by Dianna T. Kenny, John G. Carlson, F. Joseph McGuigan
and John L. Sheppard*

STRESS AND HEALTH

Research and Clinical Applications

Edited by

Dianna T. Kenny,
The University of Sydney, Australia

John G. Carlson,
University of Hawaii, USA

F. Joseph McGuigan,
International Stress Management Association,
San Diego, USA

and

John L. Sheppard,
The University of Sydney, Australia

 harwood academic publishers
Australia • Canada • France • Germany • India • Japan
Luxembourg • Malaysia • The Netherlands • Russia • Singapore • Switzerland

Amsteldijk 166
1st Floor
1079 LH Amsterdam
The Netherlands

British Library Cataloguing in Publication Data

A catalogue record for this book is available from the British Library.

ISBN 90-5702-376-8
ISSN 1029-6697

Cover artwork: Harry Pettis, *Ce n'est pas Henri, at ce ne sont pas nuages*, 1997, Sir Joseph Banks High School
Cover design: Ray Howard

DEDICATION

This book is dedicated to:

Hans Jurgen Eysenck (1916–1997), who, as one of the preeminent and most influential psychologists of the twentieth century, indelibly stamped the fields of intelligence and personality with his own, and inspired students and fellow researchers with the synergistic effects of his undaunted integrity, ceaseless but joyous mental activity, and personal courage.

and

F. Joseph (Joe) McGuigan (1924–1998), who, as founder of the International Stress Management Association, through his science and his personal warmth and generosity, devoted himself to understanding and controlling stress in the lives of his fellow man.

CONTENTS

Section 4   Management of Stress and Stress-related Disorders

Section 5   Stress, Cardiovascular Disease and Cancer

Section 6 Occupational Stress

LIST OF CONTRIBUTORS

Billie Bonevski
World Health Organisation research
scholar
General Practice Research Group
Imperial Cancer Research Fund
Radcliffe Infirmary, Oxford,
England

Richard R. Bootzin
Professor, Department of
Psychology
University of Arizona
Tucson, AZ 85721, USA
Email: Bootzin@ccit.arizona.edu

Donald G. Byrne
Professor, Division of Psychology
Australian National University
Canberra, ACT 2600, Australia
Email: Don.Byrne@anu.edu.au

John G. Carlson
Professor and Director of Health
Psychology
Department of Psychology
University of Hawaii
Honolulu, HI 96822, USA
Email: JGCInc@aol.com

John Carmody
Associate Professor
School of Physiology and
Pharmacology
University of New South Wales
Sydney, Australia
Email: j.carmody@unsw.edu.au

Claude M. Chemtob
Director, Stress Disorders
Laboratory
National Center for PTSD
Pacific Islands Division
Department of Veterans' Affairs
Honolulu, Hawaii, USA

Jan van Dixhoorn
F van Blankenhelmstraat 10
Amersfoort, The Netherlands
Fax: (31) 33461 0502

⁺Hans J. Eysenck
Professor, Department of
Psychology
Institute of Psychiatry
University of London
Denmark Hill
London SE3 SAF, UK
Fax: 017 1274 9467

Jonathan Feldman
Rutgers University
New Brunswick, NJ 08903, USA

Nicholas Giardino
Rutgers University
New Brunswick, NJ 08903, USA

Richard Gevirtz
Professor in the Health Psychology
Program
California School of Professional
Psychology
San Diego, CA 92121, USA
Email: rgevirtz@mail.cspp.edu

Jack E. James
Professor, Department of
Psychology
National University of Ireland
Galway, Ireland
Email: j.james@ucg.ie

Dianna T. Kenny
Associate Professor in Psychology
Department of Behavioural Sciences
Faculty of Health Sciences
The University of Sydney
Lidcombe, NSW 2141, Australia
Email: d.kenny@cchs.usyd.edu.au

Jerome F. Kiffer
The Cleveland Clinic Foundation
9500 Euclid Avenue
Cleveland OH 44195, USA
Fax: 216 444 8994

Paul Lehrer
Professor pf Psychiatry University
of Medicine and Dentistry New
Jersey
Robert Wood Johnson Medical
School
671 HoesLane,
Piscataway, NJ 08854, USA
Email: lehrer@umdnj.edu

Lennart Levi
Stress Research
Karolinska Institute
PO Box 220
SE 171-77, Stockhom, Sweden
Email: lennart.levi@ipm.ki.se

Marita P. McCabe
Professor, School of Psychology
Deakin University
Burwood Campus
Burwood, VIC 3125, Australia
Email: maritam@deakin.edu.au

Joe Macdonald Wallace
14 Cranleigh Avenue
Rottingdean
Brighton, Sussex BN27GT, UK

†F. Joseph McGuigan
US International University
International Stress Management
Association
San Diego, CA 92131, USA

Michael G. McKee
Department of Psychiatry and
Psychology
Head, Section of General and
Health Psychology
The Cleveland
Clinic Foundation
9500 Euclid Avenue
Cleveland, OH 44195, USA
Fax: 216 444 8894

Eric Reheiser
US Center for Research in
Behavioral Medicine and Health
Psychology
Department of Psychology
4202 E. Fowler Ave./BEH339
University of South Florida
Tampa, FL 33620-8200, USA

John Reheiser
US Center for Research in
Behavioral Medicine and Health
Psychology
4202 E. Fowler Ave./BEH339
University of South Florida
Tampa, FL 33620-8200, USA

Paul Rosch
President, The American Institute of
Stress
124 Park Avenue
Yonkers, NY 10703, USA
Email: stress124@earthlink.net

Rob Sanson-Fisher
Director, Hunter Centre for Health
Advancement
Locked Mail Bag 10
Wallsend NSW 2287, Australia
Fax: (612) 4924 6211

John L. Sheppard
Associate Professor in Psychology
Department of Behavioural Sciences
Faculty of Health Sciences
The University of Sydney
East Street
Lidcombe NSW 2141, Australia
Email: j.sheppard@cchs.usyd.edu.au

Charles Spielberger
Distinguished Research Professor
and Director, Center for Research in
Behavioral Medicine and Health
Psychology
Department of Psychology
4202 E. Fowler Ave./BEH339
University of South Florida
Tampa, FL 33620-8200, USA
Email: spielber@luna.cas.usf.edu

Johann Stoyva
Professor, Behavioral Physiology
Institute
Bainbridge Island
WA, USA
Fax: (303) 440 7307

David Tracey
Professor and Head, School of
Anatomy
University of New South Wales
Sydney, NSW 2052, Australia
Email: d.tracey@unsw.edu.au

Peter R. Vagg
Center for Research in Behavioral
Medicine and Health Psychology
Department of Psychology
4202 E. Fowler Ave./BEH339
University of South Florida
Tampa, FL 33620-8200, USA

Judith Walker
Senior Lecturer, School of
Physiology and Pharmacology
University of New South Wales
Sydney NSW 2052, Australia
Email: judy.walker@unsw.edu.au

Anthony H. Winefield
Associate Professor, Department of
Psychology
The University of Adelaide
Adelaide, SA 5005, Australia
Email: awinefield@arts.adelaide.
edu.au

Chapter 1

BACKGROUND AND OVERVIEW TO STRESS AND HEALTH: Research and Clinical Applications

John G. Carlson, PhD

BACKGROUND: THE INTERNATIONAL CONGRESS

The papers in this volume were largely drawn from contributions to the First International Congress on Stress and Health, a five-day meeting held in Sydney, Australia, in October, 1996. This meeting was in effect an amalgamation of conferences of three organizations. The International Conferences on Biobehavioral Self-Regulation and Health (formerly sponsored by the Association for Applied Psychophysiology and Biofeedback) were a series of three meetings previously held in Honolulu, Hawaii (1987), Munich, Germany (1991), and Tokyo, Japan (1993), whose stated goal was mainly 'to show the convergence and potential integration of a wide variety of related research, theory, and self-regulation techniques for disorders that respond to nontraditional medical approaches—especially from the standpoint of long-term health and prevention' (Carlson & Seifert, 1991, p. 1). It was our attempt in these meetings to bring together world-class pure and applied science researchers in the field of self-regulation and health to foster the exchange of ideas. Two related collections of papers evolved from these meetings to augment this attempt (Carlson & Seifert, 1991; Carlson, Seifert & Birbaumer, 1994).

The second major contributer to the Sydney Congress was the Department of Behavioural Sciences, Faculty of Health Sciences, at the University of Sydney, which conducted 10 highly successful conferences in Australia—again with a series of edited conference proceedings to help ensure the broad impact of the presented papers (e.g. Sheppard, 1989). The Australia conference organizer, John Sheppard (the University of Sydney), spent several years in collaboration with the organizers of the International Conferences on Biobehavioral Self-Regulation and Health in an effort to bring these two conference structures together for the Congress. In turn, his hand-picked organizer and colleague, Dianna Kenny (the University of Sydney), was given primary responsibility for developing the Sydney Congress. The Australia connection brought with it a range of eminent researchers and practitioners in the field of behavioral medicine 'down under' that greatly complemented the international focus of the meeting.

The third organization who joined with us in sponsoring the now somewhat more complex infrastructure was the International Stress Management Association, primarily under the guidance of F. J. McGuigan (US International University). This organization, too, had sponsored several previous international meetings and brought to the emerging Congress a particular thematic structure for the Sydney meeting—that of stress and its relevance for health. In short, all three organizations made unique contributions to the First International Congress on Stress and Health, and their combined visions were stated in the goal of the meeting: '... to struggle with the profound puzzle of the relationships between mind and brain, psyche and soma, stress and health ... to be more clear about the stress formulations that we adopt, and to pay more attention to the ecological context' (Kenny, 1996).

The final result obtained by these organizers was an enormously successful Congress, with 314 presenters and over 420 attendees from countries representing all five continents. The theme of the meeting, 'Stress and Health', drew an impressive array of eminent speakers and topics, as is apparent in this volume.

OVERVIEW: THE CHAPTERS

The 31 contributers to this collection of chapters give a truly global perspective on the problems of stress and health. We have attempted to overcome difficulties due to cultural, linguistic, professional, and other differences among our contributers through organization, editing, and commentary, where appropriate. At the same time, we have striven to maintain the excitement and content of the individual contributions as closely as possible. The end result, we hope, is a balance of originality in the form of the chapters themselves with enough structure and editorial summary to help achieve a unified volume.

The sections of this book that separate the topical areas are mainly to help systematize the presentations. In some cases, however, it was difficult to decide the placement of a chapter—it may have fit as well in several categories. We will leave it to the reader to find the interconnections and relatedness among specific papers that best enhances their readability and value in fostering stress research and clinical applications.

BIOLOGICAL, PHYSIOLOGICAL AND PSYCHOLOGICAL BASES OF STRESS

Chapter 2.   The Role of Oscillations in Self-Regulation: Their Contribution to Homeostasis

In this profound discussion by Nicholas Giardino, Paul Lehrer and Jonathan Feldman, we are introduced to a significant expansion of the concept of homeostasis in stress responding. The authors begin with a challenge to the doctrine of homeostasis, that departures from a normal state are corrected to maintain a constant condition. Rather, they argue that constancy is not the natural condition, but instead that bodies adjust 'broadly' to stressful demands and are never constant—no steady-state ever exists for physiological systems, even when environmental demands are constant. Further, while excessive stress may be damaging, it appears that moderate stress actually enhances the performance of bodily systems.

The authors review examples of oscillatory behaviors in living systems ranging from cell-free biochemical reactions to single-celled and multicellular life forms, pointing out that oscillations occur at multiple levels in a system and temporally throughout a wide range of time. Oscillation and self-regulation may be two aspects of a single principle, such that a system may stabilize (self-regulate) only if it oscillates. In fact, life itself may be regarded as the continuous coordination of oscillations, as in, say, the coordination of complex cardiac behavior from respiratory, baroreflex, and thermoregulatory control systems. Conversely, disease may be an alteration in the coupling of oscillations, the stopping of oscillations, or transitions to different modes of control.

The authors go on to discuss the role of interactions between the parasympathetic and sympathetic divisions of the autonomic nervous system to make the point that the simplistic antagonistic relationship once thought to exist is somewhat more complex, involving both agonistic and antagonistic activity in both divisions. In the specific realm of heart rate variability, multiple levels of oscillatory control may lend themselves to better analysis through nonlinear mathematical models and may provide insight into the workings of the autonomic system more generally. The authors hypothesize that a general disruption of self-regulation of autonomic processes is what underlies a wide range of cardiovascular and related disorders. Further, chronic stress—such as demonstrated in tasks that require high mental load—may temporarily alter heart rate variability, suggesting that stress may lead to disease through disruption of normal oscillatory processes. Clinically, one implication of these arguments is that training designed to enhance system variability may improve a disease condition.

Thus, Giardino and his colleagues leave us with an intriguing alternative to the traditional concept of homeostasis—it is variability in bodily reactions that is healthy, not a steady state—and it is clinical interventions that promote oscillatory patterns and behavioral complexity that may facilitate a return to normal functioning and enhanced resistance to stress.

Chapter 3. The Physiology of Stress

Richard Gevirtz lends to this collection of views on stress and stress management a succinct review of current knowledge on the physiological mechanisms of stress, in particular the autonomic and endocrine/immune systems. Gevirtz maintains that the human stress response has evolved in man's social environment and is not sufficiently understood in terms of primitive reactions to life threatening events.

The autonomic nervous system (ANS), in particular the sympathetic division, plays a fundamental role in stress. This 'stress nervous system' appeared to early physiologists to activate the body generally for fight or flight, but this may be a simplistic conception. There does appear to be some general activation within the sympathetic system owing partly to the effects of ganglia that serve to direct communication within the system to several end point organs simultaneously, including to the adrenal medulla and its secretions of major neurotransmitters. Most post-ganglionic fibers in the sympathetic system are activated by norepinephrine and are said to be *adrenergic* Alpha adrenergic receptors produce such end organ responses as vasodilation and intestinal bladder sphincter contraction. Beta adrenergic receptors cause vasodilation, bronchodilation, and bladder relaxation, among other effects. Conversely, many but not all *cholinergically*-mediated responses of the parasympathetic system are in the opposite direction. Some opposite and some parallel effects of the sympathetic and parasympathetics systems are seen in the regulation of various responses.

The sympathetic and parasympathetic nervous systems probably interact a great deal more than initially believed. Also, both systems appear to have many distinct subsystems, such as, distinct vasoconstrictive mechanisms for muscles and cutaneous tissue within the sympathetic neurons, and polyvagal distinctions within the parasympathetic system for bodily maintenance as well as social and other functions.

In original formulations of the endocrine stress system it was postulated that following initial sympathetic activation, release of a hormone from the hypothalamus stimulates the pituitary gland to secrete adrenocorticotropin hormone (ACTH), activating the cortex of the adrenal glands. The result is the release of glucocorticoid hormones that appear to be broadly functional in ameliorating some of the initial effects of stress (such as inflammation) and providing 'buffers to protect tissue from their overreaction'. Thus, the effects may be construed as a form of 'counter regulation' for stress reactions.

Through these and other physical mechanisms during stress, a variety of systems are affected, including the immune system (which may be suppressed following stress); the respiratory system (which, as a result of hyperventilation can alter the body's acid/base balance in the direction of heightened alkalinity and produce multiple 'stress' symptoms); and the striate musculature (which may exhibit rapid muscle contractions plus 'splinting or bracing' reactions).

Finally, Gevirtz turns to a discussion of the consequences of prolonged activity within the physiological systems he has reviewed, for example, sympathetic pathways may be important in muscle pain via 'trigger points' within muscle tissue. In such instances, muscle relaxation training may be a benefit. Parasympathetic pathways may play a role in at least some kinds of asthma and other chest symptoms as well as panic. In these cases, training in slow, diaphragmatic breathing may improve treatment outcomes.

Chapter 4. Psychological Foundations of Stress and Coping: A Developmental Perspective

Dianna Kenny has provided in this chapter an important model for understanding the development of coping in childhood and implications for dealing with stress in adulthood. Coping is defined as attaining, conserving, and minimally utilizing one's resources throughout life. Attachment, developmental, and coping experiences throughout the lifespan manifest themselves in the individual's personality and psychopathology in ways that reduce or enhance risk due to stress. Attachment for the child—in the form of relationships to parents or other caregivers—is primary as a resource upon which the development of other resources depends. The author attempts to integrate extant theories of stress and coping, development, attachment, personality, and psychopathology in this comprehensive model for understanding the processes of coping. Relationships that have been observed between stress and illness, summarized in a later section, underscore the importance of understanding the development of successful coping behaviors.

Resource models of stress and coping have emphasized multiple sources of physical, social, energy, and personal resources as critical. Kenny's model, by contrast, argues that attachment processes subsume resource processes. A second class of variables in current vogue in models of coping are broadly construed as forms of social support. In the author's view, social support takes the form of the affective quality of object representations due to early attachments. Further, a lack of social support may foretell a loss of resources (failure of coping).

Consistent with the notion of coping as a matter of resource maintenance or loss, the process of development itself has been conceptualized by some as an 'interchange' of gains and losses (growth and decline) throughout the lifespan. Another important developmental construct from Dr Kenny's perspective is that of formal operational thinking in some adolescents, which may, in turn, lead to specialization (say, an interest in music or design) and the accrual of additional resources that may aid in coping. In the extreme, combined with other vulnerabilities, formal operations may also eventuate in the ultimate failure of coping at this stage—adolescent suicide. Vulnerabilities may stem, in part, from faulty initial attachments.

Successful attachments in the child may underlie competent coping (resilience) for a number of reasons. One, a strong sense of safety may make it possible for the child to interact with the environment and develop a wide array of competencies through successful experiences. Two, evidence supports a strong relationship between very early attachment and subsequent cognitive development. Similarly, three, successful early attachment appears to be related to the later development of social competence.

Finally, Kenny reviews several approaches to the characterization of coping, including the Folkman & Lazarus attempt to categorize forms of coping in terms of efforts that are emotion-focused (such as, escape and avoidance) and those that are problem-focused (including direct confrontation). Kenny concludes that such concepts oversimplify the much more complex phenomena of coping —for example, it is probably the case that all coping involves both problem- and emotion-focused strategies— and that further efforts in this area may be best guided by a clinical-empirical approach to attachment and object relations in children.

HEALTH CONSEQUENCES OF STRESS

Chapter 5.   Chronic Pain—Neural Basis and Interactions with Stress

This chapter by David Tracey, John S. Walker, and Judith Carmody effectively dispels the common myth that chronic pain is 'all in the head' by giving us a resumé of current knowledge concerning the physical aspects of chronic pain. Tracey and his colleagues present some fascinating connections between stress and chronic pain that have immediate implications for therapeutic interventions.

While the experience of acute pain may stop when nociceptive stimulation due to a painful stimulus comes to an end, chronic pain continues beyond any useful period in terms of warning or recuperation. Chronic pain may involve both peripheral and central mechanisms that cause hyperalgesia (greater than normal sensitivity to pain stimuli) and allodynia (pain experiences due to otherwise innocuous stimuli). Tracey et al. provide insight into the sensitization of nociceptors through inflammatory mediators. Essentially the idea is that injury results in the recruitment of immune cells that, in turn, release bradykinin, other substances that are known to sensitize nociceptive afferents. The mechanism for sensitization through inflammatory mediators is an influx of ions into the neuron which heightens the excitability of the nociceptor. Another physical mechanism for chronic pain may be through upregulation of specific neurotransmitters when there is tissue damage or arthritis, specifically neuropeptides. Such neuromodulators increase the responsiveness of spinal neurons that respond to noxious stimulation.

From the standpoint of central mechanisms for chronic pain, another likely candidate for problems in the spinal cord are the WDR neurons. These neurons are responsive to both noxious and innocuous stimuli and are probably functional in conscious awareness of pain. Finally, the involvement of certain brain structures in chronic pain is suggested. There is even some suggestion that the somatosensory cortex may be reorganized in sufferers of chronic back pain.

While there are thus compelling indications for complex physical bases for chronic pain, additional complications are posed by the apparent role of stress in pain modulation. There is animal evidence for both opioid and non-opioid analgesia in stress, the former owing to mild stress (such as brief exercise) and the latter to more severe stress. The release of beta-endorphin along with ACTH in the classical pathway for stressful stimulation has a probable role in these effects. Conversely, there is evidence that stress in some forms (akin to anxiety) can also exacerbate pain so, again, the mechanisms are by no means simple ones. At the human level, there is evidence to indicate that chronic pain causes stress. In the latter case, post-traumatic stress disorder may arise out of some forms of acute pain (e.g. childbirth) and may also be correlated with chronic pain reports. Thus, therapeutic interventions for stress, such as, systematic desensitization and relaxation training, may be implicated as well for treatment of chronic pain. There is a possibility that a common pathway for therapeutic effects may be the activation of endogenous opioids. Alternatively, antidepressants may be effective. In short, given the complex nature of pain mechanisms, complex interventions including behavioral therapies as well as pharmacological approaches may be optimal.

Chapter 6. Stress, Senescence, and Longevity: How are They Connected

In this readable and stimulating essay, Paul Rosch first reminds us of a number of physical, cognitive, and emotional changes that are associated with aging, and also that there are large individual differences in which specific changes and the degree of change that can be expected. Both genetic and environmental factors contribute to the large variations in susceptibility to the inevitable consequences of aging.

Selye suggested that stress refers to 'the rate of wear and tear on the body', an idea that is close to Rosch's notions concerning biologic aging, and a definition that ties the concepts of aging and stress together in a useful way.

Some persons age biologically very rapidly—as in sufferers of

Hutchinson-Gilford Syndrome, On the other hand, authenticated records report individuals and groups who have survived to ages well over 100 years. Rosch suggests that very low levels of stress in some ancient and other not so ancient civilizations may be an anti-aging factor. Besides exceptional health in old age, the absence of cancer in certain populations from India to the Arctic Circle has impressed observers.

Rosch points out that many of the features of old age—gray hair, wrinkles, atheroslerosis—owe to oxidative stress. This is a process whereby some number of oxygen molecules, termed 'free radicals', are not utilized normally by body cells. Rather, these molecules latch onto and destroy cell membranes, oxidize cholesterol, DNA, and other material, and participate in chain reactions with similar effects. A particular problem may be the oxidation of low density lipoproteins, causing these molecules to attract other cells and release substances that increase smooth muscle cell buildup in the arterial walls. It appears that emotional stress may enhance this process dramatically. Conversely, there are a number of positive outcomes that may be attributable to low caloric intake and to at least moderate intake of a number of vitamins and other substances that tend to supply electrons that stabilize free radicals, including melatonin and vitamins C, E, and beta carotene, among others.

In Rosch's view, not enough is known regarding the role of emotional stress in free radical production, although there is evidence to relate stress to a number of destructive processes similar to those in aging. Thus, stress reduction may be another way to indirectly combat the effects of oxidation in the aging process.

Chapter 7.   Stress and Sexual Function

In this interesting chapter, Marita McCabe has reviewed both animal and human literature dealing with the role of stress in sexual function. Primate research has indicated that subordinate males show lower testosterone levels and less sexual activity than higher ranking males. It is possible that one direction for these effects is that stress due to being in a nondominant position results in lowered testosterone and, in turn, less sexual behavior. With human males, the situation is more complex. For instance, testosterone injections may improve ejaculatory function without affecting sexual desire or frequency of sex, among other indicators. Social variables probably exert a range of influences on the male sexual response. Social stress (e.g. belief that one is not attractive to females) may impair functioning, as may being unemployed, at least as measured by the erectile response. On the other hand, social support in the form of a wife's behavior may have moderating effects. Daily hassles may actually enhance sexual desire (but not behavior), possibly through a misinterpretation of the source of physiological arousal produced by the hassles.

In the absence of research, it has been suggested that the variables that control female sexual behavior are the same as for men. With regard to social stress among primates, McCabe points out that clear dominance hierarchies are not so identifiable among females, so it is more difficult to determine effects of social stress. Subordinate females remain insensitive to hormones that induce ovulation so that more dominant females appear to be more sexually active and reproduce more often. In the case of human females, unemployment does not appear to affect sexual activity (orgasms) as it does in males, but the effects of other forms of social stress are not known.

Anxiety has been identified as a major inhibitory factor in sexuality owing to changes in subjective appraisal of sexual desire based on physiological changes. In males, sexual anxiety owing to other negative emotions in sexual situations, e.g. guilt, fear, anger—may impair aspects of the sexual response. General anxiety is generally found to produce inhibitory effects on the sexually dysfunctional male but enhance sexual responses in functional males. In females, who are sexually functional, women, it appears that the enhanced physiological arousal in stress may be interpreted as enhanced sexual desire, with a positive impact on sexual experience. By contrast, sexually dysfunctional women may interpret enhanced physiological arousal negatively, resulting in a decrease in their subjective sexual arousal.

Among the implications of these data for treatment is that sexually dysfunctional males should be encouraged to perform under low stress/anxiety conditions. By contrast, there may be advantages in altering the subjective interpretation of heightened sexuality in both functional and dysfunctional women to emphasize the positive aspects of sexual arousal.

MANAGEMENT OF STRESS AND STRESS-RELATED DISORDERS

Chapter 8.   Why Might Stress Management Methods be Effective?

In this chapter, F. J. McGuigan outlines his model for developing stress controlling behavior based on Edmund Jacobson's technique of Progressive Relaxation. McGuigan begins by reviewing some types of situations to exemplify variables that may be stressful—work overload in an office, anticipating a painful medical procedure, and even dreams at night. In all these cases, an individual needs to be able to exert control over behavior in order to prevent reflexive stress reactions. Two means for controlling behavior are through control over the environment—such as restructuring the workplace or reorganizing a schedule to prevent work overload—and through more direct behavioral self-control. The latter may involve arousal reduction methods (e.g. relaxation) or cognitive restructuring (e.g. altering the perception of personal stressors).

McGuigan points out that there are both nonspecific and specific variables to be understood in the processes of behavioral control, variables that are common to many methods and those unique to a specific method, respectively. Among the former variables, suggestion is inherent in virtually all efforts to consciously manage stress. McGuigan suggests, however, that there may be a number of reasons to minimize suggestion in the process of relaxation. For example, suggestion may lead a person to think that muscles are truly relaxed when they are not. A second nonspecific stress management variable is the reduction of stimulation from the external environment. Again, however, favorable effects may be only temporary and lack generalization across everyday situations. Among specific variables for behavioral self-control are unique behavioral acts designed to calm oneself—specific forms of deep breathing, reciting a mantra, and giving self-instructions to change the environment. A problem is learning how to *implement* one's insight into stress management methods.

We may cultivate the 'muscle sense' and implement muscular control by successively contracting and relaxing subtle striated muscles, as in Jacobson's method of Progressive Relaxation. One feature of this approach is the method of Diminishing Tensions, in which the person systematically decreases the amplitude of a muscle contraction until it is very slight and becomes covert.

The next step in developing behavioral control is to 'program behavior' that controls specific desired responses, a problem of volition. McGuigan, like Jacobson, theorizes that covert activities of the speech muscles (self-instruction) and eye muscles (visual imagery) may provide the controlling stimuli for subsequent behavior. Accordingly, effective behavior control in stressful situations involves reducing bodily arousal in order to be better aware of covert motor activity. Then, self-instruction will become more salient and effective in providing the discriminative stimuli for the desired, stress-controlling response.

Chapter 9. Biofeedback and Stress

This readable chapter by Michael McKee and Jerome Kiffer outlines the role of biofeedback and applied psychophysiology in the assessment and treatment of stress-related disorders. Biofeedback is defined by the authors as the use of instruments that detect and display biological activity to enable learning of control over bodily processes. Early research and more recent outcome studies in this area suggest the usefulness of biofeedback in enabling control over a variety of 'involuntary' processes.

The most common forms of biofeedback include electromyographic (EMG) training that involves monitoring and display (feedback) of muscle potentials, especially in the treatment of tension headache, muscle re-education, and muscle relaxation training; skin temperature biofeedback involving monitoring of peripheral temperature usually in the extremities (especially the hands), as used in the treatment of Raynaud's disease and in general relaxation training; respiratory biofeedback through capnometry (measurement of CO_2 or breathing functions), sometimes useful in asthma and hyperventilation; and neurofeedback for electroencephalograpic (EEG) activity of the brain, potentially useful in the treatment of attention deficit hyperactivity disorder.

McKee and Kiffer outline two models for biofeedback training, the first in which the goal is to learn a specific bodily response, and the second in which the goal is control over physiological arousal as an aid for managing stress-related responses. Specific responses that have been shown to respond to biofeedback training include vasospastic symptoms of Raynaud's disease, fecal incontinence, neuromuscular disorders in the rehabilitation setting, and certain musculoskeletal pain symptoms. Training for low arousal has been used in the arena of anxiety disorders, performance disorders, and a host of stress-related physiological symptoms and usually targets symptoms that vary with autonomic arousal. Biofeedback is often used in conjunction with various forms of stress management and psychotherapy to enhance its range of effects, rendering it difficult to isolate the contribution of biofeedback to the therapeutic package. Biofeedback patients may develop greater awareness of bodily processes, better attention to early signs of stress responding, and changes in patterns of thinking, feeling, and acting that facilitate stress control. On the positive side, patient satisfaction with biofeedback may be high in terms of helpfulness, problem understanding, and usefulness of strategy for dealing with stress.

The authors then turn to applications of biofeedback with several stress-related disorders including hypertension, insomnia, temporomandibular disorders, and headaches. Biofeedback appears to be gaining greater acceptance among providers and patients as one part of multimodal treatment packages but outcome research is not keeping pace with this development.

Chapter 10. Stress Management: What Can We Learn from the Meditative Disciplines?

Johann Stoyva reviews two major meditative approaches in this interesting chapter, namely the Vipassana (mindfulness) tradition and the Zen tradition. In turn, Stoyva argues that three practices derived from these traditions may be used as ways to cope with adverse stress reactions: Relaxed, abdominal breathing (Vipassana), used to reduce anxiety; paying quiet attention to respiratory sensations (Zen), which may be helpful in dealing with common types of insomnia; and task absorption (Vipassana), that may also reduce anxiety as well as excessive rumination.

Relaxed, abdominal breathing is achieved in a sitting position, with a 'mental-quieting device' that consists of attending to the muscle movements that accompany the rise and fall of the abdomen. The technique is easily described, easily learned, and has the advantage that it can be used in an anxiety producing situation. For about half of a group of medical students, Stoyva found that abdominal breathing—as an adjunct to systematic desensitization for performance anxiety—was credited by the students with helping them deal with anxiety arousing situations. Several more students reported that the exercise enabled them to reduce background levels of tension and anticipatory   anxiety.

The second practice, paying quiet attention to sensations that accompany respiration, is termed the 'Mental Quieting Exercise'. It may help to reduce anxiety-related thought as well as 'mental chatter' that may relate to insomnia. This practice differs from the first in the focus of attention—on the respiratory tract rather than the muscles used in breathing. A shaping technique may also be useful in which attention is first on only several breaths, later on additional breaths. Stoyva suggests some variations on the method for insomnia, including some additional behavioral interventions.

The third practice, Mindfulness, is defined as being fully aware of what is going on in one's surroundings, including sensory and social stimuli, as well as internal cues (feelings, thoughts, etc.) while one is engaged in other activities. 'One gently lets go of each thought that occurs, then notes what comes up next on the "mental screen" ' (p. 11). The result may be total absorption in the present task or situation, plus an awareness of being absorbed. In a recent study reported by Stoyva, mindfulness techniques significantly reduced feelings of depression, anger, and mood disturbance in women walkers by comparison with walkers not using mindfulness methods. Mindfulness might also counter effects of excessive rumination in stress responding, the tendency to focus on 'how badly we feel' rather than taking action to change.

Chapter 11. Behaviour Change Following Affect Shift: A Model for the Treatment of Stress Disorders

This chapter by John Sheppard offers a theoretical perspective on the treatment of stress disorders by proposing a visuo-cognitive affect shift model derived from examining commonalities in eight therapies. The therapies include psychoanalysis, cognitive behaviour therapy, religious practices in the East, theories of brain activity, and theories of information processing. Specifically, the therapies are eye movement desensitization and reprocessing -EMDR (Shapiro), autogenic neutralization (Luthe), a Buddhist practice from Tibet of 100,000 prostrations, a phenomenon from Indian religious traditions—the kundalini, EEG biofeedback (Peniston), abreaction in psychoanalysis (Freud), neurolinguistic programming (the Bandlers, the Andreas, and Grinder), and anxiety management training (Suinn). Sheppard noticed all these approaches to the management of stress disorders had features in common, despite their considerable differences in technique and theoretical orientation.

All these therapies proceed in a sequential pattern of visualization and imagery of memories in relaxation, a repetitive meditative aspect, cognitive working of material, emotional catharsis with a numbing- neutralization-desensitization, moving from negative to positive emotions, and positive action. The preparation phase consists of repetitive meditative visualization and imagery applied to memories of trauma, while practising relaxation. This is carried out in a healing setting where the person can feel safe in a supportive atmosphere. The preparation phase leads in to a cognitive working phase and this is followed by a phase of emotional arousal and discharge. Between these phases the model allows for a feedback loop whereby emotional discharge may result in further cognitive processing. After emotional catharsis there is a shift from previously negative emotions to their more positive counterparts, and from this there ensues a final phase of behavioural mastery.

Chapter 12. Stress Management in Health Education

J. Macdonald-Wallace gives us some glimpses into his own history as an educator in the field of stress management in this chapter, as well as some insight regarding the important role of Edmund Jacobson in shaping the thought and methods that went into the author's first courses on managing stress.

Beginning with attempts to enhance performance by teaching his students to be more relaxed, the author advanced into other applications. It is Jacobson who apparently provided much of the material for the author's first course in 'stress management for education'. This evolved over time into a course on health education and stress in the individual, the term 'stress management' not having been readily accepted at academic levels even as late as the 1960s.

Then, the idea emerged in the field that stress could be managed therapeutically and a wide range of therapists, many of them self-styled, began to offer a host of relatively unresearched techniques, providing a 'stumbling block' to the development of methods for managing stress. In Macdonald-Wallace's view, biological stress is not a condition requiring 'cure'. Managing stress, on the other hand, may be enhanced through methods suggested in Jacobson's view of muscular 'tension control'. Additional training designed to enhance awareness of the involvement of covert speech and imaginal processes may also be helpful, albeit difficult.

MacDonald-Wallace concludes his paper with the arguable suggestion that research or one-on-one clinical training are not effective ways to teach the understanding of stress, its relationship to health, and the management of stress. Stress management, he believes is best brought to large numbers of people through public education, from elementary school through universities.

Chapter 13. Stress Management and Prevention on a European Community Level: Options and Obstacles

This chapter by Lennart Levi offers a very useful update on stress management and stress prevention in Europe, particularly in the workplace. In a recent large study of worksite stress, it has been reported that 30% of workers regard their health to be at risk due to work, 30% report that their work is repetitive, and about 17–20% regard their work as a source of continual pressure due to time. In response to increasing recognition of work stress as a growing threat in the labor market, the World Health Organization and International Labor Organization joined forces in the 1980s to develop programs to review the role of psychosocial factors in this area. A related report identified such variables as worktime, management practices, and technological changes and other actions to be taken. A multidisciplinary approach and national and international level interventions were encouraged.

A practical outcome of a conference of the European Foundation for the Improvement of Living and Working Conditions in 1993 was a guide for small and medium size businesses in which stress concepts are defined, causes and consequences of work stress are identified, and high risk populations are designated. Increasing work stress is cited as a problem for workers and companies, prevention is emphasized, and positive outcomes in terms of change and worker motivation are cited.

Principles of stress prevention put forth by the European Union include evaluating, combating, and avoiding risks, adapting work to the individual, and developing comprehensive prevention policies. In practice, stress management/prevention has begun to emphasize the person-environment fit. For example, in a company in Sweden, an intervention for excessive workplace stress was begun that increased the variety of work tasks through rotation, increased understanding of the nature of production links, and focused on job enrichment. Workers were also solicited for suggested improvements and encouraged to try them out. The outcome was a large decrease in personnel turnover and sick leave absenteeism, and a large increase in productivity.

The World Health Organization proposes criteria for setting goals for action with regard to stress management and prevention: Public health significance must be determined; level of public awareness must be established; modifiability of the problem by available means must be specified; economic, social, and ethical costs of action/inaction must be weighed; A target group and agent of change must be identified.

Some difficulties and constraints when attempting to effect preventive action with regard to stress management and prevention include constraints common to health services, constraints in the field of health, and separation of the health disciplines from one another.

Lastly, a number of 'supporting activities' are needed to ensure that negative psychosocial conditions that affect worker health are impacted: Occupational health workers and investigators need to be motivated and trained and terminology and methods need to be developed. Levi is optimistic that such changes are being made, not only in Europe but also in the United States.

Chapter 14. Cognitive-Behavioral Treatment of Insomnia: Knitting up the Ravell'd Sleave of Care

In this fascinating and exceptionally useful chapter by Richard Bootzin, we are updated on cognitive-behavioral research on one of the more common and problematic conditions of humankind, insomnia. The author makes the point early that short-term psychological treatments specifically targeting the disorder are supported by a large body of outcome studies, whereas general psychotherapy and psychodynamic approaches have failed to show effectiveness in the area of sleep disturbance. This chapter provides a summary of a number of effective methods for intervention.

The author first reviews the causes of sleep disturbance including substances used as sleep aids, problems with biological rhythms, physical and psychological problems, the sleep environment, and sleep habits. Among substances that may cause difficulties Bootzin includes the hypnotics which, he argues, may best be prescribed for short terms, in low doses, intermittently, and with a period of gradual withdrawal. There may be some advantages to be shown in the use of melatonin by the elderly but, as with sedative/hypnotics, the general use of melatonin over the long term is not supported by data. Biological rhythm difficulties include those due to jet lag, shift-work schedules, aging, and seasonal light changes. Such difficulties can be alleviated by timed bright light exposure and, in the case of changing work schedules, stress coping methods, sleep hygiene information, and family counseling. Bootzin provides updates on methods for treatment of a variety of physical disorders that may impair sleep, including sleep apneas, muscular disorders of the limbs, pain, and Alzheimer's disease. While some sleep hygiene methods and symptom-specific devices may help in the case of obstructive sleep apnea, for most physical disorders, specific pharmacological interventions may be required as sleep aids. Psychological conditions that exacerbate sleep may include stress in general and depression in particular. The author recommends specific attention to each of the psychological problems that accompany sleep disturbance on the assumption that there may not be generalization of treatment effects from one problem to another. Finally, among the causes for sleep disturbance Bootzin reviews aspects of the sleeper's environment and behaviors that may be problematic. In the former case, noise levels may be a particular issue. In the latter case, a variety of behaviors that exacerbate sleep disturbance may include using the bed for activities that heighten physiological arousal, using bedtime for excessive rumination regarding daytime problems, and failure to maintain a consistent sleep schedule.

Bootzin then carefully reviews cognitive-behavioral approaches to the problems of insomnia. Such approaches include adequate assessment, sleep hygiene education, stimulus control, sleep restriction, relaxation and related methods, and cognitive therapy. Multicomponent approaches that combine several of the cognitive-behavioral methods have been shown to be more effective than a single type of intervention. By contrast, the evidence is not clear as to whether pharmacological interventions can be effectively combined with behavioral therapies to treat insomnia, although the latter may help alleviate some of the negative effects on sleep due to withdrawal from medication. It does appear that patients are more positive regarding nonpharmacological approaches, that long-term gains may be maximized using cognitive-behavioral approaches alone, and that such treatments may be most effective in patients who do not use sleep medications.

Chapter 15. Cognitive-Behavioral Theory, Research and Treatment of Trauma Disorders

This chapter by John Carlson and Claude Chemtob comprehensively reviews the authors' extensive research program in the area of post-traumatic stress disorder (PTSD)—mainly in populations of combat veterans and children traumatized by a major hurricane. The authors outline their cognitive-behavioral model of stress that maintains that a challenge to the a person's physical integrity activates the 'survival system', a behavioral, physiological, and cognitive cluster of reactions designed to support biological systems in the face of severe threat. Further, within the survival system, a number of subsystems, including early warning (vigilance), defense, and arousal are potentially activated, resulting in pervasive effects of trauma on the individual, including difficulties in the regulation of both activation and inhibition of each of the component subsystems.

The implications of this model for treatment are several, including that each of the subsystems of the survival mode of trauma reaction may require specific treatment protocols that may not fully generalize to other reactions. The model is consistent with several modes of therapy, in particular those that include attention to memory processes as well as to physiological and behavioral reactions. Some forms of desensitization training may be particularly helpful, including 'eye movement desensitization and reprocessing' (EMDR). In this method, a patient is asked to hold in mind images relevant to traumatic experiences along with related bodily sensations and negative cognitive statements (such as, 'I am out of control') while tracking a therapist's hand back and forth for a short period of time. Then, the patient is asked to review immediate experiences.

The authors first review a series of experimental studies designed to provide additional insight into their multidimensional model of trauma, and then proceed to discuss several major controlled outcome studies using cognitive-behavioral interventions. In one manipulation, combat veterans with PTSD manifesting anger symptoms were randomly assigned to a multimodal anger treatment protocol or maintained in a group that received routine clinical care. Veterans receiving therapy showed reduced anger and anxiety levels on several scales and increased anger control. In a second study involving EMDR training with several groups of combat veterans presenting with PTSD, it was demonstrated that EMDR produced clinically significant effects along several parameters of the disorder, including structured interview measures of PTSD, by comparison with control and alternative treatment groups. In a later study with a group of children with severe signs of PTSD that had been shown not to be tractable to prior therapy, similar positive effects of EMDR were obtained.

This systematic attempt to integrate experimental and clinical approaches to trauma disorders demonstrates the usefulness of a systematic multimodal approach to the effects of trauma on the individual.

STRESS, CARDIOVASCULAR DISEASE, AND CANCER

Chapter 16. Personality as a Risk Factor in Cancer and Coronary Heart Disease

Hans Eysenck has bequeathed to us in this fascinating discussion a review of a broad array of recent studies that have attempted to demonstrate the role of personality factors in cancer and coronary heart disease. Eysenck points out that for the greater part of this century, the medical establishment has been skeptical especially of the idea that there is a cancer-prone personality. But, in Eysenck's view, beginning in the 1950s research began to accumulate that has tended to support the role of certain personality variables in cancer and a different set of variables in coronary heart disease.

Eysenck outlines theories of the cancer-prone personality (C-type) and the coronary heart disease (CHD) prone personality (A-type) that characterize the former as unassertive, harmony-seeking, unable to express emotions, and with difficulties in coping that may lead to helplessness and depression; the latter is especially likely to manifest easily-aroused feelings of anger, hostility, and aggression. The evidence relative to these theories is presented in the form of studies that compare cases with controls, prospective studies, and studies involving interventions designed to alter C-type and A-type characteristics, noting effects on mortality.

Among case-control studies, Eysenck cites several that showed a 6 to 1 difference in development of cancer between low scorers on Eysenck's neuroticism scale (emotion repressors/deniers) and those with high scores. Moreover, cancer-prone persons who smoked were even more likely to develop cancer (a synergistic effect). Using inventories to measure specific disease-related traits as well as disease-prone (or healthy) 'types', Grossarth-Maticek independently conducted research in this area demonstrating, in part, the importance of establishing 'trust' and providing explanations of test items when distinguishing between cancer-prone and CHD-prone individuals. Careful work by Fernandez-Ballesteros and her colleagues have also shown that breast cancer patients are higher on a scale for rational/ emotional defensiveness and another for need for harmony compared with healthy women.

Among prospective studies, Eysenck and Grossarth-Maticek identified the characteristic, 'self-regulation', with such positive attributes as self-acceptance, purpose in life, and autonomy, and showed positive correlations with 'health' as measured generally. Other studies by the latter researcher followed for 30 years large number of persons classified by personality testing as cancer-prone, CHD-prone, and healthy. Grossarth-Maticek's model accurately predicted significant percentages of cancer and CHD victims.

Finally, among international studies, those by Grossarth-Maticek demonstrating the effectiveness of interventions for cancer and CHD are cited to help support a causative link between personality variables and disease. In particular, a method called 'autonomy training' is reviewed, a technique designed to shift personality characteristics away from the C-type and A-type to healthier features.

Chapter 17. Psychosocial Aspects of Cancer Control

In this constructive chapter, Rob Sanson-Fisher and B. Bonevski discuss a number of ways in which psychosocial outcomes for cancer patients can be improved. Despite treatment advances in some areas, it is likely that cancer will increase in the next 25 years. In the arena of tertiary care (minimizing the impact of the disease), in particular, it is becoming increasingly important to focus on minimization of the psychosocial impact of cancer and its treatments. However, a search by the authors revealed that less than 20% of related literature was devoted to studies evaluating the effectiveness of psychosocial interventions.

Measuring instruments in this area should include valid and reliable assessment of anxiety and depression, quality of life, and patient needs/satisfaction with care. Measures should focus on self-reports and take the patient's perspectives on psychosocial outcomes into account.

Establishing a baseline for burden of suffering is necessary before a system is changed to allow for evaluation of impact. Considerable research has provided evidence of the psychosocial morbidity experienced by cancer patients, including anxiety and depression. Patients also report needs for more information (e.g. for test results), and for more services and resources.

Quality assurance with regard to technical aspects of cancer care is less of a problem than patient satisfaction with regard to psychosocial aspects of their care (e.g. communication and information). There is evidence that physicians are not accurately detecting patients with high psychological and emotional distress relative to their cancer or treatment.

With respect to the cost-effectiveness of psychosocial interventions, In the absence of data, an effort was made by the first author and a colleague to develop guidelines for breaking 'bad news' to a patient, which led to the discovery of some large discrepancies between patients and physicians in their views of the importance of different guidelines. Research using randomized controlled trials in this area is needed.

Psychosocial data from cancer patients can provide a basis for feedback for providers that will help them identify groups needing enhanced care, and identify areas of treatment or care that may require improvement.

Finally, specific training is needed designed to teach skills to providers suggested by the feedback they receive. Interactional skills are effectively taught through providing a rationale, rehearsal, practice, and feedback.

Chapter 18. Caffeine and Stress

In this unique review, Jack James discusses the role of caffeine, both in terms of increased usage during stress and on the effects of caffeine in terms of bodily and psychological reactions. Of all psychoactive substances, caffeine is the most used, reaching 80 percent of the world's population every day, mainly by way of tea and coffee. The substance is absorbed into the body rapidly and thoroughly, and exerts its effects by way of blockage of adenosine receptors during most of the waking hours. Chronic use causes physical dependence and a variety of withdrawal symptoms.

Cardiovascular effects due to caffeine ingestion are notable. In particular, substantial blood pressure increases due to 'drug challenge' (relatively large amounts), even in habitual users, have been obtained in a number of studies. Research challenges the notion that habitual use produces complete cardiovascular tolerance. The implications of these data are that caffeine may be a contributor to cardiovascular disease owing to its pressor effects.

There may also be a synergistic effect of caffeine and stress. The ingestion of large amounts of caffeine when under stress may exacerbate symptoms, in some documented cases. The evidence with respect to anxiety is unclear, in part because people appear to ingest more caffeine when under stress, for reasons unknown. In one study by the author, increased anxiety in a group of psychiatric patients was found among very heavy.

The relationship between caffeine and cognitive effects has been studied in the area of insomnia, again yielding inconsistent support. Studies in which caffeine is consumed prior to sleep in a laboratory setting generally show disruptive effects especially in terms of sleep onset. James suggests that attention should be given to the relationship between patterns of caffeine consumption and sleep onset, since most people ingest less coffee prior to bedtime.

There have been very few studies of the impact of caffeine on children, with some evidence of emotional and attentional effects in 'low consumers' and some anxiety effects in 'high consumers' undergoing withdrawal. More important may be the effects of caffeine on neonates.

When caffeine use is treated, a fading technique may be useful. A problem with assessment of caffeine use during treatment also noted with other drugs is reliance on self report and a lack of quantitative bioanalytic analyses. Overall, the dearth of research in the area of caffeine effects is reason enough for more attention to adverse effects of this potentially powerful stimulant.

Chapter 19. Implementation of Relaxation Therapy within a Cardiac Rehabilitation Setting

Jan van Dixhoorn makes the point early in this useful chapter that relaxation instruction is seldom a distinctive part of cardiac rehabilitation methods, although it may be one component of a patient exercise or education program. On the other hand, relaxation has been shown to have applications to numerous other health problems, and it may have potential for helping cardiac patients deal with recovery.

A review of uncontrolled studies relating autogenic training, relaxation, and a form of meditation suggest positive effects on several indicators of cardiovascular response. Among controlled studies, only two investigated effects of relaxation training by itself, while the remainder demonstrated added effects to other rehabilitation methods. A particularly optimistic result of prior research using relaxation training is that outcome variables demonstrate both physiological-medical and psychological effects. A study by the author and his colleagues have also shown significant reductions of cardiac events and rehospitalizations after five years in patients given relaxation instruction.

Psychosocial interventions in cardiac patients often include relaxation training. A meta-analysis of 12 studies in this area showed impressive reductions of cardiac mortality (51%), but Dixhoorn points out that such interventions are often complex and perhaps not cost-efficient for all patients. Moreover, the additional effects of psychosocial programs beyond exercise has not been established.

To implement a relaxation program for the cardiac patient, Dixhoorn recommends incorporating it into an exercise component, but to be prepared to limit exercise as necessary and to tailor the program to individual patient needs. He also recommends starting with a short training period. Further, it is proposed that relaxation classes be offered to all patients at the start of rehabilitation, that it be a distinctive method by itself.

Finally, Dixhoorn offers several general rules for instructing relaxation in cardiac patients that be believes apply irrespective of the specific technique that is applied.

OCCUPATIONAL STRESS

Chapter 20. Occupational Stress: Reflections on theory and practice

In this timely discussion, Dianna Kenny reviews several current models of occupational stress and proposes a treatment intervention based on a systemic approach. Kenny begins with a critique of the predominant, medical model for occupational stress in which the focus is directed at the individual worker, rather than on modifying the structure of the workplace in the direction of creating more healthy working environments. In this model, personality factors are identified as key to understanding occupational stress. Kenny maintains that empirical support for the role of personality characteristics in moderating stress is mixed. Moreover, it is not clear that manipulating personality will lead to improvement without changes in extrinsic such as relationships at work, career role, and organizational structure. Related interventions including counseling, and stress management again emphasize the individual as the focus for intervention and responsibility.

By contrast, sociological models have countered that the social organization of work is the primary determinant of stress in the workplace. The causes of occupational illness and distress lie in power structures, safety/productivity conflicts, the division of labor, industrial relations, and related factors. Despite the apparent emphasis on factors endemic to the organization, however, traditional solutions are still focused on the individual.

Systemic theories or social systems theories of occupational stress refer to a number of models, including the Demand-Control theories, Dynamic Equilibrium theory, and General Systems Theory and Cybernetics, all of which have the capacity to address current shortcomings in the conceptualisation of occupational stress and its management. The latter models are based on similar theoretical principles. In Dynamic Equilibrium Theory, the focus is on the system as a whole, rather than on its component parts. In this model, occupational stress arises when there is either individual or organizational change that creates disequilibrium between the worker's personal values and those of the organization. The Cybernetics model emphasizes feedback as the process by which homeostatic adjustments are made when disequilibrium occurs. Coping is understood as behavior aimed at discrepancy-reduction.

Turning to rehabilitation in the area of occupational stress, Kenny notes that practices are based on a medical model that attaches a medical or psychological label to the claimant and thus focuses on that one component of the entire occupational system – the so-called psychopathology of the individual worker. The system supports victim blaming and interferes with successful rehabilitation. By contrast, applying the systemic model the case manager should play a central role in the rehabilitation process and cannot effectively take either an advocacy or adversarial role with respect to the client, but rather must advocate for the process of rehabilitation itself. The focus of the intervention must be on the relationship between the illness behavior and the system. Kenny concludes with a call for the empirical testing of this model together with some ideas for facilitating research in the systems approach to rehabilitation.

Chapter 21. Measuring Stress in the Workplace: The Job Stress Survey

The recently developed Job Stress Survey (JSS) is the main focus of this useful and timely contribution by Charles Spielberger and his colleagues. Workplace stress is becoming an increasingly significant problem for the individual, for employers, and for the society. The proportion of workers complaining of stress and those complaining of stress-related illnesses both doubled in a recent five year period. This is a increasingly costly problem as well.

Guided by Lazarus's Transactional Process Theory and Spielberger's own State-Trait Anxiety Inventory. In the JSS, Individuals respond to queries concerning both the severity (on a 10-point scale) and the frequency of experience (number of days, from 0 to 9+ in the past six months) of each potentially stressful event. Two strong factors emerged in corporate, university, and military settings: job pressure and lack of organizational support.

In the study reported in detail in this chapter, Spielberger et al. compared reported stress among managerial/professional (professor and engineers) and clerical/maintenance workers and between males and females using the JSS instrument. Again, two factors identified in an overall factor analysis were job pressure and lack of support. No significant effects were found for gender, or occupational level. However, the JSS job *pressure* index showed higher levels for the managerial/professional group than for the clerical/maintenance group. Pressure stressor severity scores were higher for females than for males in both occupational groups. Lack of support severity scores were also higher in the managerial/professional group than in the clerical/maintenance group.

Thus, whereas the JSS scale failed to show differences between these occupational groups in overall stress levels and in lack of support, occupational level did interact with job pressure. Also, lack of support in the severity scale differentiated groups of workers. One notable difference between males and females was higher reported pressure-severity of stress in the latter group among all workers irrespective of occupational level.

Thus the JSS is a useful device for showing levels of severity and frequency of stress in different occupational groups and additional differences between groups attributable to job pressures and lack of organizational support.

Chapter 22. The Frustration of Success: Type A Behavior, Occupational Stress and Cardiovascular Disease

Don Byrne has given us in this important chapter what is likely to become a frequently cited reconstruction of the model for Type A Behavior Pattern (TABP) with notable implications for predictions in the area of cardiovascular disease. Byrne provides definition: That TABP is an 'action-emotion complex' that includes a variety of behaviors among which are predispositions towards aggressiveness and competitiveness, specific responses such as muscle tension and more rapid activities, and emotional reactions including irritation and hostility.

The fact that a body of studies only partially support a link between occupations and risk of cardiovascular disease suggests to Byrne that it is an *interaction* between occupational situations and TABP that is the risk factor. In a large study of TABP and the occupational environment by Byrne and colleagues, it was found that associations between TABP and occupational level appeared to be mediated by features of the occupational environment over which the worker exerted personal control, in particular, discretionary time commitment to the job.

A large body of evidence supports relationships between levels of occupational stress and coronary heart disease both within and across occupational groups. For example, some categories of physicians (e.g. surgeons) are at greater risk than others, and self-employed persons have double the risk compared with those not self-employed. Less clear are such relationships among women and between work demands and coronary heart disease, although in the latter case better measures of workload may help to establish effects.

Recent research by the author and his colleagues also supports a relationship between TABP and the experience of emotional discomfort. For example, significant correlations between some measures of TABP and state anxiety have been reported. On the one hand, this may mean that autonomic arousal associated with TABP may be experienced as, say, anxiety. On the other hand, these findings may also mean that there is a link between TABP and interpretation of stressful events. People with TABP may both expose themselves more to stress and interpret the impact of stress more personally.

The link between TABP and cardiovascular disease is by no means perfect, indicating that there is no causal association involved. Therefore, a more sophisticated explanation is needed and to this end Byrne proposes competitiveness as one possible basic cognitive set. However, Byrne contends that, for several reasons, competitiveness by itself is an insufficient basis for the pathophysiological pathway that leads to cardiovascular disease, and that rather it is the frustration of behaviors evoked within the cluster defining the TABP that provides the key to the destructive impact of the TABP. Two consequences of frustration typically are aggression and anxiety. Accordingly, Byrne presents some data to show a greater likelihood of angina pectoris in blue collar workers by comparison with white collar workers presenting with TABP, suggesting greater 'toxicity' of the work environment for the former. This analysis has some implications for interventions in the workplace that may be best directed toward modifying the TABP and to issues of occupational control.

Chapter 23. Stress in Academe: Some Recent Research Findings

Anthony Winefield updates us on a number of variables related to reports of stress among university academics in Australia, the United Kingdom, and the United States, and argues that increased workloads are at fault with serious implications along a number of dimensions. The author begins by citing two theories that are consistent with the traditionally low stress nature of university academic positions—the demands-control theory that relates high levels of demand plus low autonomy/control with stress and the person-environment fit model that relates stress to a misfit between job requirements and personal aspirations. Winefield maintains that the nature of academic work has changed in recent years to increase work-related stress from either of these perspectives; for example, workload, demands to publish, and levels of 'scrutiny' via audits have increased owing to such influences as budget cuts and higher enrollment levels.

Among the most cited sources of stress perceived by faculty are high self expectations, financial support for research, inadequate time, deadlines, and interruptions to work. Some data indicates that rank (higher stress among junior faculty) and gender (higher stress among female faculty) may play a role in degree of reported stress.

Most recent studies have shown that stress levels in academia compare unfavorably to certain other occupations, including academic administration and working in the transport arena. There is some suggestion that stress levels for academics in Australian universities may be higher than those for their counterparts in schools in the United Kingdom and the United States.

Winefield concludes, in part, that academics are increasingly vulnerable to 'burnout', that quality of teaching and research may decline, and that academics may become increasingly unattractive to able young people. He recommends interventions to reduce demands associated with academic work and the introduction of stress management courses.

References

Carlson, J. G. & Seifert, R. (eds.) (1991) *International Perspectives on Self-regulation and Health.* New York: Plenum Press.

Carlson, J. G., Seifert, R. & Birbaumer, N. (eds.) (1994) *Clinical Applied Psychophysiology.* New York: Plenum Press.

Kenny, D. (ed.) (1996) *Proceedings of the International Congress on Stress and Health.* Sydney, Australia: University of Sydney.

Sheppard, J. (ed.) (1989) *Advances in Behavioural Medicine*, vol. 6. Sydney, Australia: Cumberland College of Health Sciences.

Chapter 2

THE ROLE OF OSCILLATIONS IN SELF-REGULATION:
Their Contribution to Homeostasis

Nicholas D. Giardino, Paul M. Lehrer PhD and Jonathan M. Feldman

INTRODUCTION

Stress is an inescapable but also necessary part of life. Our world presents us with challenges and obstacles, as well as the resources and motivation to flourish. Life has organized itself to adapt and prosper in our environment and to maintain its identity in the face of external and internal demands. In doing so, humans and other complex organisms sense and respond to environmental pressures and opportunities with coordinated physiological and behavioral activity. And we remain healthy to the extent that we can maintain this organization. Oscillations in both physiology and behavior play a major role in this balance between stability and adaptivity. In the following pages, we will demonstrate how variability in both domains reflects the degree of coordination within and between biological systems, and, more fundamentally, enables an organism to maintain more precise self-regulation. In addition we will explore how under certain conditions stress may actually enhance regulation and well-being. In order to describe the role of oscillations and stress in self-regulation, however, we must first modify the long held notion of homeostasis to account for the fact that variability, rather than a steady state, is the hallmark of a healthy organism; and that variability may be a hallmark of the healthy limits of physiological function as well as healthy adaptation to environmental demand.

ADDITIONS TO THE CONCEPT OF HOMEOSTASIS

The principle of homeostasis, first developed by Bernard (1878) and Cannon (1929), typically involves the maintenance of a constant interior milieu in the face of external and internal perturbations. In healthy organisms deviations from normal may occur in response to environmental demand, but they are quickly corrected in order to maintain a constant state. Our revision to this theory is one of emphasis: Under normal conditions our bodies are far from static and adjust broadly to current demands. For example, while at quiet rest, blood pressure may be maintained around 110/70 mm Hg (though even then it is not actually static, as we will discuss later). Climbing a flight of stairs is normally accompanied by a sharp increase in blood pressure in response to increased demand for blood supply to organ and muscle tissues. However, those with healthier cardiovascular systems will exhibit *greater* increases in blood pressure during such activity!

The term *allostasis* has been introduced in one effort to take into account the more dynamic conditions under which physiological systems typically operate (Sterling & Eyer, 1988). Allostasis describes the operating range of healthy systems and their ability to increase or decrease vital functions to new levels in response to changing demands. Allostasis acknowledges that physiological variables are *not* maintained at a steady state, but that regulation is achieved through change. Extending this concept over the dimension of time, McEwen and Stellar (1993) describe the potentially damaging effects of repeated strain and elevated activity levels on organs and tissues, which they define as the state of *allostatic load*. Excessive allostatic load is the 'hidden price' that the body pays for anticipatory and compensatory control of stressful events. Thus, these new conceptualizations extend the notion of homeostasis to account for the dynamic quality of physiological regulation.

However, the picture is still not complete. Still unaccounted for in these explanations of physiological control is that, for virtually all physiologic variables, no steady-state exists—ever. That is, even under unchanging environmental demand, levels of physiological activity change over time (i.e. they oscillate). Secondly, while excessive strain or unyielding high levels of activity are likely to have damaging effects on any system, a moderate amount of stress is likely to enhance system performance. In this chapter we will describe how normal oscillations, i.e. those present even in the absence of challenge, are associated with healthy functioning systems. The term *homeokinetics* has been used (Yates, 1982) to express the fact that regulation in the body is associated with oscillatory processes. In addition we will show how reduced variability at rest may indicate a predisposition to dysregulation and a vulnerability to the deleterious effects of stress.

To use another example from the cardiovascular system, the heart rate of a healthy individual is far from stable. Even at rest, complex variability characterizes heart rate over time—even very brief periods of time. With each breath, for example, heart rate increases with inhalation and decreases with exhalation, a phenomenon known as respiratory sinus arrhythmia. Multiple slower oscillations have also been detected, yielding a highly complex pattern of variability. Attenuation of this normal complexity is seen in many disease states and is associated with decreased cardiac control. In fact, a decline in complex variability is a reliable marker of increased susceptibility to sudden cardiac death and mortality following myocardial infarction (Goldberger, Rigney, Mietus, Antman & Greenwald, 1988; Kleiger, Miller, Bigger & Moss, 1987). But, cardiovascular parameters are not the only operations that oscillate over normal conditions. Thus, we will now turn our attention to the more general notion of rhythms in biological control.

OSCILLATIONS IN BIOLOGICAL SYSTEMS

Oscillations are defined here as systematic rhythms in physiological variables. Although they may vary somewhat from pure sine waves in amplitude and/or frequency, they are similar to such waves. Oscillatory behaviors are ubiquitous in living systems. Biological rhythms can be found in cell-free biochemical reactions, in single-celled organisms, and throughout the entire spectrum of multicellular life. The specific functions they serve vary widely, yet, not surprisingly, similar physiological mechanisms appear to generate oscillations that give rise to rhythmic behaviors in marine mollusks and in mammals (Cohen, Rossignol & Grillner, 1988;Roberts & Roberts, 1983). In virtually all life forms, for example, variability in the behavior of controlled functions may arise as a result of inherent delays in regulatory feedback loops. Many rhythmic behaviors are most easily observed at the organ-system or organism level, but, as William Harvey discovered long ago when he noticed that small pieces of heart continued to beat spontaneously long after they were excised, many are also intrinsic to the tissues and cells of which they are composed. In fact, in the same system, oscillations can be observed at multiple levels, from the periodic movement of ions at cell membranes, to oscillations in systemic parameters such as blood pressure or lymphocyte counts, to cyclic variations in the behavior of the organism as a whole.

Rhythms in living systems span a wide temporal range as well. Biological oscillations have been identified with periods that last from milliseconds to days, months, even years. Many seem to have evolved with periods synchronous to external environmental stimuli (e.g. tidal, circadian, lunar, and annual rhythms), while others appear to be related to internal regulatory functions. Of course, there is some overlap between these two groups. Most internal regulatory functions are linked at some level to cyclic environmental changes, such as the circadian cycle. However many, and those that will be the main focus of this chapter, are not merely epiphenomena of regulatory mechanisms that evolved in a periodic environment. Rather, they seem to be inextricably linked to an organism's ability to self-regulate in the face of changing, unpredictable environmental demands. In terms of stress and disease, these oscillatory behaviors enable the individual to effectively 'cope' with stressful stimuli through more efficient organization and processing.

In fact, oscillation and self-regulation may be just two different aspects of one general principle. Wever (1964), for example, demonstrated in his mathematical model of biological rhythms that control systems become more stable if the instantaneous controlled value (e.g. hormone levels, heart rate, etc.) oscillates. In fact, for a controlled biological function, the mean value, but not the instantaneous value, remains stable *only* if the system oscillates. Thus, for example, average concentrations of a hormone will be stable over time only if endocrine activity fluctuates systematically over time. If it ceases to oscillate, or if it deviates far from its normal oscillation function, the control system becomes unstable. Using *in vivo* data, Hyndman (1973) determined that the system structures responsible for oscillations in blood pressure and vasomotor activity also enable precise control of blood pressure and core body temperature, respectively. Likewise Rapp, Mees and Sparrow (1981) have shown that, in a biochemical control network, information encoded in a frequency (versus amplitude-encoded information) is more resistant to interference from noise (i.e. a more accurate reflection of the input signal) and provides enhanced precision of control, especially in the absence of immediate feedback.

If physiological oscillations are characteristic of healthy biological systems, then disordered states, such as those brought about by chronic stress and/or disease which places strain on physiological control mechanisms and alters the operating range of the system, would likely be marked by alterations in these oscillations. In addition, since the stressful nature of any given stimulus resides less in its objective characteristics and more in the organism's ability to cope with it, the integrity of such rhythms should also reflect the ability to successfully manage environmental challenge. Indeed, this seems to be the case.

VARIABILITY AS AN INDEX OF HEALTHY FUNCTIONING

For all complex biological systems (e.g. cardiovascular, immune, neuroendocrine), the controlled output (e.g. blood pressure, heart rate, or lymphocyte activity) represents the sum activity of several mechanisms and involves the interaction of internal feedback mechanisms and external inputs from other systems. As a result, the complexity of the system output is often a good indicator of the health of the system. So, healthy functioning systems generally exhibit a high degree of complexity, while illness is often characterized by a loss of system complexity, indicating a decoupling of system components as well as a decrease in external inputs (Goldberger, 1991; Lehrer, in press; Pincus, 1994; Pincus & Goldberger, 1994). The rules that govern the interaction, or *coupling*, within and between system components can be fairly complicated. For instance, the exact output of multiple oscillatory mechanisms depends on the intrinsic frequency and phase of each component oscillator and the strength of the coupling between them (Winfree, 1980). However, for our purposes, it is not an oversimplification to say that a certain amount of coupling allows an organism to more effectively respond to changing environmental challenges (see also Goldberger, Rigney & West, 1990; Hyndman, 1973). Conversely, rigid coupling (resulting in stereotypic periodicity) or complete decoupling (resulting in 'white noise', or complete absence of directed behavior) often underlies pathology in disordered systems (Goldberger & Rigney, 1990). Thus, a system of loosely coupled bio-oscillators provides for an adaptive organism by allowing it to identify and implement adaptive responses to internal and external demands (West, 1990; Lehrer, in press).

Healthy coupling is often exhibited as increased complexity in the behavior under examination. Thus, behavioral variability is often associated with normal functioning, both physiological *and* psychological (Lehrer, in press). For a variety of functions studied, including respiration, heart rate, blood pressure, white blood cell count, hormone secretion, ion channel activity, EEG, and psychological mood, complexity of output patterns are associated with healthy states.

Again, while the classical principle of homeostasis states that physiological systems operate to reduce variability and achieve an equilibrium-like state (Cannon, 1929), such evidence indicates that under normal (healthy) conditions adaptive systems exhibit a behavior typical of dynamical systems far from equilibrium (Peng et al., 1994). Thus, the existence of oscillations in normal processes necessitates a more sophisticated explanation than the intuitive descriptions adequate for homeostasis (Garfinkel, 1983). Basic to this understanding is the notion that biological systems organize themselves into collective forms in which the component parts act synergetically to produce some global activity. These organizations produce stable adaptive systems that persist in form and function even with the loss of some functional units or under the pressure of external demands. The stability of systems of weakly coupled oscillators may be a central organizing principle for the operation of biological systems. Pathology arises when a physiological system loses the stability of its normal operating mode. Thus, the strength or complexity of an oscillating behavior would be indicative of the integrity of the underlying system's regulatory capacity and stability. We must now ask why this is so. Why do oscillations exist as part of normal functioning systems? And why is the complexity of oscillation associated with health and adaptiveness?

THE ROLE OF OSCILLATIONS

Cyclic behaviors have been observed in living organisms since antiquity. In earlier times, these rhythms were believed to be a consequence of a 'vital force' present only in biological organisms (Bunning, 1973). In 1958, however, the observation by Belousov (1958; translated in Field & Burger, 1984) of oscillations in a simple chemical reaction (the oxidation of citric acid by bromate in the presence of cerium ions) stimulated research in such phenomena in the biological realm in order to provide an alternative to the vitalist hypothesis. These investigations uncovered similar oscillations in biochemical reactions as well, and eventually led to material physiological explanations for even gross behavioral variability. But, while it is now recognized that most biological oscillations are due to the presence of physiological feedback loops (e.g. positive, negative, or mixed) with delays[1] (Friesen & Block, 1984), it is often suggested that the resulting variability is merely an artifact of 'imperfect' control mechanisms for which the energy required to suppress would not be worthwhile.

Take for example the interaction of heart rate and blood pressure in cardiovascular control. Under normal conditions, a decrease in blood pressure leads to a decrease in the firing rate of arterial baroreceptors, which signals cardiovascular control centers in the brainstem to increase heart rate and vascular tone to compensate accordingly. However, due to certain properties of the sympathetic innervation, there is roughly a 5-second delay from the time that baroreceptors detect a change in blood pressure to the time that the cardiac pacemaker cells at the sinoatrial node respond to sympathetic nerve traffic to cause an increase in heart rate (Madwed, Albrecht, Mark & Cohen, 1989). Increased cardiac output then leads to an increase in blood pressure, which, sensed by baroreceptors, leads to a decrease in heart rate and peripheral vascular tone. But again there is a 5-second delay in transmission time, so that heart rate will continue to increase for five seconds until it is finally signaled to slow down. Thus, what results is a pattern of heart rate that increases for 5 seconds, then decreases for 5 seconds, and so on, creating an oscillatory pattern in heart rate with a period of 10 seconds. It might be said that even though the control of blood pressure by this mechanism is imperfect (i.e. a more efficient system might reduce or eliminate the 10-second oscillation), it is good enough for the organism and improving it would confer no significant evolutionary advantage. In fact, however, just the opposite seems to be true. It is oscillatory behavior, rather than its elimination, that is advantageous to the organism. The oscillating state is not dysfunctional, nor even benign (Hyndman, 1973; Rapp et al., 1981).

Rapp (1987) has described five areas in which oscillations confer positive functional advantages to an organism. First, they aid in temporal organization. Automatic mechanisms, such as entrainment and synchronization, help keep biological processes in step with the demands of

---

[1] Oscillations are also observed when system components show non-linear kinetics (e.g. certain enzyme reactions) and when they are far from equilibrium and thermodynamically open (Peng et al., 1994).

a periodic environment. Second, they establish and maintain spatial organization, such as the temporal sequence (sino-atrial node $\to$ Pukinje fibers $\to$ ventricles) of coupled oscillators that maintain the correct spatial contraction sequence in the heart. Third, they may be used to predict repetitive events. For example, circadian rhythms may permit preparation for physiological activities that occur on a daily basis. Fourth, oscillatory processes appear to be more energy efficient (Richter & Ross, 1981). And fifth, frequency encoded information (versus amplitude dependent control), which is made possible by biochemical and biophysical oscillators, is especially resistant to distortion by random noise in the input signal and enhances the precision of control mechanisms (Rapp et al., 1981).

Most definitions of biological oscillations imply that organisms have acquired, through natural selection, cyclic behaviors as part of their adaptive strategies. However, it may be that biological rhythms do not merely assist organisms to become more adaptive, rather, more fundamentally, they *constitute* living organisms. According to this view, life is seen as a process that consists of the continuous coordination of molecular and physical oscillations according to principles that will help maintain them in mutually supporting or synergetic relationships (Fraser, 1990; Winfree, 1980). In a similar manner, disease may be conceptualized in terms of alterations in the coupling of these oscillations, which may result in the genesis of new rhythms, the abolition of existing rhythms, or, perhaps more commonly, the transition of oscillations to different modes (Glass & Mackey, 1988; Wever, 1988). Diseases characterized by abnormal temporal organization have been termed *dynamical diseases* (Mackey & Glass, 1977).

For example, in Cheyne-Stokes respiration, a breathing pattern that often occurs in congestive heart failure, obesity, or after brainstem lesions, the normal oscillations in inspiration and expiration time and tidal volume are replaced by alternating patterns of hyperventilation and apnea (temporary stopping of breathing). This change in temporal pattern may be caused by an increased delay in circulation time from the lungs to the brain, an increased sensitivity to blood CO_2 levels, or changes in CO_2 production or storage rates, all of which could lead to unstable respiratory oscillations (Cherniack & Longobardo, 1973; Glass & Mackey, 1979; Mackey & Milton, 1987).

The benefits of relatively simple oscillations for regulatory control are clear. Analysis of the behavior and interaction of multiple 'simple' oscillations has progressed our understanding of many relatively complex physiological control systems. For most systems there seems to be an ideal range of oscillatory activity. Deviations from this normal range result in regulatory deficits, usually either system hyperresponsivity or hyporesponsivity, depending upon the direction of change. Yet, explanatory efforts based on simple linear models of coupling fail to account for a substantial portion of the output variance is these systems. While this may simply be due to the influence of unmeasured inputs, growing evidence points to the contribution of system nonlinearities and physiological 'noise' (Saul, 1992).

One way to account for the behavior of a system in which the constituent parts are not wholly understood or accounted for, either because they are not all known or too complex to model, is to measure the overall *complexity* of the system output. Complexity represents the combined activity of multiple regulatory oscillations. Figure 2.1 illustrates how three simple regulatory oscillations in heart rate interact to produce complex cardiac behavior. Respiratory, baroreflex and thermoregulatory control systems each influence interbeat intervals on different time scales. However, their combined inputs result in increasing complexity. Notice that, even with only this simple idealized oscillatory model, actual cardiac behavior can be reasonably approximated. Differences between panels E and F can be attributed to unrepresented inputs, system nonlinearities, and physiological noises.

Since multiple overlapping periodic oscillations will typically result in nonperiodic variability, complexity is the extent to which a process generates aperiodic fluctuations. Most direct measures of complexity have been based on concepts from chaos theory. One such method estimates the number of variables needed to reproduce the output of a system (Grassberger & Procaccia, 1983). Another is related to the amount of information needed to predict the future behavior of the system (Pincus, 1991). Several studies to date have shown that overall complexity of a system's output is a reliable measure of healthy functioning, and that a loss of complexity is associated with a loss or impairment of functional components and/or altered coupling between constituent component (Kaplan et al., 1991; Lipsitz & Goldberger, 1992; Mandell & Shlesinger, 1990; Ryan, Goldberger, Pincus, Mietus & Lipsitz, 1994). In all cases loss of complexity reflects impaired ability to adapt to stress.

In addition to deterministic influences on the behavior of control systems, random processes may also be important for healthy regulation. Recent evidence supports the counterintuitive notion that 'noise'—random background fluctuations—enhances the sensitivity of control processes. The effect, called *stochastic resonance*, occurs when a signal that is normally undetectable interacts with an optimal level of random noise, which acts to boost the signal to detectable levels (Wiesenfeld & Moss, 1995). For example, small periodic movements of a surface that are imperceptible to tactile sensation become distinguishable when mechanical or electrical noise is added to the surface (Collins, Chow & Imhoff, 1995). Likewise, the ability to sense very small muscle movements are enhanced by mechanically jiggling the muscle (Cordo, Gurfinkel, Bevan & Kerr, 1995). During exercise, increased sensitivity of a muscle's sensory neurons is associated with increased electrical noise levels in the exercising muscle

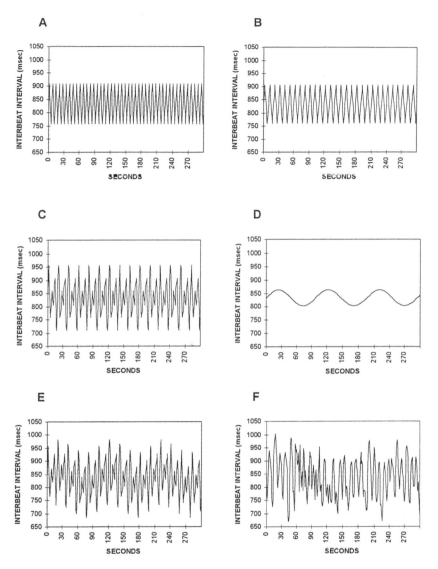

Figure 2.1 Increasingly complex cardiac behavior emerges from the interaction of simple periodic oscillations. Panels depict changes in interbeat intervals over a 5 minute period. (A) Respiratory sinus arrhythmia (12 cycles per minute). (B) Baroreflex-mediated oscillations (6 cycles per minute). (C) Combination of A and B waveforms. (D) Thermoregulatory oscillations (0.6 cycles per minute). (E) Combination of A, B & D waveforms. (F) Data from a typical healthy human recording.

(Chiou-Tan et al., 1997). It is interesting to speculate that moderate stress and exercise may have beneficial effects due at least in part to the introduction of noise to regulatory processes.

INDIVIDUAL DIFFERENCES IN DISEASE SUSCEPTIBILITY

It is often noted that there is great individual variability of response to stressful stimuli. This is attributed to such diverse factors as genes, developmental stage and past experience, which may lead some individuals to be more or less resilient to stressful events (Rutter, 1988). The exact mechanisms by which this differentiation occurs, however, remain to be clearly elucidated. Given that stressful stimuli are mediated by the nervous and endocrine systems, it is likely that *neuro-endocrine* structures serve as a locus for such differences. While much important work has been done in the study of end-organ pathology associated with exposure to stress, more general processes, and likely the source of individual differences in susceptibility, may be gleaned by exploring differences in central systems, which may contribute to diverse pathologies via similar physiological mechanisms.

Great advances have been made in identifying changes in the activity of several endocrine hormones associated with stressful exposure and the mechanisms by which they may contribute to disease. A detailed review of these compounds and processes is beyond the scope of this chapter. However, as mentioned briefly earlier, the endocrine system fits well within our model of coupled oscillating complex systems. Oscillatory behavior in hormone secretions are crucial to the regulatory processes carried out by the endocrine system. In addition, alterations in normal fluctuations have been identified in several disease processes (Greenspan, Klibanski, Rowe & Elahi, 1991). The central nervous system, of course, plays a major role in the control of almost all bodily process, and the contribution of oscillations in higher brain (i.e. psychological) processes to health, as well as mental and physical illness, will be discussed in a later section. First we will consider the role of the autonomic nervous system in the development of disease, an area of interest that stems from the fact that many of the body's regulatory activities are controlled by feedback systems mediated by autonomic processes.

THE AUTONOMIC NERVOUS SYSTEM

At the same time that Cannon proposed the concept of homeostasis he also introduced the idea of *negative feedback-regulation* of body states, which he proposed to be largely mediated by the autonomic nervous system through the hypothalamus (Cannon, 1928). Two divisions of the autonomic nervous system, the sympathetic and parasympathetic, were traditionally thought to operate antagonistically in regulating the internal environment. The sympathetic division governs the *fight-and-flight* reaction, whereas the parasympathetic branch is responsible for *rest-and-digest*. Changes brought about by increased sympathetic outflow, including increased cardiac output, changes in peripheral vasculature and blood glucose, and pupillary dilation, permit rapid response to potentially threatening environmental conditions. Parasympathetic activity, on the other hand, maintains basal heart rate, respiration and metabolism under normal conditions. We now know, however, that this division of labor is not so simple. Sympathetic and parasympathetic branches both mediate emergency responses and are tonically active, operating in conjunction with the somatic motor system to regulate normal behavior as well as altering the internal environment in the face of changing external conditions. In addition, these two branches do not always operate antagonistically. Complex interactions between the two have been observed, for example, at the sinoatrial node (Bernston, Cacioppo & Quigley, 1991, 1993; Koizumi & Kollai, 1992).

The autonomic nervous system, as perhaps all biological systems, is a nonlinear system. As such it involves several factors with nonlinear and coupled actions, and can be interpreted in terms of forced nonlinear oscillators, which appear in many branches of science, including physics and chemistry. The notion of *agonistic-antagonistic equilibrium* has been used to give structure to the nonlinear oscillators in many biological systems. One important processes described in this framework is that two forces may converge in a limit cycle[2] around a critical value, as is the case of cortisol-vasopressin or acetylcholine-epinephrine coupling (Bernard-Weil, 1986). An important characteristic of such a system is that its agents (e.g. sympathetic and parasympathetic neurotransmitters) can act by agonistic *and* antagonistic means. Thus, the dynamics of the system represented by the couple is simultaneously controlled by changes in both its agonistic and antagonistic activity. These characteristics give a biological system 1) more stability in a steady-state and 2) more adaptive control to change limit cycles when necessary.

Partly as a result of the mediating role of the autonomic nervous system, the targets of many physiological control systems exhibit complex fluctuations, rather than being maintained at a constant level (Lipsitz et al., 1997). The assessment of these resulting oscillations appears to be a useful way to measure the integrity of the underlying physiological control mechanisms (Saul, 1990). This has been studied most thoroughly in the cardiovascular system.

CARDIOVASCULAR HOMEODYNAMICS

As briefly mentioned earlier, the normal heart rhythm is not regular; but, rather, the intervals between successive contractions vary from beat to beat.

---

[2] A limit cycle is a period limit set for a system. In a stable limit cycle, values return to an original periodic limit after the introduction of a perturbation.

When the average heart rate is 60 beats per minute, the interbeat interval can change as much as 20 beats per minute every few heartbeats. In the course of day the heart rate of a healthy person may typically vary from 40 to 180 beats per minute, and will fluctuate considerably even in the absence of external stimuli (Yeragani, 1995). Changes in heart rate and its variability pattern comprise the cardiovascular response to a broad range of stimuli, including physical, psychological and environmental. Since the cardiovascular system is primarily a pressure controlled system, factors that alter blood pressure play a dominant role in heart rate fluctuations, though heart rate at any one instant in time represents the resultant of many influences on vagal and sympathetic centers, including baroreceptors, atrial receptors, chemoreceptors, muscle receptors and lung inflation (Hainsworth, 1995). Some reflexes may increase heart rate through a decrease in vagal tone, an increase in sympathetic activity, or both. Others exert opposite effects. Typically, several reflexes will operate simultaneously, often with very complex interactions.

Although variability in heart rate has been studied for over two centuries (Hales, 1733; von Haller, 1760), it is only fairly recently that the utility of this phenomenon has been explored in much detail. Before then, heart rate variability per se, though sometimes tediously analyzed by hand, was not often the focus of research. With the widespread availability of digital computing, however, these often subtle changes in heart rate became more easy to study and characterize. Today it is generally accepted that the beat-to-beat variability in cardiovascular function reflects the action of reflexes whereby the cardiovascular regulatory systems optimize responses to exogenous and endogenous perturbations (Appel et al., 1989; Hyndman, 1973). Thus, the study of variability in heart rate provides a useful window into the dynamic processes involved in homeodynamics.

Originally, spectral analysis[3] of heart rate variability revealed the existence of three rhythmic oscillations, all with periods (i.e. one complete cycle) of less than 1 minute: a high-frequency (HF) component corresponding to respiratory activity (normally between 10 and 24 cycles per minute) and referred to as respiratory sinus arrhythmia (RSA); a low-frequency (LF) component, also known as Mayer waves, with a period of about 10 seconds; and a very low frequency (VLF) component, with each cycle lasting about a minute or more (Akselrod et al., 1981; Hyndman, Kitney & Sayers, 1971; Pomeranz et al., 1985; Sayers, 1973). More recent studies, in addition to demonstrating the existence of even lower frequency

---

[3] Spectral analysis is a mathematical transformation that decomposes a complex signal into a sum of individual sine waves of various amplitudes and frequencies. The amplitude of each sine wave (called the *spectral power*) is a measure of the variability of the signal at that frequency.

oscillations in heart rate (up to, and possibly beyond, 24 hours), have shown that, although there is a tendency for oscillations to occur in these three frequency ranges, the frequency and amplitude of these oscillations are constantly changing in responses to internal and external perturbations (Kobayoshi & Musha, 1982; Saul, Albrecht, Berger & Cohen, 1988).

In short-term recordings (e.g. 5-minutes) it is widely accepted that the HF component is mediated solely by changes in vagal activity (Grossman & Wientjes, 1986; Porges, 1986; Saul et al., 1991). While there is still some dispute over the interpretation of the LF band, most available evidence seems to indicate that heart rate fluctuations in this range can be mediated by changing levels of both vagal and sympathetic activity (Akselrod et al., 1981; Pomeranz et al., 1985). The VLF component, while less studied, is thought to be related to thermoregulatory activity (Kitney, 1980) and, possibly, local adjustments of resistance in individual vascular beds matching blood flow to local metabolic demand (Akselrod et al., 1981). In addition to sympathetic influences, heart rate fluctuation at very low frequencies may also be mediated by changing levels of circulating hormones (for a more detailed discussion of heart rate variability mechanisms, see Saul, 1990).

One important point is that although variability in heart rate is a direct result of changing levels or modulation of cardiac autonomic activity it is not necessarily related to the mean firing rates of neural inputs. Although cardiac responses to modulation will usually be larger when the mean neural activity levels are higher, it is also possible for mean vagal or sympathetic activity to be elevated without any significant modulation, or for modulation to occur without any significant cardiac response. Therefore, the various components of heart rate variability are interpreted as quantifiers of autonomic responsiveness rather than autonomic activity (Saul, 1990).

Although spectral analysis of heart rate has proven useful, large intra- and inter-individual variance in spectra leading to relatively poor sensitivity and specificity when used as a test of autonomic function in individuals have led to the exploration of more complex linear as well as nonlinear techniques. As with all biological systems, significant nonlinearities exist in the cardiovascular regulatory system. For example, analysis of associations between low frequency fluctuations in heart rate and changes in respiratory tidal volume indicates that the mode of transmission between respiratory and cardiovascular control loops have a nonlinear component, though their exact mechanisms are not yet known (Saul, Kaplan & Kitney, 1989).

Since the initial identification of nonlinear behavior in cardiac tissue (Guevara, Glass & Shrier, 1981), the applications of nonlinear mathematics to cardiovascular variables have been numerous, and may provide certain advantages over linear methods. For example, measures of fractal dimension[4] and approximate entropy[5] appear to be not only more consistent (Yeragani et al., 1993), but also provide an independent evaluation of the integrity of the autonomic nervous system and cardiovascular control than can be established from linear measures (Kaplan et al., 1991; Landry, Bennett & Oriol, 1994).

CLINICAL APPLICATIONS OF HEART RATE VARIABILITY ANALYSIS

In addition to their usefulness in understanding cardiovascular regulation in normal individuals, changes in heart rate variability have been characterized in many cardiovascular disorders, including hypertension (Mancia et al., 1983), sudden cardiac death (Goldberger & Rigney, 1990), ventricular arrhythmia (Rosenbaum et al., 1994), severe heart disease (Peng et al., 1995), and myocardial infarction (Bigger et al., 1992). Heart rate variability and spectral analysis have also been used to predict mortality after myocardial infarction (Kleiger, Miller, Bigger & Moss, 1987) and congestive heart failure (Saul et al, 1988), during coronary angiography (Rich et al., 1988), as well as to determine the risk of rejection after cardiac transplantation (Binder et al., 1992). In general, pathology is associated with a decrease in heart rate variability or complexity and decrease in cardiovascular control.

After myocardial infarction (MI) total heart rate variability and individual absolute power[6] of spectral components (e.g. HF, LF, VLF) are reduced (Appel et al., 1989; Bigger et al., 1991; Malliani et al., 1991), probably reflecting an alteration in cardiac autonomic reflexes and/or decreased responsivity at the sinoatrial node to autonomic neural modulation (Schwartz et al., 1988). In addition LF seems to increase relative to total power and HF, suggesting that autonomic control of the heart may shift to sympathetic predominance (Lombardi et al., 1987) after MI. In addition, nonlinear analyses reveal reduced complexity (e.g. fractal dimension or approximate entropy) of heart rate time series in individuals with postoperative ventricular dysfunction (Fleisher, Pincus & Rosenbaum, 1993), severe heart failure and after transplantation and acute myocardial infarction (Lombardi et al., 1996).

---

[4] Fractal dimension is an estimate of the lower bound of the number of independent control variables needed to model the behavior of complex system (Grassberger & Procaccia, 1983).
[5] Approximate entropy (ApEn) is a 'regularity statistic' that quantifies the predictability of fluctuations in a given variable (e.g. heart rate) (Pincus, 1991). Higher ApEn indicates greater complexity in system output.
[6] Absolute power refers to the total amount of variability within a particular frequency range (e.g. RSA). In contrast, normalized power is the amount of variability in a frequency range relative to the total variability across all (VLF and higher) frequency ranges.

Similar alterations in heart rate variability are seen in many non-cardiac pathologies as well, including diabetic neuropathy (Kitney, Byrne, Edmonds, Watkins & Roberts, 1982; Lischner et al., 1987), asthma (Lehrer et al., 1996), sudden infant death syndrome (Pincus, Cummins & Haddad, 1993), chronic fatigue syndrome (Pagani, Lucini, Mela, Langewitz & Malliani, 1994), nonclinical panic and blood phobia (Thayer & Friedman, 1993), generalized anxiety disorder (Lyonfields, Borkovec & Thayer, 1995), anorexia nervosa (Kreipe, Goldstein, De King, Tipton & Kempski, 1994), panic disorder (Yeragani et al., 1993) and major depression (Rechlin, Weis, Spitzer & Kaschka, 1994). Changes in variability have also been well documented in aging (variability decreases with age) (Lipsitz & Goldberger, 1992; Schwartz, Gibb & Tran, 1991; Shannon, Carley & Benson, 1987;), and between men and women (complexity and HF are normally higher and LF lower in women) (Liao et al., 1995; Ryan et al., 1996). Taken as a whole, the wide range of conditions that exhibit predictable alterations in heart rate variability suggest that these cardiovascular dynamics may be reflective of more general autonomic control.

To simplify, what these studies show is that an inability to adapt well to stress (either physiological or psychological) is associated with deviations from the normal oscillatory mode and decreased complexity of the cardiac signal. Because oscillation and complexity are an index of cardiac autonomic responsivity, and because the types of illness associated with altered cardiac variability extend well beyond cardiovascular diseases, we can hypothesize that a more general disruption of autonomic self-regulation underlies these diverse disorders.

Recall earlier we explained how loosely coupled systems result in an ideal level of regulatory control, and how the complexity of system output is an index of this healthy coupling. For heart rate variability, there is an optimal range of oscillation that is associated with increased signal complexity and healthy regulatory control. Alterations in these normal oscillations are associated with abnormalities in reactivity or regulation of arousal, such that individuals may respond to harmless stimuli or fail to respond when a response is required. In asthma, for example, increased heart rate variability is associated with parasympathetic hyperreactivity and greater airway irritability (Hashimoto, Maeda & Yokoyama, 1996; Lehrer et al., 1996). Hypertensives, who show decreased baroreflex control of blood pressure (i.e. the baroreceptors are hyporesponsive to changes in blood pressure), exhibit smaller than normal oscillations heart rate and blood pressure (Mancia et al., 1983; Novak, Novak, de Champlain & Nadeau, 1993). In panic disorder, decreased heart rate variability is associated with dysregulation of arousal, while subsequent increases in cardiac oscillations are associated with clinical recovery following cognitive therapy or imiprimine treatment (Middleton & Ashby, 1995). The notion that heart rate variability reflects healthy autonomic regulation is further supported by independent studies that show autonomic hyper- or hyporesponsivity that are consistent with the patterns of changes observed in heart rate variability in many of the above disorders (e.g. Bristow, Honour, Pickering, Sleight & Smyth, 1969; Van Brummelen, Buhler, Kiowski & Amman, 1981) In addition, it is well known that extensive connections exist between cardiovascular regulatory components and the central nervous system, resulting in complex interactions between behavioral activation and cardiovascular feedback systems (Langhorst, Schulz, Schulz & Lambertz, 1983). For example, reticular activation leads to a decrease in baroreceptor efficiency, while baroreceptor afferents exert a dampening effect of the central nervous system. Chemoreceptors act in a similar manner, but in the reverse direction.

Finally, heart rate variability is altered temporarily by acute stressful mental activity in healthy individuals, causing changes similar to those observed in disease. In studies employing mirror tracking, arithmetic calculations, Stroop color word conflict and reaction time tasks, absolute HF and LF power typically decrease, while LF relative to HF and total power increases, with increasing mental load (Grillot et al., 1995; Hyndman & Gregory, 1975; Langewitz and Rüddel, 1989; Pagani et al., 1989; 1991). These findings suggest that chronic stress may lead to disease by long-term suppression of autonomic self-regulation.

CONTROLLING BIOLOGICAL OSCILLATIONS

Given the ubiquity of biological oscillations and the association of certain types of rhythms with healthy functioning, one might ask whether the induction of such rhythms can serve to restore health in disorders characterized by the alteration of normal oscillations.

Alterations in heart rate variability have been associated with increased autonomic reactivity and declining pulmonary function in asthma (Kallenbach et al., 1985; Lehrer et al., 1996). Recently in our laboratory we tested the hypothesis that increasing short-term cardiac variability through biofeedback would lead to an improvement in pulmonary function and asthma symptoms. In a controlled pilot study of 20 subjects it was found that heart rate variability biofeedback, but not the control intervention (EMG biofeedback), lead to an improvement in pulmonary function and a reduction in the report of certain important asthma symptoms (Lehrer et al., 1997). Importantly, these improvements were associated with increases in LF heart rate variability. Thus, it appears that the stimulation of healthy oscillations in disordered systems may strengthen and help restore normal regulatory mechanisms.

While the therapeutic utility of HRV biofeedback may prove to be useful in a wide range of pathologies associated with autonomic dysregulation, a similar principle has been applied to other physiological processes. To use a very simple illustration, dysregulated physiological systems characterized by oscillatory behavior can be viewed as a seesaw with a sticky balance support. Traditional interventions have had the effect of pushing down on one side of the balance to correct what appears to be either too high or too low levels of activity. The approach we have presented here suggests that a more effective treatment involves exerting force on *both* sides, in keeping with the system's natural oscillatory tendency.

To give another concrete example, we know that two hormones play a major role in hydroelectrolytic metabolism control, adrenal cortical hormones (ACH) and vasopressin (VP). ACH, in general, lead to a decreasing water content of the cell compartment in favor of the extracellular space, by different action on renal tubules and cell membranes (Elliot & Yrarrazaval, 1952). VP, on the other hand, leads to an increasing water content of the cell compartment. But, while these effects can be seen reliable *in vitro*, they are not always observed as such *in vivo*. The water diuresis provoked by ACH is not constant and an escape from the action of VP has been observed. Similarly, the therapeutic effects of ACH on cerebral edema (partially due to an overhydration of glial cells) does not correspond to what one would expect from experimental data (Kleeman, Koplowitz, Maxwell, Cutler & Dowling, 1960). This may be due to VP hypersecretion after cortisol loading, which may cancel the expected effects of ACH. These observations have lead to the exploration of 'paradoxical' therapies, such as the administration of both corticoids *and* vasopressin for conditions previously treated with only corticoids (e.g. subdurnal hematoma, astrocytomas, thalamic space-occupying lesion, and metastatic tumors from breast cancer origin), with significant improvement in treatment outcome (Bernard-Weil, 1983, 1986).

PSYCHOLOGICAL VARIABILITY IN MENTAL AND PHYSICAL ILLNESS

Not surprisingly, psychological behavior appears to be governed by many of the same concepts used to describe oscillatory behavior in physiological processes. As with physiological systems, organized complexity is the hallmark of healthy psychological behavior, while hyperstabilities and hyperinstabilities may characterize a breakdown in normal mental functioning and leave the *person-system* vulnerable to the deleterious effects of stress, much as they do in other systems. The formal quantitative use of this paradigm is relatively recent in the study of psychopathology, but seems to be supported in recent clinical reports.

On an intuitive level, it has been noted (Lehrer, in press) that the diagnostic definitions of mental illness, for example as laid out in DSM-IV, rely on the functional stereotypies characteristic of most psychiatric disorders. The hyperstable modes observed in bipolar disorder moods or

OCD thoughts and rituals, or the hypostable cognitive processes of schizophrenia or ADHD help define these disorders for clinicians. While concepts from nonlinear dynamics and related fields almost certainly will advance our understanding of psychopathology on a heuristic level, only time will tell if more quantitative assessments will be possible. Early efforts seem to indicate that they will.

Gottschalk, Bauer and Whybrow (1995) analyzed daily mood ratings over the course of a year or more from patients with bipolar disorder and normal controls. They found that while bipolar subjects showed some brief periods of fairly well-defined 'cycling' in mood, their overall pattern of mood changes were *less* complex[7] than normal controls. That is, the mood of bipolar patients was more predictable over the course of a year than psychologically healthy control subjects. While this finding may not be surprising in the context of the material presented above, it is contrary to 'common wisdom' regarding bipolar disorder. That is, psychologists typically think of persons with this illness as exhibiting *greater* variability in mood than healthy individuals—cycling extremes of mood. But, according to Gattschalk et al., it is *healthy* people who exhibit more variability in mood over time.

Electroecephalogram (EEG) studies may also reveal differences in complexity between psychopathology and healthy states. In schizophrenia, for example, EEG patterns were able to be modeled with a smaller number of variables than healthy controls (Roschke & Aldenhoff, 1993). Similar differences in EEG were found between sons of alcoholics and those of non-alcoholic parents (Ehlers, Havstad & Schuckit, 1995). While the interpretation of these EEG data can be tricky, they suggest a reduction in the coupling of oscillatory brain activity in those with psychological disorders, and, interestingly, even those at high risk for the development of disease.

THE INTERACTIONS OF OSCILLATIONS AT MULTIPLE LEVELS

Finally, we will close with an example of how oscillations at very different levels of analysis may affect and be affected by one another in psychopathology.

It is now widely accepted that relationships exist between stress and immune function (e.g. Glaser, Kiecolt-Glaser, Speicher & Holliday, 1985), stress and depression (Irwin, Daniels, Bloom, Smith & Weiner, 1987), and depression and immune function (e.g. Kronfol, Silva, Greden, Gardner &

---

[7] The measure used in this and the EEG studies in the following paragraph is the fractal dimension (D). D provides an estimate of the lower bound of the number of variables necessary to describe the behavior under study. There may be reason to be cautious, however, about the application of this measure to biological data (see, for example, Theiler & Rapp, 1996).

Carrol, 1983). Stressful life-events have consistently been linked to immunosuppression and often precede the onset of major depressive episodes, and altered immune activity and reduced responsivity is observed in major depression[8]. Changes in neuronal calcium activity has been in recorded in depression and during immunosuppression. Vollmayr, Sulger, Gabriel and Aldenhoff (1995) looked at intracellular free calcium concentrations in T-lymphocytes in response to mitogen stimulation in depressed and non-depressed subjects. They found that stimulation of lymphocytes triggered an oscillatory calcium signal in individual T-cells, the strength of which was associated with the percentage of T-cells responding. However, both calcium oscillations and T-cell responses were significantly attenuated in depressed patients. After treatment with interpersonal psychotherapy, calcium oscillations and lymphocyte responses in remitted subjects resembled those in the normal group, and were inversely proportional to Hamilton Depression scores in all subjects. Thus, psychotherapy, which, not incidentally, may be viewed as helping the person increase their cognitive and behavioral repertoire (i.e. increasing variability of response to stressors), resulted in a restoration of disordered calcium oscillations, which appear to mediate an important component of the immune response.

SUMMARY

In summary, health, both physiological and psychological, requires an ability to self-regulate in the face of internal and external demands. In the preceding chapter we have emended the classical principle of homeostasis to account for our current understanding of physiological and psychological control processes, and to explain the behavior of controlled variables in these systems. Instead of maintaining a constant interior milieu, our bodies capitalize on the advantages offered by oscillatory dynamics to enable more adaptive and precise control in self-regulation. The oscillating state, rather than the steady state, is the norm for nearly all bodily functions. It was shown that it is possible to measure the integrity of physiological and psychological control systems by quantifying the variability of controlled variables, and that in diverse bodily systems and at multiple levels of analysis, oscillatory patterns and complexity of behavior are associated with healthy functioning and resiliency to stress. Finally, we demonstrated that the induction of healthy functions through biofeedback or the pharmacological application of agonistic-antagonistic equilibrium may be able to restore normal activity to disordered systems.

---

[8] It is important and interesting to note that stress cannot simply be equated here with psychiatric distress. The changes in immune function seen in depression, for example, are not found in anxiety disorders, such as social phobia (Rapaport & Stein, 1994).

References

Akselrod, S., Gordon, D., Ubel, F. A., Shannon, D. C., Barger, A. C. & Cohen, R. J. (1981) Power spectrum analysis of heart rate fluctuation: a quantitative probe of beat-to-beat cardiovascular control. *Science*, **213**, 220–222.

Appel, M. L., Berger, R. D., Saul, J. P., Smith, J. M. & Cohen, R. J. (1989) Beat to beat variability in cardiovascular variables: music or noise? *Journal of the American College of Cardiology*, **14**, 1139–1148.

Belousov, B. P. (1958) *Collections of Abstracts on Radiation Medicine*. Moscow: Medgiz.

Bernard, C. (1878) *Les phenomenes de la vie*, vol. 1. Paris: Librarie J-B Bailliere et Fils.

Bernard-Weil, E. (1983) Mathematical model for hormonal therapy in cerebral collapse and malignant tumors of the brain. *Neurological Research*, **5**, 19–35.

Bernard-Weil, E. (1986) A general model for the simulation of balance, imbalance and control by agonistic-antagonistic biological couples. *Mathematical Modeling*, **7**, 1587–1600.

Bernston, G. C., Cacioppo, J. T. & Quigley, K. S. (1991) Autonomic determinism: The modes of autonomic control, the doctrine of autonomic space, and the laws of autonomic constraint. *Psychological Review*, **98**, 459–487.

Bernston, G. C., Cacioppo, J. T. & Quigley, K. S. (1993) Cardiac psychophysiology and autonomic space in humans: Empirical perspectives and conceptual implications. *Psychological Bulletin*, **114**, 296–322.

Bigger, J. T., Fleiss, J. L., Steinman, R. C., Rolnitzky, L. M., Kleiger, R. E. & Rottman, J. N. (1992) Frequency domain measures of heart period variability and mortality after myocardial infarction. *Circulation*, **85**, 164–171.

Binder, T., Frey, B., Porenta, G., Heinz, G., Wutte, M., Kreiner, G., Grossinger, H., Schmidinger, H., Pacher, R. & Weber, H. (1992) Prognostic value of heart rate variability in patients awaiting cardiac transplantation. *Pacing & Clinical Electrophysiology*, **15**, 2215–2220.

Bristow, J. D., Honour, A. J., Pickering, G. W., Sleight, P. & Smyth, H. S. (1969) Diminished baroreflex sensitivity in high blood pressure. *Circulation*, **39**, 48–54.

Bunning, E. (1973) *The Physiological Clock. Circadian Rhythms and Bological Chronometry*, (3rd edn). London: The English Universities Press.

Cannon, W. B. (1928) The mechanism of emotional disturbance of bodily function. *The New England Journal of Medicine*, **198**, 877–884.

Cannon, W. B. (1929) Organization for physiological homeostasis. *Physiology Reviews*, **9**, 399–431.

Cherniack, N. S. & Longobardo, G. S. (1973) Cheyne-Stokes breathing: An instability in physiologic control. *New England Journal of Medicine*, **288**, 952–957.

Chiou-Tan, F. Y., Magee, K. N., Tuel, S. M., Robinson, L. R., Krouskop, T. A., Nelson, M. R. & Moss, F. (1997) Augmented sensory nerve action potentials during distant muscle contraction. *American Journal of Physical Medicine & Rehabilitation*, **76**, 14–18.

Cohen, A. H., Rossignol, S. & Grillner, S. (1988) *Neural Control of Rhythmic Movements in Vertebrates*. New York: Wiley.

Collins, J. J., Chow, C. C. & Imhoff, T. T. (1995) Stochastic resonance without tuning. *Nature*, **376**, 236–238.

Cordo, P., Gurfinkel, V. S., Bevan, L. & Kerr, G. K. (1995) Proprioceptive consequences of tendon vibration during movement. *Journal of Neurophysiology*, **74**, 1675–1688.

Ehlers, C. L., Havstad, J. W. & Schuckit, M. A. (1995) EEG dimensions in the sons of alcoholics. *Alcoholism: Clinical and Experimental Research*, **19**, 992–998.

Elliot, K. A. C. & Yrarrazaval, S. (1952) An effect of adrenalectomy and cortisone in tissue permeability *in vitro*. *Nature*, **169**, 416–417.

Field, R. J. & Burger, M. (1984) *Oscillations and Traveling Waves in Chemical Systems*. New York: Wiley.

Fleisher, L. A., Pincus, S. M. & Rosenbaum, S. H. (1993) Approximate entropy of heart rate as a correlate of postoperative ventricular dysfunction. *Anesthesiology*, **78**, 683–692.

Fraser, J. T. (1990) *Of Time, Passion and Knowledge*. Princeton, NJ: Princeton University Press.

Friesen, W. O. & Block, G. D. (1984) What is a biological oscillator? *American Journal of Physiology*, **246**, R847–R853.

Garfinkel, A. (1983) A mathematics for physiology. *American Journal of Physiology*, **245**, R455–R466.

Glaser, R., Kiecolt-Glaser, J. K., Speicher, C. E. & Holliday, J. E. (1985) Stress, loneliness, and changes in herpesvirus latency. *Journal of Behavioral Medicine*, **8**, 249–260.

Glass, L. & Mackey, M. C. (1979) Pathological conditions resulting from instabilities in physiological control systems. *Annals of the New York Academy of Sciences*, **316**, 214–235.

Glass, L. & Mackey, M. C. (1988) *From Clocks to Chaos: The Rhythms of Life*. Princeton, NJ: Princeton University Press.

Goldberger, A. L. (1991) Is the normal heartbeat chaotic or homeostatic? *News in Physiological Science*, **6**, 87–91.

Goldberger, A. L. & Rigney, D. R. (1990) Sudden death is not chaos. In *The Ubiquity of Chaos*, edited by S. Krasner. Washington, DC: American Association for the Advancement of Science.

Goldberger, A. L., Rigney, D. R., Mietus, J., Antman, E. M. & Greenwald, S. (1988) Nonlinear dynamics in sudden cardiac death syndrome: Heart rate oscillations and bifurcations. *Experientia*, **44**, 983–987.

Goldberger, A. L., Rigney, D. R. & West, B. J. (1990) Chaos and fractals in human physiology. *Scientific American*, **262**(2), 43–49.

Gottschalk, A., Bauer, M. S. & Whybrow, P. C. (1995) Evidence of chaotic mood variation in bipolar disorder. *Archives of General Psychiatry*, **52**, 947–959.

Grassberger, P. & Procaccia, I. (1983) Measuring the strangeness of strange attractors. *Physica D*, **9**, 189–208.

Greenspan, S. L., Klibanski, A., Rowe, J. W. & Elahi, D. (1991) Age-related alterations in pulsatile secretion of TSH: Role of dopaminergic regulation. *American Journal of Physiology*, **260**, E486–E491.

Grillot, M., Fauvel, J. P., Cottet-Emard, J. M., Laville, M., Peyrin, L., Pozet, N. & Zech, P. (1995) Spectral analysis of stress-induced change in blood pressure and heart rate in normotensive subjects. *Journal of Cardiovascular Pharmacology*, **25**, 448–452.

Grossman, P. & Wientjes, K. (1986) Respiratory sinus arrhythmia and parasympathetic cardiac control: some basic issues concerning quantification, application and implications. In *Cardiorespiratory and Cardiosomatic Psychophysiology*, edited by P. Grossman, K. Janssen & D. Vaitl. New York: Plenum Press.

Guevara, M. R., Glass, L. & Shrier, A. (1981) Phase locking, period doubling bifurcations, and irregular dynamics in periodically stimulated cardiac cells. *Science*, **214**, 1350–1353.

Hainsworth, R. (1995) The control and physiologic importance of heart rate. In *Heart Rate Variability*, edited by M. Malik & A. J. Camm. Armonk, NY: Futura.

Hales, S. (1733) *Statistical Essays: Containing Haemastaticks*. London: Innys, Manby and Woodward.

Hashimoto, A., Maeda, H. & Yokoyama, M. (1996) Augmentation of parasympathetic nerve function in patients with extrinsic bronchial asthma—evaluation by coefficiency of variance of R-R interval with modified long-term ECG monitoring system. *Kobe Journal of Medical Sciences*, **42**, 347–359.

Hyndman, B. W. (1973) The role of rhythms in homeostasis. *Kybernetic*, **15**, 227–236.

Hyndman, B. W. & Gregory, J. R. (1975) Spectral analysis of sinus arrhythmia during mental loading. *Ergonomics*, **18**, 255–270.

Hyndman, B. W., Kitney, R. I. & Sayers, B. McA. (1971) Spontaneous rhythms in physiological control systems. *Nature*, **233**, 339–341.

Irwin, M., Daniels, M., Bloom, E. T., Smith, T. L. & Weiner, H. (1987) Life events, depressive symptoms, and immune function. *American Journal of Psychiatry*, **144**, 437–441.

Kallenbach, J. M., Webster, T., Dowdeswell, R., Reinach, S. G., Millar, S. & Zvi, S. (1985) Reflex heart rate control in asthma: Evidence of parasympathetic overactivity. *Chest*, **87**, 664–648.

Kaplan, D. T., Furman, M. I., Pincus, S. M., Ryan, S. M., Lipsitz, L. A. & Goldberger, A. L. (1991) Aging and complexity of cardiovascular dynamics. *Biophysics Journal*, **59**, 945–949.

Kitney, R. I. (1980) An analysis of the thermoregulatory influences on heart rate variability. In *The Study of Heart Rate Variability*, edited by R. I. Kitney & O. Rompelman. Oxford: Oxford University Press.

Kitney, R. I., Byrne, S., Edmonds, M. E., Watkins, P. J. & Roberts, V. C. (1982) Heart rate variability in the assessment of autonomic diabetic neuropathy. *Automedica*, **4**, 155–167.

Kleeman, C. R., Koplowitz, J., Maxwell, R., Cutler, R. & Dowling, J. T. (1960) Mechanisms of impaired water excretion in adrenal and pituitary insufficiency IV: Interrelationship of adrenal cortical steroids and antidiuretic hormone in normal subjects and in diabetes insipidus. *Journal of Clinical Investigation*, **39**, 1472–1480.

Kleiger, R. E., Miller, J. P., Bigger, J. T. & Moss, A. J. (1987) Decreased heart rate variability and its association with increased mortality after acute myocardial infarction. *American Journal of Cardiology*, **59**, 256–262.

Koizumi, K. & Kollai, M. (1992) Multiple modes of operation of cardiac autonomic control: Development of the ideas from Cannon and Brooks to the present. *Journal of the Autonomic Nervous System*, **41**, 19–30.

Kreipe, R. E., Goldstein, B., DeKing, D. E., Tipton, R. & Kempski, M. H. (1994) Heart rate power spectrum of autonomic dysfunction in adolescents with anorexia nervosa. *International Journal of Eating Disorders*, **16**, 159–165.

Kronfol, Z., Silva, J., Greden, J., Gardner, R. & Carrol, B. J. (1983) Impaired lymphocyte function in depressive illness. *Life Sciences*, **33**, 241–247.

Landry, D. P., Bennett, F. M. & Oriol, N. E. (1994) Analysis of heart rate dynamics as a measure of autonomic tone in obstetrical patients undergoing epidural or spinal anesthesia. *Regional Anesthesia*, **19**, 289–295.

Langewitz, W. & Rüddel, H. (1989) Spectral analysis of heart rate variability under mental stress. *Journal of Hypertension*, **7**, S32–S33.

Langhorst, P., Schulz, B., Schulz, G. & Lambertz, M. (1983) Reticular formation of the lower brainstem. A common system for cardiorespiratory and somatomotor functions: discharge patterns of neighboring neurons influenced by cardiovascular and respiratory afferents. *Journal of the Autonomic Nervous System*, **9**, 411–432.

Lehrer, P. M. (in press) Book review and essay: Chaos, catastrophe, oscillation, and self-regulation. *Applied Psychophysiology and Biofeedback*.

Lehrer, P., Carr, R. E., Smetankine, A., Vaschillo, E., Peper, E., Porges, S., Edelberg, R., Hamer, R. & Hochron, S. (1997) Respiratory sinus arrhythmia versus neck/trapezius EMG and incentive inspiratory biofeedback for asthma: A pilot study. *Applied Psychophysiology and Biofeedback*, **22**, 91–105.

Lehrer, P. M., Hochron, S., Carr, R., Edelberg, R., Hamer, R., Jackson, A. & Porges, S. (1996) Behavioral task-induced bronchodilation in asthma during active and passive tasks: a possible cholinergic link to psychologically-induced airway changes. *Psychosomatic Medicine*, **58**, 413–422.

Liao, D., Barnes, R. W., Chambless, L. E., Simpson, R. J., Sorlie, P. & Heiss, G., for the ARIC Investigators (1995) Age, race, and sex differences in autonomic cardiac function measured by spectral analysis of heart rate variability: the ARIC study. *American Journal of Cardiology*, **76**, 906–912.

Lischner, M., Akselrod, S., Mor Avi, V., Oz, O., Divon, M. & Ravid, M. (1987) Spectral analysis of heart rate fluctuations. A non-invasive, sensitive method for the early diagnosis of autonomic neuropathy in diabetes mellitus. *Journal of the Autonomic Nervous System*, **19**, 119–125.

Lipsitz, L. A. & Goldberger, A. L. (1992) Loss of 'complexity' and aging: Potential applications of fractals and chaos theory to senescence. *Journal of the American Medical Association*, **267**, 1806–1809.

Lipsitz, L. A., Pincus, S. M., Morin, R. J., Tong, S., Eberle, L. P. & Gootman, P. M. (1997) Preliminary evidence for the evolution in complexity of heart rate dynamics during autonomic maturation in neonatal swine. *Journal of the Autonomic Nervous System*, **65**, 1–9.

Lombardi, F., Sandrone, G., Mortara, A., Torzillo, D., La Rovere, M. T., Signorini, M. G., Cerutti, S. & Malliani, A. (1996) Linear and nonlinear dynamics of heart rate variability after acute myocardial infarction with normal and reduced left ventricular ejection fraction. *American Journal of Cardiology*, **77**, 1283–1288.

Lombardi, F., Sandrone, G., Pernpruner, S., Sala, R., Garimoldi, M., Cerutti, S., Baselli, G., Pagani, M. & Malliani, A. (1987) Heart rate variability as an index of sympathovagal interaction after acute myocardial infarction. *American Journal of Cardiology*, **60**, 1239–1245.

Lyonfields, J. D., Borkovec, T. D. & Thayer, J. F. (1995) Vagal tone in generalized anxiety disorder and the effects of aversive imagery and worrisome thinking. *Behavior Therapy*, **26**, 457–466.

Mackey, M. C. & Glass, L. (1977) Oscillation and chaos in physiological control systems. *Science*, **197**, 287–289.

Mackey, M. C. & Milton, J. G. (1987) Dynamical diseases. *Annals of the New York Academy of Sciences*, **504**, 16–32.

Madwed, J. B., Albrecht, P., Mark, R. G. & Cohen, R. J. (1989) Low-frequency oscillations in arterial pressure and heart rate: a simple computer model. *American Journal of Physiology*, **256**, H1573–H1579.

Malliani, A., Pagani, M., Lombardi, F., Furlan, Guzzetti, S. & Cerutti, S. (1991) Spectral analysis to assess increased sympathetic tone in arterial hypertension. *Hypertension*, **17**, III-36–III-42.

Mancia, G., Ferrari, A., Gregorini, L., Parati, G., Pomodossi, G., Bertinieri, G., Grassi, G., di Rienzo, M., Pedotti, A. & Zanchetti, A. (1983) Blood pressure and heart rate variabilities in normotensive and hypertensive human beings. *Circulation Research*, **53**, 96–104.

Mandell, A. J. & Shlesinger, M. F. (1990) Lost choices, parallelism and topological entropy decrements in neurobiological aging. In *The Ubiquity of Chaos*, edited by S. Krasner. Washington, DC: American Association for the Advancement of Science.

McEwen, B. S. & Stellar, E. (1993) Stress and the individual: Mechanisms leading to disease. *Archives of Internal Medicine*, **153**, 2093–2101.

Middleton, H. C. & Ashby, M. (1995) Clinical recovery from panic disorder is associated with evidence of changes in cardiovascular regulation. *Acta Psychiatrica Scandinavica*, **91**, 108–113.

Novak, V., Novak, P., de Champlain, J. & Nadeau, R. (1993) Altered cardiorespiratory transfer in hypertension. *Hypertension*, **23**, 104–113.

Pagani, M., Furlan, R., Pizzinelli, P., Crivellaro, W., Cerutti, S. & Malliani, A. (1989) Spectral analysis of R-R and arterial blood pressure variabilities to assess sympatho-vagal interaction during mental stress in humans. *Journal of Hypertension*, **7**, S14–S15.

Pagani, M., Lucini, D., Mela, G. S., Langewitz, W. & Malliani, A. (1994) Sympathetic overactivity in subjects complaining of unexplained fatigue. *Clinical Science*, **87**, 655–661.

Pagani, M., Rimoldi, O., Pizzinelli, P., Furlan, R., Crivellaro, W., Liberati, D., Cerutti, S. & Malliani, A. (1991) Assessment of the neural control of the circulation during psychological stress. *Journal of the Autonomic Nervous System*, **35**, 33–42.

Peng, C. K., Buldyrev, S. V., Hausdorff, J. M., Havlin, S., Mietus, J. E., Simons, M., Stanley, H. E. & Goldberger, A. L. (1994) Non-equilibrium dynamics as an indispensable characteristic of a healthy biological system. *Integrative Physiological and Behavioral Science*, **29**, 283–293.

Peng, C. K., Havlin, S., Hausdorff, J. M., Mietus, J. E., Stanley, H. E. & Goldberger, A. L. (1995) Fractal mechanisms and heart rate dynamics. Long-range correlations and their breakdown with disease. *Journal of Electrocardiology*, **28**(Suppl.), 59–65.

Pincus, S. M. (1991) Approximate entropy as a measure of system complexity. *Proceedings of the National Academy of Sciences*, **88**, 2297–2301.

Pincus, S. M. (1994) Greater signal regularity may indicate increased system isolation. *Mathematical Biosciences*, **122**, 161–181.

Pincus, S. M., Cummins, T. R. & Haddad, G. G. (1993) Heart rate control in normal and aborted-SIDS infants. *American Journal of Physiology*, **264**, R638–R646.

Pincus, S. M. & Goldberger, A. L. (1994) Physiological time series: what does regularity quantify? *American Journal of Physiology*, **266**, H1643–H1656.

Pomeranz, B., Macaulay, R. J. B., Caudill, M. A., Kutz, I., Adam, D., Gordon, D., Kilborn, K. A., Barger, C., Shannon, D. C., Cohen, R. J. & Benson, H. (1985) Assessment of autonomic function in humans by heart rate spectral analysis. *American Journal of Physiology*, **248**, H151–H153.

Porges, S. W. (1986) Respiratory sinus arrhythmia: physiological basis, quantitative methods, and clinical implications. In *Cardiorespiratory and Cardiosomatic Psychophysiology*, edited by P. Grossman, K. Janssen & D. Vaitl. New York: Plenum Press.

Rapaport, M. H. & Stein, M. B. (1994) Serum interleukin-2 and soluble interleukin-2 receptor levels in generalized social phobia. *Anxiety*, **1**, 50–53.

Rapp, P. E. (1987) Why are so many biological systems periodic? *Progress in Neurobiology*, **29**, 261–273.

Rapp, P. E., Mees, A. I. & Sparrow, C. T. (1981) Frequency encoded biochemical regulation is more accurate than amplitude dependent control. *Journal of Theoretical Biology*, **90**, 531–544.

Rechlin, T., Weis, M., Spitzer, A. & Kaschka, W. P. (1994) Are affective disorders associated with alterations in heart rate variability? *Journal of Affective Disorders*, **32**, 271–275.

Rich, M. W., Saini, J. S., Kleiger, R. E., Carney, R. M., te Velde, A. & Freeland, K. E. (1988) Correlation of heart rate variability with clinical and angiographic variables and late mortality after coronary angiography. *American Journal of Cardiology*, **62**, 714–717.

Richter, P. H. & Ross, J. (1981) Concentration oscillations and efficiency: Glycolysis. *Science*, **211**, 715–717.

Roberts, A. & Roberts, B. L. (1983) *Neural Origins of Rhythmic Movements*. London: Cambridge University Press.

Rosenbaum, D. S., Jackson, L. E., Smith, J. M., Garan, H., Ruskin, J. N. & Cohen, R. J. (1994) Electrical alterans and vulnerability to ventricular arrhythmia. *New England Journal of Medicine*, **330**, 235–241.

Rischke, J. & Aldenhoff, J. B. (1993) Estimation of the dimensionality of sleep-EEG data in schizophrenics. *European Archives of Psychiatry and Clinical Neuroscience*, **242**, 191–196.

Rutter, M. (1988) Resilience in the face of adversity. *British Journal of Psychiatry*, **147**, 598–611.

Ryan, S. M., Goldberger, A. L., Pincus, S. M., Mietus, J. & Lipsitz, L. A. (1994) Gender- and age-related differences in heart rate dynamics: Are women more complex than men? *Journal of the American College of Cardiology*, **24**, 1700–1707.

Saul, J. P. (1990) Beat-to-beat variations of heart rate reflect modulation of cardiac autonomic outflow. *News in Physiological Sciences*, **5**, 32–37.

Saul, J. P. (1992) Cardiorespiratory variability: Fractals, white noise, nonlinear oscillators, and linear modeling. What's to be learned? In *Rhythms in Physiological Systems*, edited by H. Haken & H. P. Koepchen. Berlin Heidelberg: Springer-Verlag.

Saul, J. P., Albrecht, P., Berger, R. D. & Cohen, R. J. (1988) Analysis of long term heart rate variability: methods, 1/f scaling and implications. *Computers in Cardiology*, **14**, 419–422.

Saul, J. P., Arai, Y., Berger, R. D., Lilly, L. S., Colucci, W. S. & Cohen, R. J. (1988) Assessment of autonomic regulation in chronic congestive heart failure by heart rate spectral analysis. *American Journal of Cardiology*, **61**, 1292–1299.

Saul, J. P., Berger, R. D., Albrecht, P., Stein, S. P., Chen, M. H. & Cohen, R. J. (1991) Transfer function analysis of the circulation: unique insights into cardiovascular regulation. *American Journal of Physiology*, **261**, H1231–H1245.

Saul, J. P., Kaplan, D. T. & Kitney, R. I. (1989) Nonlinear interactions between respiration and heart rate: classical physiology or entrained nonlinear oscillators. *Computers in Cardiology*, **15**, 299–302.

Sayers, B. McA. (1973) Analysis of heart rate variability. *Ergonomics*, **16**, 17–32.

Schwartz, J. P., Gibb, W. J. & Tran, T. (1991) Aging effects on heart rate variation. *Journal of Gerontology*, **46**, M99–M106.

Schwartz, P. J., Zaza, A., Pala, M., Locati, E., Beria, G. & Zanchetti, A. (1988) Baroreflex sensitivity and its evolution during the first year after myocardial infarction. *Journal of the American College of Cardiology*, **12**, 629–636.

Shannon, D. C., Carley, D. W. & Benson, H. (1987) Aging of modulation of heart rate. *American Journal of Physiology*, **253**, H874–H877.

Sterling, P. & Eyer, J. (1988) Allostasis: a new paradigm to explain arousal pathology. In *Handbook of Life Stress, Cognition and Health*, edited by J. Fisher & J. Reason. London: John Wiley and Sons.

Thayer, J. F. & Friedman, B. H. (1993) Assessment of anxiety using heart rate nonlinear dynamics. In *Chaos in Biology and Medicine*, edited by W. Ditto. Bellingham, WA: SPIE—the International Society for Optical Engineering.

Theiler, J. & Rapp, P. E. (1996) Re-examination of the evidence for low-dimensional structure in the human electroencephalogram. *Electroencephalography and Clinical Neurophysiology*, **98**, 213–222.

Van Brummelen, P., Buhler, F. R., Kiowski, W. & Amann, F. W. (1981) Age-related decrease in cardiac and peripheral vasculature responsiveness to isoprenaline: studies in normal subjects. *Clinical Science*, **60**, 571–577.

Vollmayr, B., Sulger, J., Gabriel, P. & Aldenhoff, J. B. (1995) Mitogen stimulated rise of intracellular calcium concentration in single T lymphocytes from patients with major depression is reduced. *Progress in Neuro-Psychopharmacology & Biological Psychiatry*, **19**, 1263–1273.

von Haller, A. (1760) *Elementa Physiologica*. Lausanne, Switzerland:

West, B. J. (1990) *Fractal Physiology and Chaos in Medicine*. Teaneck, NJ: World Scientific.

Wever, R. (1964) Pendulum versus relaxation oscillation. In *Circadian Clocks*, edited by J. Aschoff. Amsterdam: North Holland Publishing Company.

Wever, R. A. (1988) Order and disorder in human circadian rhythmicity: Possible relations to mental disorders. In *Biological Rhythms and Mental Disorders*, edited by D. J. Kupfer, T. H. Monk & J. D. Barchas. New York: The Guilford Press.

Wiesenfeld, K. & Moss, F. (1995) Stochastic resonance and the benefits of noise: From ice ages to crayfish and SQUIDS. *Nature*, **373**, 33–36.

Winfree, A. T. (1980) *The Geometry of Biological Time*. New York: Springer-Verlag.

Yates, F. E. (1982) Outline of a physical theory of physiological systems. *Canadian Journal of Physiology and Pharmacology*, **60**, 217–248.

Yeragani, V. K. (1995) Heart rate and blood pressure variability: Implications for psychiatric research. *Neuropsychobiology*, **32**, 182–191.

Yeragani, V. K., Pohl, R., Berger, R., Balon, R., Ramesh, C., Glitz, D., Srinivasan, K. & Weinberg, P. (1993) Decreased heart rate variability in panic disorder patients: A study of power-spectral analysis of heart rate. *Psychiatry Research*, **46**, 89–103.

Yeragani, V. K., Srinivasan, K., Vempati, S., Pohl, R. & Balon, R. (1993) Fractal dimension of heart rate time series: An effective measure of autonomic function. *Journal of Applied Physiology*, **75**, 2429–2483.

Chapter 3

THE PHYSIOLOGY OF STRESS

Richard Gevirtz, PhD

PART I: PHYSIOLOGICAL RESPONSE TO STRESS

The Transactional Model of Stress

Modern definitions of 'stress' are primarily based on the transactional model originally described by Lazarus and Folkman (1984). In essence, '... potentially stressful events are appraised as either stressful or benign in the context of an individual's own values, beliefs, experiences, and coping resources' (Cohen, 1992, p. 110).

With this general model in mind, this chapter describes basic concepts and some recent developments in the physiology and biology of stress. Because this is an enormous topic, I will focus primarily on the autonomic nervous system and secondarily on the endocrine system/immune system.

Throughout, it is useful to conceive of the stress response as one that has evolved in humans in a highly social context. Our perception of acceptance or rejection in our social interactions determines a good deal of what we mean by stress in an everyday context. This is a departure from earlier works (e.g. Selye, 1956) which emphasised the endocrine response in much more primitive and directly life threatening situations and interpolated findings from these extreme settings to 'everyday' stressors. Thus, endocrine and pituitary medullary responses to parachute jumping (Ursin, Baade & Levine, 1978) were thought to constitute a model for all stressors, rather than for only dramatically threatening events. Modern conceptualizations have made this distinction and have emphasized the more transient and responsive autonomic systems. Endocrine-based measures may not be sufficiently sensitive to measure the effects of daily stressors and hassles (e.g. Cummins & Gevirtz, 1992), whereas autonomic measures contain a wealth of information for these more common stressors.

The Autonomic Nervous System

Guyton and Hall (1995) offer an excellent overview of the medical physiology in the major stress systems. Guyton (1976) provides more detailed coverage. The nervous system is divided into two main divisions, the central nervous system (CNS) consisting of the brain and spinal cord and the peripheral nervous system consisting of the Somatic/Sensory system and the autonomic nervous system (ANS). The ANS has two branches, the sympathetic (SNS) and the parasympathetic (PNS). Most traditional work has centred on the ANS for understanding the physiology of stress. The ANS functions with visceral and other organ systems in the body. In many systems it functions as the sole regulatory pathway, while in others it shares regulatory functions with other systems. The ANS is activated mainly by centres in the spinal cord, the hypothalamus, and the brain stem. While these centres are important, it is worth noting that the cerebral cortex can also exert an influence. Recent work on developmental psychobiology has revealed relationships between late developing brain centers, such as the orbitofrontal cortex, and the down regulation of the ANS. This material was recently compiled in a fascinating book by Allan Schore (1994).

The Sympathetic Branch

The SNS has long been thought of as the 'Stress Nervous System' since it seems to mobilize resources in the body for emergency situations such as 'fight or flight'. While this conceptualization is generally correct, it has been shown to be too simplistic in many ways. The name, itself, implies that the system works as an orchestra, with all parts in 'sympathy' to all other parts, thus creating a unified mass action response to perceived threats, physiological trauma, or other types of dysregulation. This idea is based partly on the anatomy of the system itself. The sympathetic nerves originate in the spinal column between T-1 and L-2 and travel to paravertebral sympathetic chains. From there, they travel to target organs: the heart, the bronchi, the gut, the adrenal medulla, the kidney, and to other sites. In this organization the system is unique, in that there is a distinctive preganglionic fiber to the chain and a postganglionic fiber to the target organ. By setting up this chain-like way station, communication among the elements of the system is greatly enhanced. The preganglionic fibers can synapse with the postganglionic fibers and innervate the target organs directly. They can travel up and down in the chain to influence other organs. In this way, complicated communication is possible. Many of the postganglionic fibers pass back to become spinal nerves and radiate throughout the body as skeletal nerves which can influence blood vessels, sweat glands, and piloerector muscles.

One group of preganglionic sympathetic nerves passes through the chain, through the splanchnic nerves, and finally synapses at the adrenal medullae. They stimulate specialized nerve endings that secrete epinephrine (adrenaline) and nor-epinephrine (nor-adrenaline) into the circulating blood. These hormones are carried to almost all parts of the body where they have an effect similar to the direct sympathetic innervation, except that the effect is much longer acting (up to 10 times). Thus, as various effects on target organs occur, the adrenal medullary pathway recreates almost the same response, but with a much longer duration.

The overall architecture of the SNS allows for specificity or mass action depending on the environmental demands. The pre-ganglionic/post-ganglionic split with up and down connections ensures this flexibility.

Neurotransmitters are the chemical communicators in the nervous system. The neurotransmitters in the sympathetic system are more complicated than in the other peripheral systems. In both the SNS and PNS there are two basic synaptic transmitters: norepinephrine and acetylcholine. Fibers that secrete the former are called adrenergic, and those secreting the latter are labelled cholinergic. All preganglionic fibers (those going from the spinal cord to the paravertebral ganglionic chain) are cholinergic. This is true in both the SNS, where the distinction between pre and post-ganglionic fibers is dramatic, and also in the PNS where the postganglionic fibers are quite short and primarily located at the target organ site, itself. This is the reason that any acetcholine-like substance can trigger both PNS and SNS target organs when applied at the ganglia.

The post-ganglionic fibers in the PNS are all cholinergic, but in the SNS they are mostly adrenergic. The primary exception to this rule is the sweat glands, which along with a few blood vessels, are cholinergically innervated. Thus a great deal of pharmacological interest has centred on adrenergic blockers or, conversely, on reducing cholinergic reactions to psychoactive drugs.

Research with cholinergic and adrenergic drugs has shown that there is a variety of receptor types within both the PNS and SNS. The two main acetylcholine receptors have been classified as 'muscarinic' since they are activated by only muscarine (a poison found in toadstools), and 'nicotinic' (stimulated by nicotine only). Acetylcholine stimulates both of them. Several adrenergic receptor types have been found and more are anticipated. These receptors have been classified as 'Beta' and 'Alpha' types. 'Beta1' and 'Beta2' subtypes are firmly established; other types have been detected, but not yet established. Both alpha and beta receptors can be excitatory or inhibitory.

Alpha receptors produce vasodilation, iris dilation, intestinal relaxation, intestinal sphincter contraction, pilomotor contraction, bladder sphincter contraction, and (recently discovered) muscle spindle activation.

Beta receptors produce vasodilation, cardioacceleration, increased myocardial strength, intestinal relaxation, bronchodilation, calorigenesis, glycogenolysis, lipolysis, and bladder relaxation. Many drugs which are agonists or antagonists of these systems exist. For example, propranolol is a well-known beta blocker that produces a kind of 'peripheral relaxation'. Because of this effect it is sometimes used by performing artists or athletes.

The organs targeted by the ANS are well known. In reviewing the major targets we will be setting the stage for what is currently known about various disorders that have been thought to be mediated by sympathetic pathways.

Table 3.1 shows the target organ and the effects of sympathetic and parasympathetic stimulation. In addition to the direct SNS pathways to target organs, the adrenals are also recruited by the SNS by way of direct pathways to the adrenal medulla and through indirect hypothalamic-pituitary-adrenocortical pathways.

Recently, sympathetic pathways to the muscle spindle have been documented in several species. The spindle is the sensory organ for muscle, regulating length and stretch. It has also been shown to contain nociceptive afferents (Barker & Banks, 1986; Passatore, Fillipi & Grassi, 1985). This discovery of sympathetic enervation may explain the long observed relationship between 'muscle tension' and stress. Our group has found that the myofascial trigger point 'hyperirritable spots, usually within a taut band of skeletal muscle or in the muscle's fascia, that is painful on compression can give rise to characteristic referred pain, tenderness, and autonomic phenomena' are quite responsive to stimuli thought to stimulate the SNS. These myofascial trigger points can be blocked only by sympathetic blockers. EMG activity in the trigger point generates activity at high levels while a needle, at the same depth in adjacent non-tender muscle is essentially quiet (Hubbard & Berkoff, 1993). It is our belief that trigger points are muscle spindles that have been over-activated by emotional stresses, physical demands on the muscle, trauma, or combinations of the above. This discovery may open up new avenues to the study of SNS activation of target organ activity (Gevirtz , Hubbard & Harpin, 1996; McNulty, Gevirtz, Hubbard & Berkoff, 1994;).

The gastrointestinal (GI) system is heavily influenced primarily by the parasympathetic system, though it contains an intrinsic nervous system of its own, the intramural plexus. The PNS increases overall GI tract activity which involves prolonged peristalsis (kneading-like slow contractions) and sphincter relaxation. The SNS has the effect of rapidly halting GI activity by way of the greater, lesser and least splanchnic nerves which emerge from the spinal column at T5/T6, T9, and T11, respectively.

Blood vessels in the viscera and skin are constricted by sympathetic activity but they are little affected by parasympathetic activity. Facial areas such as the cheeks, one notable exception, can be dilated by PNS enervation (e.g. blushing). The work of Robert Freedman (1991; Freedman, Sabharwal et al., 1988) has clearly demonstrated that finger blood flow is reduced under sympathetic influence. In contrast, voluntary increases, such as

Table 3.1   Autonomic effects on various organs of the body

Organ	Effect of Sympathetic Stimulation	Effect of Parasympathetic Stimulation
Eye: Pupil	Dilated	Constricted
Cillary muscle	Slight relaxation	Contracted
Glands: Nasal	Vasoconstriction and slight	Stimulation of thin, copious
Lacrimal	secretion	secretion (containing many
Paroid		enzymes for enzyme-
Submaxillary		secreting glands)
Gastric		
Pancreatic		
Sweat glands	Copious sweating (cholinergic)	None
Apocrine glands	Thick, odoriferous secretion	None
Heart Muscle	Increased rate	Slowed rate
	Increased force of contraction	Decreased force of atrial contraction
Coronaries	Dilated (β_2); constricted (α)	Diluted
Lungs: Bronchi	Dilated	Constricted
Blood vessels	Mildly constricted	? Dilated
Gut: Lumen	Decreased peristalsis and tone	Increased peristalsis and tone
Sphincter	Increased tone	Relaxed
Liver	Glucose released	Slight glycogen synthesis
Gallbladder and bile ducts	Relaxed	Contracted
Kidney	Decreased output	None
Bladder: Detrusor	Relaxed	Excited
Trigone	Excited	Relaxed
Penis	Ejaculation	Erection
Systemic blood vessels: Abdominal	Constricted	None
Muscle	Constricted (adrenergic α)	None
	Dilated (adrenergic β)	
	Dilated (cholinergic)	
Skin	Constricted	None
Blood: Coagulation	Increased	None
Glucose	Increased	None
Basal metabolism	Increased up to 100%	None
Adrenal cortical secretion	Increased	None
Mental activity	Increased	None
Pilocrector muscles	Excited	None
Skeletal muscle	Increased glycogenolysis	None
	Increased strength	

Source: Guyton, A. + Hall, J.E. (1981) *Textbook of Medical Physiology* (6th edn), p. 715. W. B. Saunders, with permission from W. B. Saunders Company.

biofeedback based finger temperature elevations, are mediated by blood borne beta-adrenergic compounds. Thus, the role of the SNS in relaxation type interventions is probably more complicated than may have been previously thought. When someone is taught to warm their hands to 94°, we can assume that systemic factors that transcend the ANS are at work.

Arterial blood pressure is also influenced by SNS activity in that it is the result of increased cardiac output and increased peripheral resistance. PNS pathways have a mild effect because they slow down heart rate and indirectly lower blood pressure.

In addition to these modes of control, blood pressure is also influenced by autonomic reflexes, primarily the baroreceptor reflex. Stretch receptors in the aorta and carotid arteries, when stimulated by high blood pressures, signal the brainstem, which inhibits sympathetic action and promote parasympathetic action to the heart and blood vessels. This system is keenly sensitive to acute changes but quickly adapts to long-term levels. The baroreceptor system has an oscillating rhythm of about 10 seconds. This phenomenon is called the Traube-Hering-Mayer wave. Recently much work has centered on understanding of the baroreceptor sensitivity (BRS). Hypertensives or even those with a family history of hypertension show lower BRS than normotensives (Eckberg & Sleight, 1992). Measurement of BRS may turn out to be of interest to psychophysiological disorders since it is a sensitive indicator of ANS/PNS feedback coherence and may be affected by 'stress' over time.

Dual control by the SNS and PNS is seen in the lungs where bronchodilation is sympathetically controlled and bronchoconstriction is parasympathetically controlled. Many more examples of this reciprocal relationship probably exist and await further research.

The Sympathetic/Adrenal Medullae

As mentioned above, parts of the sympathetic response are backed up by a blood-borne system secreted by the core or medulla of the adrenal glands. Sympathetic stimulation causes large quantities of epinephrine and nor-epinephrine to be released into the blood stream. As noted earlier, these circulating hormones have similar effects on the target organs described above, except that the effects are of much greater duration (up to 10 times longer). The two hormones differ from each other slightly. Epinephrine produces more dramatic cardiovascular effects and greatly increases metabolism (up to 100%), while nor-epinephrine has a more potent effect on peripheral resistance and, therefore, blood pressure. The sympathetic/adrenal medullary system is one of many examples of redundant systems built into the body. Failure of either the SNS system at the target organs, or of the adrenal medullae, have little effect on the overall organism.

The Parasympathetic System (PNS)

As was mentioned earlier and shown in Table 3.1, the PNS is simpler in structure than the SNS and has always been presumed to have more organ specificity. This system is characterized as facilitating restoration and maintenance of the organism. However, withdrawal of the system during stress may also play an important role.

Most research has been aimed at the reciprocal relationship between the SNS and PNS in the functioning of the cardiac system.

Porges (1995) has added much to our knowledge of the PNS with regard to conceptualizations of stress. He describes the PNS as a Polyvagal system with two branches. The first, the vegetative vagal system is older in an evolutionary sense. The second labeled the 'smart vagus', originates in the nucleus ambiguous of the brain stem. The more primitive vegetative vagus acts to preserve resources as one would expect in reptiles. That is, it greatly shuts down cardiac activity as exemplified in the primitive diving reflex. This system is balanced by the mammalian 'smart' vagus that regulates more social functions such as facial muscle flexibility, vocal functions, swallowing, and also controls the respiratory modulation of the heart. These PNS pathways are often ignored in the study of stress, but may be of great importance in facial EMG studies and in understanding how social hierarchies can be stimuli for a stress response.

A respiratory oscillator in the medulla has a periodicity of about 8–12 seconds (.12 to .30 Hz) and when seen in the heart period is called respiratory sinus arrhythmia (RSA). Many observers have described the RSA system as 'withdrawing' during stress. Thus, you may see vagal tone as a measure in stress studies. Psychophysiologists have been especially interested in PNS activity here because of the airway constriction occurring in asthma. Porges (1995) presents an in depth theoretical review and Bernston, Cacciopo & Quigley (1993) a review of the physiology of this response system. By measuring the power or amplitude of frequencies around the breathing rhythm (.12 to .30 Hz), one can discern the parasympathetic or 'vagal tone' influencing the heart rate. In this way, it might be possible to get a more integrated view of how the two branches of the ANS may interact to control organ systems and thus disorders of those systems.

SNS and PNS Complex Interactions

While the SNS and PNS can be thought of as separate, like almost all aspects of the nervous system, they often work in complex interactive ways. A great deal of recent physiological research has tried to better understand these functions. For example, Bernston, Caccioppo & Quigley (1991) have constructed 'topological' maps that show how PNS/SNS reciprocity and co-activity might work at various levels of each. They advance an alternative to the 'single vector model' of the autonomic continuum. While simple linear response curves representing the relationship between psychological and physiological variables have often failed, with '...independent measures of the relative activity of both ANS divisions within an organ state, or its reactive change, in the dimensions of autonomic space' (p. 482), a more complete description is possible.

It seems clear that psychophysiology will be greatly enriched by the technological advances that allow non-invasive monitoring of subtle autonomic functions. Many psychophysiological and anxiety disorders are probably associated with subtle autonomic dysfunction or breakdown of homeostasis in the ANS . Better understanding of the nuances of ANS functioning could promote improved diagnosis and treatment.

General Considerations
An important feature of the ANS is the concept of 'tone'. Both the SNS and PNS maintain an adequate frequency rate to keep the target organ at a mid range value. In this way excitation or inhibition can be used for regulation. Beyond this, the two branches interact in several organ systems to further complicate the picture.

Modern research of the ANS has emphasized the complexity of the system. As an example, Jänig and McLachlan (1992) talk about 'functional pathways' as the 'building blocks of the autonomic nervous system'. They trace the history of the ANS conceptualization from Langley to Cannon to Hess and to the present. 'The idea that the sympathetic outflow to the cardiovascular and visceral systems is always activated in parallel remains firmly ensconced in modern textbooks, usually contrasted with the so-called specificity of the parasympathetic system ...' (Jänig & McLachlan, 1992, p. 5). Actually, modern recording techniques have elucidated many very distinct systems within the SNS. Among the examples cited are distinct vasoconstrictor systems (muscle vs. cutaneous) and visceral organs regulated completely independently of cardiovascular systems. Jänig and McLachlan (1992) state, 'It is therefore quite clear that 'sympathetic tone' as such simply does not exist ...' (p. 8). In fact, the SNS must be studied as a complex system with differentiation throughout the peripheral and central nervous systems.

Likewise, the PNS has recently been described as having distinct branches which may have evolved in mammals to better adapt to complex environmental demands (Porges, 1995). 'The behavioral derivatives of the two branches of the vagus suggest a typology in which one branch of the vagus deals with unconscious reflexive vegetative function and the other is involved in more conscious, voluntary, flexible and often social activities' (p. 309). The vegetative vagus contains only visceral efferents, while the smart vagus innervates the somatic musculature of the palate, larynx, pharynx, and esophagus.

During stress, the two branches can be thought of as in conflict, with the vegetative vagus trying to shut down the cardiovascular system (as in the diving reflex) while the smart vagus withdraws vagal tone as an adaptation to '... novelty in the environment while coping with the need to maintain metabolic output and continuous social communication' (p. 310).

This 'polyvagal' model may lead us to a much richer knowledge of the relationships among the branches and among specific classes of stressors and their distinct physiological patterns. Since the smart vagus can be seen in the light of evolutionary adaptations, it leads us to reemphasize the social context of stress.

Endocrine Stress Responses

Hans Selye (1956, 1973) has elucidated a comprehensive homeostatic model of stress, centered mostly around the endocrine response systems. With the conceptualization of the 'Generalized Adaptation Syndrome' (GAS), he postulated that the normal adaptation process maintains healthy homeostasis and enhances the organism's ability to meet threats, but that prolonged stressors would lead to a physiological 'exhaustion' state that would lead to organ pathology. Ulcers served as the prototypical disease for the model.

This model was formulated primarily on observations of animals in physiological laboratories. It had been shown that a cortical interpretation of a threat to homeostasis leads to hypothalamic activation with neural control of the posterior lobe of the pituitary gland (through corticotropin-releasing hormone, CHA). The pituitary, in turn, releases adrenocorticotropin hormone (ACTH) into the blood stream where it targets the adrenal cortex. The adrenal cortex releases glucocorticoids, anti-inflammatory substances that try to control the consequences of trauma. This response is much slower and occurs in the aftermath of the initial sympathetic or even the adreno-medullary response. Selye (1936) had noted the non-specificity of the pituitary-adrenocortical system. A great number of physical, chemical, and psychological stimuli seem to be able to accelerate the production of glucocorticoids by the adrenal cortex. This is unusual in biology where specificity of innervation is the rule. This led Selye to conclude that the system evolved to be responsive to a wide variety of stressors (Saffran & Dokas, 1983). While many other hormones are affected by stress (insulin, prolactin, thyroid hormones, epinephrine, glucagon, endorphins, and enkephalins), the adrenal hormonal response has been the major focus of research on the physiology of stress. Studies with adrenalectomized animals have shown that the heightened anxiety and stress response that occurs after surgery, can be reversed with corticosterone (a glucocorticoid), (File, Vellucci & Wendlandt, 1979).

Modern versions of the GAS emphasize the biphasic role of the adrenal steroids, first to counteract inflammation, and then to set up buffers to protect tissue from their overreaction (Munck, Guyre & Holbrook, 1984). Moreover, we now know that stress hormones can affect virtually every organ system in the body, especially the brain (McEwen & Mendelson, 1993). The key concept here is 'counter regulation'. Adrenal steroids seem to play an important role in countering many of the body's initial responses to stress, maintaining a critical balance. For example, glucocorticoid helps to keep the noradrenergic arousal system in check. This may serve an anti-depressive function since it has been shown that a hyperactive or dysregulated noradrenergic system is associated with depression (Gold, Goodwin & Chrousos, 1988). No doubt future research will uncover many complex interactions between stress hormones and neurotransmitter systems.

Taken as a whole it appears likely that stress hormones play an important role in depressive disease. Prolonged exposure to uncontrollable stressors seems to dysregulate seratonergic receptor sites. Benzodiazapine and seratonergic systems also seem to exhibit complex bi-phasic responses to stress hormones (McEwen & Mendelson, 1993). With the rapid advances in psychopharmacology, these relationships should emerge and broaden the scope of the physiology of stress.

Respiratory Response Systems

Until recently respiratory responses were rarely mentioned in coverage of stress physiology. However, there is an extensive literature on this and related topics which goes back almost 100 years (c.f. Han et al., 1997). The basic idea in this literature is that stress or more importantly, prolonged stress, can lead to hyperventilation (breathing at a faster rate than metabolically needed) which, by altering the acid/base balance, can lead to a constellation of symptoms such as, dyspnea, panic, fatigue, anxiety, dizziness, muscle weakness, and so on. Several recent books have emphasized the importance of these syndromes in a variety of disorders (Fried, 1993; Timmons & Ley, 1994).

To briefly summarize, it has been shown that there exists a transient response to stress, characterized by rapid, shallow breathing which leads to a slight elevation in the acid-base balance of the body (that is in the direction of alkalinity). While this response seems to produce short-term anxiolytic and analgesic effects, when the response is prolonged it can lead to the symptoms described above. For example, cortical blood flow is reduced, vasoconstriction can occur, the cardiovascular system is activated, muscle tone increased, gastrointestinal disruption can occur, and even the coronary artery can become constricted.

The bases for these changes are complex and multi-faceted. One important system that has been understood for many years is the oxygen dissociation curve. The oxygen dissociation curve is a well known physiological law that shows the relationship between blood pH and the ability of oxygen to be released from hemoglobin. As blood pH becomes more alkaline, the oxygen becomes overbound to the hemoglobin molecule. This means that oxygen is not as available to organs in the body (including the cerebral cortex). There is evidence (though this is controversial) that prolonged over-breathing can become homoeostatically set in such a manner as to create the symptoms above, yet allow ostensibly normal physiological function. This state of affairs has been labeled the 'hyperventilation syndrome'. It is a diagnostic entity that has been popular in Europe.

The Striate Musculature

The striate musculature, independent of the spindle/sympathetic interactions described earlier, does play a reactive role in the stress response. This may be seen in two ways: very short latency muscle contractions (under 100 msec) and muscle bracing or splinting. McGuigan has described these responses (1978) in various locations. It is clear from the timing sequences that a rapid muscular contraction is among the body's first responses to a stressful stimulus. Speech muscles respond to both words and letters with latencies of 44 to 85 ms. (Davis, 1983). Similarly, Bickford et al. (1964) reported very rapid response latencies in arms and legs (25 to 50 ms.). Latencies this rapid can be viewed as automatic and 'hard wired' and are probably the most rapidly responsive components to the perception of a stressor.

Another pathway that has been postulated is that of a stress- induced muscular patterning often called splinting or bracing. The most thorough description of this theoretical perspective was given by Whatmore and Kohli (1974) who coined the term 'disponisis' for maladaptive muscular bracing in functional disorders. In light of the current knowledge of muscle described in Part II below, the automatic nature of the muscle patterns must be re-examined. However, even if the cortex can override specific muscular patterning, the splinting or bracing response may still be of importance.

PART II: CONSEQUENCES OF PROLONGED ACTIVATION OF THE STRESS RESPONSE SYSTEMS

In this section, we focus on the consequences of prolonged activation in a few of the above described systems. This topic has been extensively explored, but often with insufficient data to confirm strong conclusions. The emphasis here is on the basis for models of psychophysiological disorders, that is disorders where we have evidence for a pathway starting with psychological or emotional constructs interacting with physiological mediators and finally influencing physical symptoms. A related pathway may exist for psychological symptoms such as panic, anxiety, or depression. These will be considered when some peripheral mechanism is thought to be involved.

Disorders Related to Sympathetic Pathways

As noted, the sympathetic pathways have become the focus of attention for most psychophysiologic disorders. It is only recently, however, that concrete evidence for physiological mediators between symptoms and psychological factors has been found. Two groups of disorders are worth emphasis, muscle pain disorders and irritable bowel syndrome (IBS).

Muscle pain has been presumed to be related to stress in the environment, but the presumed mechanisms were either unknown or systematically eliminated. Factors such as fatigue, micro-trauma, spasm, or posture have been thought to be the target as the pain mediator. Evidence for these pathways has been absent or at least not convincingly confirmed. Starting with the pioneering work of Janet Travell and David Simons (1983), it has been increasingly recognized that 'trigger points' represent a good candidate for muscle pain mechanisms. Trigger points (TPs) are small nodules embedded in the muscle body that are tender to touch and refer pain to a characteristic area, sometimes distant from the TP itself. As mentioned earlier, our group has been able to show electromyographically that the trigger points are activated (or shut down) by alpha sympathetic pathways. This then paves the way for a true psychophysiological model of chronic muscle pain. Various emotional or stressful stimuli drive the activity in the TP for a long enough time to create the conditions for pain. We have hypothesized that this occurs in the muscle spindle, the sensory component of the muscle, but this remains speculative (see Simons, 1996). The role of bracing or splinting (disponesis) in this model is still unclear. Muscle response in the form of extrafusal contraction in the face of a stressor has been commonly observed (e.g. Whatmore & Kohli, 1974). In the experimental environment used in our needle TP studies, this response is not consistently seen. Perhaps the presence of a needle in the muscle overrides the usual motor reactions.

Our current efforts involve tracing the pathway to determine the psychological or perceptual stimuli most often involved, to fleshing out the exact physiological pathways. We suspect that situations involving interpersonal conflict, fear of negative self-evaluation, and lack of assertiveness play an important role. At this point the work points the way to understanding muscle pain, at least partly as a psychophysiological disorder. This view of course has treatment (Gevirtz, Hubbard & Harpin, 1996) as well as research implications.

Another disorder that appears to be a sympathetically mediated psychophysiological disorder is Irritable Bowel Syndrome (IBS). This disorder accounts for almost 50% of all gastroenterology referrals. Since there is typically no evidence of medical pathology, it is often thought to be a psychological disorder by physicians. However, studies by Drossman's group (Drossman et al., 1990) and others have found no real sign of psychopathology in most IBS sufferers. They do note that there is a subgroup of 'medical seekers' who do appear to have significant psychosocial problems with frequent histories of abuse. A research group at UCLA led by Emeran Mayer (Bernstein et al., 1996; Lembo et al., 1994) have pioneered a psychophysiological model that emphasises brain-gut interactions. Using balloon distension techniques in the colon, they have been able to show that IBS patients have hypersensitivity mediated by splanchnic afferents. Blanchard and Malamood (1996) have recently reviewed data that show that treatment of chronic worry or rumination in IBS patients is quite effective in reducing symptoms. These studies suggest a mediator path which would begin to explain IBS as another psychophysiological disorder. Processes associated with ruminative worry seem to disrupt the normal brain-gut regulation and, in addition, potentiate pain amplification through sympathetic splanchnic afferents. Interventions which help to re-regulate these systems seem to alleviate symptoms. For example, over sixty years ago Jacobson (1938) reported using 'progressive relaxation', a well known means of reducing sympathetic activity, to successfully treat IBS.

The SNS is undoubtedly involved in many other disorders as well. Research identifying mediators is just beginning, however. Disorders that are good candidates are: migraine headache, dermatological conditions, flare-ups of diseases such as inflammatory bowel disease or Lupus, aspects of cardiovascular disease, panic disorder, etc.

Treatment Implications
The specificity of sympathetic pathways may imply that distinctive psychosocial stimuli may be involved for each organ system. This would lead to treatment protocols that target the specific psychophysiologic pathway. The two examples above have evolved as our knowledge of the disorders has increased. For muscle pain, treatment relies on the pathway reaching back from the 'spindle spasm' to the sympathetic innervation to psychological/emotional factors such as difficulty with assertion, avoidance of conflict, or fear of criticism. For IBS, we have noted that autonomic pathways to the gut are interrupted by chronic stressors such as worry or rumination. As other distinct pathways emerge, treatment protocols will become more specific and thus more effective. This conceptualization may be distinct from mass action arousal syndromes.

Disorders Related to Parasympathetic Nervous System Dysregulation

While the PNS is probably involved in many aspects of health and disease, it is of primary interest in two major areas: life sustaining cardio-pulmonary regulation, and bronchial asthma. Several authors have documented the role of the vagal systems in sudden respiratory failure (Fox & Porges, 1985), recovery of acute myocardial infarction (Bigger et al., 1988), and hypertension (Malliani, Pagani, Lombardi & Cerutti, 1991). In this regard, Porges' idea of the reciprocal relationship between the smart and vegetative vagus is salient. The idea that more subtle influences may be at work in other disorders underlies the role of the PNS in bronchial asthma.

Asthma is characterised by excessive bronchial airway reactivity, usually in response to an allergen or external irritant. A great deal is now known about the histamine and mast cell mechanisms at the end point of the reaction. Much less is known about the autonomic systems involved. We do know that the SNS plays only a minor role in actual airway regulation and that the bronchospastic reaction is mediated by the PNS. It has been recognized that there is a subset of asthmatics that can have an attack triggered by emotional or stressful situations. It is assumed that the PNS plays a role, but the mechanism had been unclear (Lehrer, Eisenberg & Hochron, 1993). Most research is pointing toward subtle dysregulation of the SNS/PNS balance especially following prolonged stress. We (Heeren, Gevirtz & Seltzer, 1997) have found that asthmatics with emotionally triggered attacks show a more pronounced RSA response after a stressor than do asthmatics with non-emotionally triggered attacks. Similarly Sturani, Sturani & Tosi (1985) found that intrinsic asthma patients (those without common allergies), showed an exaggerated bradycardia (heart rate decrease) response to a cold stimulus on the face (diving reflex) compared to non-asthma patients. This would seem to indicate a dominance in the vegetative vagus possibly through smart vagal withdrawal. In any case, this research points the way towards including autonomic responses to stress in our understanding of asthma.

Treatment Implications

Lehrer (1997) has recently written an essay describing the possible advantages of using nonlinear models (chaos analysis) in assessing ANS homeostasis or lack thereof. It may be that our newfound interest in PNS will lead to more productive treatment models for disorders such as panic, asthma, hypertension, motion sickness, etc. than was possible with more linear models. Lehrer's emphasis on 'oscillators' may be generalizable to disorders such as chronic fatigue or fibromyalgia where evidence exists for stress having a long term effect on disrupting chronobiological oscillations. Treatments in this instance would be targeted to restoring the proper mix of rhythms, be they circadian, utradian, or very low frequency cardiovascular oscillations. As an example, Lehrer et al. (1997) describe a form of RSA biofeedback long used in Russia for asthma treatment. The underlying rationale is daily recalibration of low frequency cardiac cycles through the biofeedback exercises. In this pilot study, this training produced dramatic lung function improvements compared to a normal relaxation type treatment. Similarly, Herbs and Gevirtz (1994) found that RSA biofeedback training was as effective as finger temperature training in reducing blood pressure in hypertensives. In this model the training is conceptualized not as only enhancing vagal tone, but as a method of restoring disordered dynamic homeostatic systems.

Respiratory Factors as Mediators of Psychophysiological and Anxiety Disorders

Respiratory responses to stress are emerging as good candidates for mediators of symptoms in a variety of stress related and anxiety disorders. The mechanisms of subtle hyperventilation and the systemic sequelae which affect a wide variety of organ systems appear to explain at least some of the variance in a number of disorders such as functional cardiac disorder, panic, some phobias, and general somatization disorders.

Functional cardiac disorder is a common classification used by cardiologists and internists to describe patients with symptoms such as chest pain, dyspnea, dizziness, etc. but without measurable medical pathology. We have shown that these patients, often with low normal End Tidal Carbon Dioxide ($ETCO_2$) and rapid respiration rate, decrease symptoms dramatically when trained in slow diaphragmatic breathing. The rate of symptom reduction is highly and significantly correlated with normalization of breathing parameters (r = .59) indicating the probable role of respiration as a mediator of chest symptoms (DeGuire, Gevirtz, Kawahara & Maguire, 1992; DeGuire et al, 1996).

Breathing anomalies may help explain some aspects of anxiety disorders such as Panic Disorder (PD). The role of hyperventilation in PD has been hotly debated (c.f., Papp, Klein & Gorman, 1993). Some of the contradictory findings could be explained by the existence of sub-groups among these patients. Ronald Ley (1992) has proposed three such sub-groups ranging from heavy respiratory and physiological involvement to mostly cognitive distortion. Of interest here is the proposed existence of a respiratory sub-group with frequent 'out of the blue' attacks. We (Moynihan & Gevirtz, 1996) have found that the 'out of the blue' or spontaneous sub-type patients had lower $ETCO_2$ indicating a possible mechanism through which frequent over breathing could produce symptoms.

Fried (1993) describes many other disorders with possible respiratory mediation.

Treatment Implications
Treatment implications connected with respiratory psychophysiology have been discussed for many years. Robert Fried (1993) discusses the far ranging physical and psychological consequences of hyperventilation (both acute and chronic) in great detail. An international organisation has focussed on respiratory psychophysiological topics for over 10 years (International Society for the Advancement of Respiratory Psychophysiology, ISARP). Timmons and Ley (1994) also have many chapters devoted to clinical applications of respiratory phenomena.

A consensus of most clinicians in this area is that almost all psychophysiological and some anxiety disorder treatment protocols should start with breathing retraining. As this has been the basis of virtually every Eastern meditative art for thousands of years, this seems to be a safe recommendation.

Disorders Related to Endocrine Dysregulation

It has long been assumed that prolonged secretion of glucocorticoids has deleterious health consequences. This was the primary implication of the concept of the 'exhaustion' stage of Selye's GAS (1974). Ulcers were noted as the prototypical disease that results from this prolonged "exhaustion" of the endocrine system. Since this early conceptualisation, many other diseases and syndromes have been hypothesised to be the result of excessive glucocorticoid production in response to environmental demands. For example corticosteroids have been postulated to be involved in the development of atherosclerosis, elevated serum lipids, increased proportion of dead or injured endothelial cells (Henry, 1983). This pathway is proposed over and above a sympathoadrenal medullary involvement in lipid mobilization (Havel & Goldstein, 1959). More recent efforts have focussed on hostility as the active ingredient in cardiovascular disease, with glucocorticoids playing an important, but not exclusive role (Suarez & Williams, 1992).

It has long been recognised that stress, especially if chronic and uncontrollable, can affect immune function. From these early observations the field of psycho immunology has emerged. Humoral and cellular immune responses have been extensively studied in laboratory and naturalistic settings. Findings have generally been interpreted to indicate that a lowered immune function after stress will occur. Though most people under stress do not become ill, when other vulnerabilities and risk factors exist, the stress/hormonal/ immune connection becomes important. This topic is beyond the scope of the present chapter but has been recently covered in a book entitled *Human Stress and Immunity*, edited by Ronald Glaser and Janice Kiecolt-Glaser (1994).

SUMMARY

This chapter described the fundamental physiological responses to stress. We have emphasised the autonomic, endocrine and immune systems in an effort to understand the pathways that especially prolonged stress might have in affecting the body because these might help us understand psychophysiological disorders. This is a significant task from a public health point of view, since the disorders described above account for a large proportion of health care resource utilisation. With the dwindling resources available, it is clear that improving our understanding of the impact of stress on the body will produce large dividends both from a humane and financial point of view.

References

Barker, D. & Banks, R. (1986) The muscle spindle. In *Myology*, edited by A. Engel & B. Banker, pp. 309–341. McGraw-Hill: New York.

Bernstein, C., Niazi, N., Robert, M., Mentz, H., Kodner, A., Munakata, J., Naliboff, B. & Mayer, E. (1996) Rectal afferent function in patients with inflammatory and functional intestinal disorders. *Pain*, **66**, 151–161.

Bernston, G., Cacioppo, J. & Quigley, K. (1993) Respiratory sinus arrhythmia: Autonomic origins, physiological mechanisms and psychophysiological implications. *Psychophysiology*, **30**, 183–196.

Bickford, R., Jacobson, J. & Cody, D. (1964) Nature of average evoked potentials to sound and other stimuli in men. *Annals of the New York Academy of Sciences*, **112**, 204–210.

Bigger, J., Kleiger, R., Fleiss, J., Rolnitzky, L., Steinman, R. & Miller, J. (1988) Components of heart rate variability measure during healing of acute myocardial infarction. *American Journal of Cardiology*, **61**, 208–215.

Blanchard, E. & Malamoud, H. (1996) Psychological treatment of irritable bowel syndrome. *Professional Psychology*, **27**, 241–244.

Cohen, S. (1992) Stress, social support & disorder. In *The Meaning and Measurement of Social Support*, edited by H. Veieland & V. Baumann. New York: Hemisphere Publishing Corp.

Cummins, S. & Gevirtz, R. N. (1992) The relationship between daily stress and urinary cortisol in a normal population: An emphasis on individual differences. *Behavioral Medicine*, **19**, 129–134.

Davis, W. (1983) The degree of perceptual salience and perceptual difficulty on covert oral responses. Unpublished doctoral dissertation, University of Lousville, Kentucky.

DeGuire, S., Gevirtz, R., Hawkinson, D. & Dixon, K. (1996) Breathing retraining: A three-year follow-up study of treatment for hyperventilation syndrome and associated functional cardiac symptoms. *Biofeedback and Self-Regulation*, **21**, 191–198.

DeGuire, S., Gevirtz, R. N., Kawahara, Y. & Maguire, W. (1992) Hyperventilation syndrome and the assessment of treatment for functional cardiac symptoms. *American Journal of Cardiology*, **70**, 673–677.

Drossman, D., Thompson, G., Talley, N., Funch-Jensen, P., Jansens, J. & Whitehead, W. (1990) Identification of subgroups of functional gastrointestinal disorders. *Gastroenterology International*, **3**, 159–172.

Eckberg, D. & Sleight, P. (1992) *Human Baroreflexes in Health and Disease*. Oxford: Clarendon Press.

File, S., Velluci, S. & Wendlandt, S. (1979) Corticosterone-an anxiogenic or anxiolytic agent? *Journal of Pharmacy of Pharmacology*, **31**, 300–305.

Fox, N. & Porges, S. (1985) The relation between neonatal heart period patterns and developmental outcome. *Child Development*, **56**, 28–37.

Freedman, R. R. (1991) Physiological mechanisms of temperature biofeedback. *Biofeedback and Self-Regulation*, **16**, 95–115.

Freedman, R. R., Sabharwal, S. C., Ianni, P., Nagaraj, D., Wenig, P. & Mayes, M. D. (1988) Nonneural beta-adrenergic vasodilating mechanism in termperature biofeedback. *Psychosomatic Medicine*, **50**, 394–401.

Fried, R. (1993) *The Psychology and Physiology of Breathing*. New York: Plenum.

Gevirtz, R., Hubbard, D. & Harpin, R. E. (1996) Psychophysiologic treatment of chronic lower back pain. *Professional Psychology: Research and Practice*, **27**, 561–566.

Glaser, R. & Kiecolt-Glaser, J. (eds.) (1994) *Human Stress and Immunity*. San Diego: Academic Press.

Gold, P., Goodwin, F. & Chrousos, G. (1988) Clinical and biochemical manifestations of depression. Part 1. *New England Journal of Medicine*, **319**, 348–353.

Guyton, A. (1976) *Structure and Function of the Nervous System*. Philadelphia, PA: W. B. Sanders Co.

Guyton, A. (1981) *Textbook in Medical Physiology*, 6th ed. Philidelphia, PA: W. B. Saunders Co.

Guyton, A. & Hall, J. (1995) *Textbook of Medical Physiology*, 9th ed. Philadelphia, PA: W. B. Sanders Co.

Han, J. N., Stegan, K., Simkens, K., Canberghs, M., Schepers, R., Van den Bergh, D., Clement, J. & Van de Woestijne, K. (1997) Unsteadiness of breathing in patients with hyperventilation syndrome and anxiety disorders. *European Respiratory Journal*, **10**, 167–176.

Havel, R. & Goldstein, A. (1959) The role of the sympathetic nervous system in the metabolism of free fatty acids. *Journal of Lipid Research*, **1**, 102–108.

Heeren, M., Gevirtz, R. & Seltzer, J. Psychophysiological response patterns in emotionally triggered asthma. Poster presented at the 28th annual meeting of the Association for Applied Psychophysiology and Biofeedback, San Diego, CA, March, 1997.

Henry, J. (1983) Coronary heart disease and arousal of the adrenal cortical axis. In *Bio-behavoral Basis of Coronary Heart Disease*, edited by T. M. Dembrowski & T. Schmidt. Basel, Switzerland: Karger.

Herbs, D. & Gevirtz, R. (1994) The effect of heart rate pattern feedback for the treatment of essential hypertension. Presented at the 25th annual meeting of the Association for Applied Psychophysiology and Biofeedback, Atlanta, GA.

Hubbard, D. & Berkoff, G. (1993) Myofascial trigger points show spontaneous needle EMG activity. *Spine*, **18**, 1803–1807.

Jacobson, E. (1938) *Progressive Relaxation* (revised edn), Chicago: University of Chicago Press.

Jänig, W. & McLachlan, E. (1992) Specialized functional pathways are building blocks of the autonomic nervous system. *Journal of the Autonomic Nervous System*, **41**, 3–14.

Lazarus, R. & Folkman, S. (1984) *Stress, Appraisal, and Coping*. New York: Springer.

Lehrer, P. (1997) Book review and essay: Chaos, catastrophe, oscillation, and self-regulation. *Applied Psychophysiology and Biofeedback*, **22**, 215–223.

Lehrer, P., Eisenberg, S. & Hochron, S. (1993) Asthma and emotion: A review. *Journal of Asthma*, **30**, 5–21.

Lehrer, P., Carr, R., Smetankine, E., Vaschillo, E., Peper, E., Porges, S., Eckberg, R., Hamer, R. & Hochron, S. (1997) Respiratory sinus arrhythmia versus neck/ trapezious EMG and incentive inspirometry biofeedback for asthma: a pilot study. *Applied Psychophysiology and Biofeedback*, **22**, 95–109.

Lembo, T., Munakata, J., Mentz, H., Niazi, N., Kodner, A., Nikas, V. & Mayer, E. (1994) Evidence for the hypersensitivity of lumbar splanchnic afferents in irritable bowel syndrome. *Gastroenterology*, **107**, 1686–1696.

Ley, R. (1992) The many faces of pain: Psychological and physiological differences among three types of panic attacks. *Behavior Research and Therapy*, **30**, 347–357.

Malliani, A., Pagani, M., Lombardi, F. & Cerutti, S. (1991) Clinical and experimental evaluation of sympatho-vagal interaction: Power spectral analysis of heart rate and arterial pressure variabilities. In *The Reflex Control of Circulation*, edited by I. H. Zucker & J. P. Gilmore, pp. 937–964. Boca Raton, FL: CRC Press.

McEwen, B. & Mendelson, S. (1993) Effects of stress on the neurochemistry and morphology of the brain: Counterregulation versus damage. In *Handbook of Stress*, (2nd edn), edited by L. Goldberger & S. Breznitz. New York: The Free Press.

McGuigan, F. J. (1978) Cognitive Psychophysiology: Principles of Covert Behavior. Englewood Cliffs, New Jersey: Prentice Hall.

McNulty, W., Gevirtz, R., Hubbard, D. & Berkoff, G. (1994) Needle electromyographic evaluation of trigger point response to a psychological stressor. *Psychophysiology*, **31**, 313–316.

Moynihan, J. & Gevirtz, R. (1996) Towards identifying subtypes of panic using respiratory and psychophysiologic factors: a preliminary investigation. *Biological Psychology*, **43**, 253 (abstract).

Munck, A., Guyre, P. & Holbrook, N. (1984) Physiological function of glucocorticoids in stress and their relation to pharmacological actions. *Endocrinology Review*, **5**, 25–44.

Papp, L., Klein, D. & Gorman, J. (1993) Carbon dioxide hypersensitivity, hyperventilation and panic disorder. *American Journal of Psychiatry*, **150**, 1149–1157.

Passatore, M., Filippi, M. & Grassi, C. (1985) Cervical sympathetic nerve stimulation can induce an intrafusal muscle fibre contraction in the rabbit. In *The Muscle Spindle*, edited by I. Body & M. Gadden. London: Macmillan.

Porges, S. (1995) Orienting in a defensive world: Mammalian modifications of our evolutionary heritage. A polyvagal theory. *Psychophysiology*, **32**, 301–318.

Saffran, M. & Dokas, L. (1983) Sites of nonspecificity in the response of the adrenocortical system to stress. In *Selye's Guide to Stress Research*, vol. 3, edited by H. Selye. New York: Scientific and Academic Editions.

Schore, A. (1994) *Affect Regulation and the Origin of the Self*. Hillsdale, New Jersey: Lawrence Erlbaum Assoc.

Selye, H. (1936) Non-specificity of the pituitary-adrenocortical system to stress. *Nature*, **138**, 32.

Selye, H. (1956) *The Stress of Life*. New York: McGraw-Hill.

Selye, H. (1973) The evolution of the stress concept. *American Scientist*, **61**, 692–699.

Selye, H. (1974) *Stress without Distress*. Philidelphia: J. P. Lippincott.

Simons, D. (1996) Clinical and etiological update of myofascial pain from trigger points. *Journal of Musculoskeletal Pain*, **4**, 93–121.

Sturani, C., Sturani, A. & Tosi, I. (1985) Parasymathetic activity assessed by diving reflex and by airway response to methacholine in bronchial asthma and rhinitis. *Respiration*, **48**, 321–328.

Suarez, E. & Williams, R. (1992) Interactive models of reactivity: The relationship between hostility and potentially pathogenic physiological responses to social stressors. In *Perspectives in Behavioral Medicine—Stress and Disease Process*, edited by N. Schneiderman, P. McCabe & A. Baum. Hillsdale, N.J.: Lawrence Erlbaum Associates.

Timmons, B. & Ley, R. (eds.) (1994) *Behavioral and Psychological Approaches to Breathing Disorders*. New York: Plenum Press.

Travell, J. & Simons, D. (1983, 1992) *Myofascial Pain and Dysfunction: The trigger point Manual*, vols. 1 & 2. Baltimore: Williams & Wilkins.

Ursin, H., Baade, E. & Levine, S. (1978) *Psychobiology of Stress: A Study of Coping Man*. New York: Academic Press.

Whatmore, G. & Kohli, D. (1974) *The Physiopathology and Treatment of Functional Disorders*. New York: Grune & Statton.

Chapter 4

PSYCHOLOGICAL FOUNDATIONS OF STRESS AND COPING: A Developmental Perspective

Dianna T. Kenny, PhD

INTRODUCTION

In 1985, a massive earthquake devastated Mexico City. The physical and psychological ravages of the earthquake were mitigated briefly by the report of the astonishing survival of 23 newborn babies who were rescued between four and eight days after the earthquake from the rubble of collapsed maternity hospitals. What can account for the extraordinary resilience displayed by these neonates, some of whom had survived without food, warmth, or contact comfort for up to eight days? A follow up investigation of eight of these infants 15 months after the earthquake did not reveal any overt signs of pathology as a result of their experience (Lopez & Leon, 1989).

Studies of 55 Mexican school children aged 6–12 years who had survived the earthquakes revealed very different cognitive representations of earthquakes depending on their age and level of cognitive development (Vega, Ollinger, Zimmerman & Figueroa, 1987). Among the adult survivors aged 18–64 years, a number of researchers reported very different crisis-response patterns depending on age, past losses, and pre-existing psychosocial problems at the time of the earthquake (de la Fuente, 1990; Dufka, 1988).

In this chapter, I will address some key questions highlighted in the above vignette pertaining to coping in children and adolescents. For example, how does coping change over the course of development? Is coping in childhood continuous with adult coping or are there qualitative differences? How does development affect coping? What are the critical precursors of coping in children, and how does coping affect development? In attempting to address these issues, I will draw on a range of theories in the developmental psychology and stress literature. Bodies of knowledge related to development, attachment, stress and coping, personality, and developmental psychopathology initially pursued essentially parallel courses, and developed their own models, descriptors, theories, and research paradigms. As each body of knowledge matured, main effect models gave way to more interdisciplinary, interactive, and transactional models (Compas, Hinden & Gerhardt, 1995). This paper represents a further attempt to integrate theories in each of these domains and to present a heuristic, unitary model that incorporates the fundamental principles of each of these domains into a coherent and testable framework.

The Model

In this paper, I propose that coping be defined as the acquisition and conservation of resources throughout the lifespan, and the utilisation of these resources in such a way that a net loss of resources is minimised. Attachment is conceptualised as a key resource that is necessary but not sufficient for adequate coping. Both personality and psychopathology represent the outcomes of developmental, attachment, and coping experiences that can either intensify or reduce the risk of adverse consequences. The interplay of risk reducing and risk enhancing experiences may produce either resilient or vulnerable individuals. The development of psychopathology is conceptualised as an outcome of a major imbalance between risk reducing (i.e. prevention of resource loss) and risk enhancing (i.e. acceleration of resource loss) factors. Such an imbalance may occur at any stage of the lifespan, and may be brought about by the interaction of intra-personal, interpersonal, and environmental factors. Psychopathology itself may be viewed as a resource conserving strategy, whereby the pathology, for example, depression, reduces the physical and social demands on an individual whose resources have been seriously depleted by preceding life stresses and/or everyday challenges. A schematic representation of the model is contained in Figure 4.1.

The model is predicated on the view that the quality of attachment, which influences the development of either adequate or inadequate object relations (i.e. internal working models or mental representations of relationships), is the key resource upon which the development of other resources depends. Attachment quality is multi-determined, and includes the social context into which both parents and their children are born. Innate characteristics of parents, their early life experiences, including relationships with their caregivers, interact with current life experiences, such as a supportive or abusive partner and financial status to influence the level of psychosocial adjustment achievable, their ability to cope, and the emergence of psychopathology. All of these factors contribute to the quality of parenting that they are able to provide to their children. The quality of attachment is determined by the quality of parenting and by the presence and quality of compensatory relationships that are available to the child.

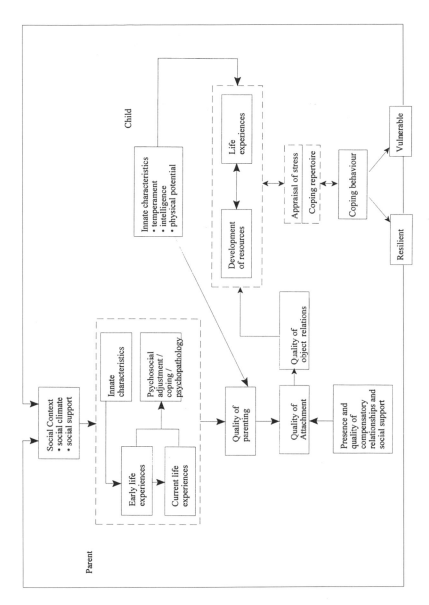

Figure 4.1 A model of the generational transmission of coping

Object relations and available resources, both material and personal, determine the way in which experiences are appraised, and these factors underpin the coping repertoire of the individual. From this repertoire, behavioural attempts to cope with challenges emerge, and the outcome of this coping behaviour is either resilience (positive coping under conditions of risk) or vulnerability (maladaptive coping, including the development of psychopathology). The child then transfers these experiences into their parenting of the next generation of children.

This model draws on theory and research into stress and coping, lifespan development, attachment, personality, psychopathology, and the related concepts of vulnerability and resilience. In the following sections, each of these theories will be described, their commonalities elucidated, and their unique contributions to the proposed model highlighted.

THEORIES OF STRESS

Over the past twenty years, there has been a shift in the focus of stress theories from the identification of stressors that cause ill health and psychopathology to the identification of resources that promote health and well-being (Antonovsky, 1979; Bandura, 1995; Dohrenwend & Dohrenwend, 1981; Hobfoll, 1988). According to Hobfoll (1989), resources are 'the single unit necessary for understanding stress' (p. 516). His proposed model of stress, i.e. *Conservation of Resources (COR)*, posits that 'people strive to retain, protect, and build resources and that what is threatening to them is the potential or actual loss of these valued resources' (p. 516). He further states that 'loss is the key element of stress and that loss spirals are especially likely under chronic stress conditions because of the ongoing depletion of resources' (Lane & Hobfoll, 1992, p. 935). In other words, 'stress occurs when resources are lost, threatened with loss, or where resources are invested without subsequent resource gain' (Hobfoll, Schwarzer & Chon, 1996, p. 14).

A number of resource models of stress propose that key resources, that is, resources that control, promote, or organise the interaction of other resources are central to understanding coping (Hobfoll, Schwarzer & Chon, 1996). Bandura's (1995) concept of self-efficacy, or Kobasa's (1979) concept of hardiness are examples of key resource models. In this paper, I will argue that attachment quality is the key resource on which people's ability to mobilise and utilise other resources is based, including their capacity to develop self-efficacy and hardiness, and to obtain social support.

In contrast to key resource models, Hobfoll (1988, 1989) and Holahan and Moos (1986, 1987) propose multiple resource models in which a number of resources interact to deal with stressors. Hobfoll proposes four types of resources which people strive to develop and enhance. These are object resources such as houses and cars, that meet basic physical needs and provide status to the individual. The degree to which the second group of resources, that is, conditions such as marriage, job security, or seniority exert a stress buffering effect on individuals may be related to the extent to which such conditions are valued by the individual. The third group of resources are personal characteristics. A large number of personal characteristics have been associated with stress resistance and physical and psychological well-being. These include positive self-regard (Jalajas, 1994; Kreger, 1995; Medvedova, 1995), internal locus of control (Abouserie, 1994; Kliewer & Sandler, 1992), optimism (Scheier & Carver, 1992, 1993), resourcefulness (Garmezy, 1983; Kobasa & Puchetti, 1983; Rutter, 1989), self-efficacy (Bandura, 1995, Schwarzer, 1994), and mastery (Felston, 1991; Hobfoll & Lerman, 1988; Younger, 1991). I will argue that quality of attachment and subsequent quality of object relations subsumes all of these personal characteristics.

Although Hobfoll's theory pertains to adult stress and coping, one can readily describe these resources as they relate to children. Children, like adults, value object resources, such as bicycles, computers, swimming pools, and the latest clothes. Conditions such as class captain, captain of the football team, dux of the school, or having a best friend serve the same stress buffering effect that adult conditions described above exert on adults. All of the personal characteristics described for adults have been reported in children. Children displaying such characteristics are frequently described as resilient (Brown & Harris, 1986; Rutter, 1985, 1986, 1987).

The fourth group of resources are called energies, and include money, time, and knowledge. Energies facilitate the acquisition of other resources. Social relationships may be energies if they are self-enhancing, that is, if they provide needed social support. They can also challenge resources and result in net loss of other valued resources. If the quality or type of social support offered is inappropriate, the recipient may be worse off emotionally from having experienced this type of support than had they received no support at all. For example, grieving individuals benefit most from the opportunity to ventilate their feelings of loss. If support people discourage this behaviour in favour of giving advice or encouraging future orientation in the grieving person, the result is increased anger and anxiety, and other complicated grief reactions (Meyerowitz, 1996).

Hobfoll's model represents an expansion and refinement of a model proposed by Lazarus and Folkman (1984), in which six key areas are identified from which an individual's capacity to cope is derived. These are health and energy; positive beliefs; material resources; problem-solving skills; social skills; and social support. Both models assign a significant role to social support.

Social Support

The complexity of the construct of social support creates problems in both definition and measurement, (Kessler, 1992; Turner, 1992; Vaux, 1992; Veiel & Baumann, 1992) but is so central to theories of stress and coping that it deserves special attention. Social support has been conceptualised in several ways the most common of which is social integration. Social integration is defined as the number, strength, and type of connections of individuals to significant others in their social environment (Antonucci, 1985; Rook, 1984). There is substantial evidence demonstrating the important role of social embeddedness in health outcomes. Moreover, its absence, that is, social isolation, has been strongly implicated in morbidity and mortality (Berkman, Leo-Summers & Horwitz, 1992; Williams et al., 1992). Conversely, Hobfoll (1985) has argued that it is not the number of relationships that is important. Rather, it is the presence of one or two intimate relationships that protects against psychosocial and health risk. The importance of at least one intimate, confiding relationship to later mental health in children has been stressed by a number of researchers, and is discussed in more detail below, in the section on attachment. Social support has also been described as relationship quality (Gentry & Kobasa, 1984), as perceived helpfulness and supportiveness (Sarason & Sarason, 1985), or as the enactment of supportive behaviours (Thoits, 1985; Winnubst, Buunk & Marcelissen, 1988).

From the foregoing, it is clear that social support as a construct is multi-determined, emanating both from the environment (Cohen & Syme, 1985; Thoits, 1986) and from perceptions within the person ie from object relations (Shumaker & Brownell, 1984); multi-faceted, incorporating social relationships, social attachments, social assistance, and the perception of the availability and quality of support; and multi-dimensional, in that support can be instrumental, tangible, informational, or emotional (House, 1981). I argue that perceived social support is the affective quality of object representations that have arisen from early attachment experiences. It is the perception of the availability of positive social support that makes real supportive relationships possible. This view has been expressed in a number of different ways by others (e.g. Cohen & Wills, 1985; Sarason, Sarason & Pierce, 1990). Whatever the definition, social support is a transactional process that may emanate as much from within the individual as from the social environment. That is, social support is both given and received.

Individuals differ widely in relational or social competence (i.e. those behaviours and skills that facilitate the acquisition and maintenance of satisfying relationships), a skill which has been found to be deficient in lonely individuals (Hansson, Jones & Carpenter, 1984). Significant differences have been reported between individuals who can muster a great deal of social support compared to those who receive very little support. Accordingly, Winnubst, Buunk and Marcelissen (1988) described social support as a personality characteristic. These differences include attractiveness, sociability, assertiveness, extroversion, emotional stability, sensitivity, and low social anxiety, among others (Heller, Swindle & Dusenbury, 1986; Sarason & Sarason, 1985). Adverse temperamental characteristics combined with poor quality attachments may combine to reduce the social competence of individuals who most need social support yet who are least capable of obtaining it. From the perspective of a resource theory of stress, lack of social support would result in further loss of resources, making the individual increasingly vulnerable to further stressful experiences (Lane & Hobfoll, 1992). When it comes to psychological resources, the rich get richer and the poor, poorer.

THEORIES OF DEVELOPMENT

Paul Baltes (1987) conceptualises lifespan development as the interchange of gains (growth) and losses (declines) throughout life. He notes that 'the nature of what is considered a gain or a loss can change with age: it involves objective in addition to subjective criteria; and is conditioned by theoretical predilection, standards of comparison, cultural and historical context, as well as by criteria of functional fitness or adaptivity' (Baltes, 1997, p. 367).

According to Baltes, an individual's field of developmental potential is dependent on age (i.e. lifespan stage and the status of the gain/loss ratio), genetic endowment (i.e. plasticity, innate characteristics), the prevailing historical, cultural, and economic conditions (i.e. historical embeddedness), and the context in which the individual is developing (contextualism). These factors, if present on the gains side of the ledger, are identifiable resources described by Hobfoll in the previous section. Clearly, the goal of development is to maintain an optimal gains/loss ratio throughout the lifespan in the same way that an individual strives to enhance and maintain resources in Hobfoll's theory.

According to Baltes's model, lifespan development is characterised by an age-related increase in specialisation (selection) of resources and skills. A balance between gains and losses is achieved through the process of *selective optimisation with compensation.* That is, limits to functioning in any developmental domain as a result of age or other limiting processes, such as illness or injury, is compensated by increasing specialisation and the development of substitute or compensatory mechanisms. For example, young infants can perceive very fine speech contrasts that occur in languages other than the one to which they are exposed (i.e. their native language environment). As they develop and are increasingly exposed to only one language environment, they lose the perceptual capacity to distinguish phonologically irrelevant contrasts due to lack of exposure to particular speech sounds (Burnham, 1986). Perception of speech contrasts diverges with age, increasing for the native language and decreasing for non-native languages between the ages of two and six years. Hence, the developmental loss of speech perception for all languages is offset by greater specialisation in the native language (Burnham, Earnshaw & Clark, 1991). Similarly, as children become more efficient in the use of their first language, they experience increasing difficulty in learning a second language (Davies, Criper & Howatt, 1994; Kellerman & Smith, 1986).

Cognitive development also lends itself to a similar gains/loss explanation. For example, during the preschool years, children slowly develop the capacity to monitor their own thought processes and performances, a skill that Flavell (1979) called metacognition. The same capacity has been labelled 'reflective-self function' by attachment theorists and will be discussed in the next section. For now, we will focus on the gains/loss dichotomy for this attribute. The emergence of metacognition is associated with improved impulse control and delay of gratification, which is related to the coping strategies used during the waiting period. Hence, development of metacognition is closely linked to the development of coping, and the ability to verbalise the coping strategies adopted to deal with frustration (Maccoby, 1983). Other gains from the emergence of metacognition include the adoption of more mature problem-solving strategies, the capacity to plan, and the development of future orientation. Metacognition, however, makes children more aware of risks, more vulnerable to negative self-evaluation, more vulnerable to being humiliated (since they have become more sensitive to the reactions of others to the self), and more anxious.

During adolescence, a cognitive shift occurs in which some concrete-operational children become formal operational adolescents (Piaget, 1970). The formal operational thinker is able to think logically about a number of interconnected variables, to develop and test hypotheses, to think abstractly, to connect past experience with future possibilities and to become aware that concrete reality is just one of many hypothetical possibilities. Not all children develop the capacity for formal operational thought once they reach adolescence, and of those who do, they tend to demonstrate another Baltian developmental characteristic, that is, specialisation. Formal operations may only develop in areas in which the adolescent exhibits great interest and involvement in, for example, physics, music, fashion design, social relationships, or literary appreciation (Piaget, 1972). These capacities constitute the gains of this period of development. Good cognitive development includes the capacity to problem-solve, to perform well academically, and to develop functional coping strategies. These skills have been identified as key resources in resilient adolescents that protect them against adversity (Werner, 1995).

However, the attainment of formal operations may also constitute a vulnerability factor, and may hinder an adolescent's attempts to deal with the many demands of this stage of development. The losses from formal operations are the development of two unique forms of adolescent self-consciousness, or adolescent egocentrism, that Elkind (1967) termed the imaginary audience and the personal fable. The cognitive skill of formal operations that allows adolescents to imagine other people's thoughts, lead them to mistakenly believe that others are as preoccupied with their thoughts and appearance as the adolescents themselves. This can create anxiety and self-criticism in the developing adolescent that may paralyse action and make communication with adults difficult. This in turn may preclude adolescents from an important source of potential social support, the adult world. Further, formal operational thinking enables adolescents to speculate about a range of philosophical, moral, social, and religious dilemmas. Some formal operational adolescents develop grandiose plans for solving all the ills of the world and assign themselves a central role in these solutions (Inhelder & Piaget, 1958), while others may become depressed and overwhelmed by the enormity of the dilemmas confronting humanity and themselves, and become frozen by self-deprecation and feelings of hopelessness into inaction. In extreme cases, in conjunction with other serious vulnerabilities, this process may lead to suicide, which is one of the leading causes of death in adolescence (Kenny & Waters, 1995).

Let us return for a moment to our Mexican neonates trapped under the rubble of an earthquake. Since they survived, apparently with no discernible ill-effects, can they be said to have 'coped' with this extraordinary life event? An analysis focused on the gains/loss ratio theory of development may provide some insight into this question. On the loss or debit side, the newborns were unfamiliar with the event and had no reservoir of coping strategies to deal with it. This combination of factors would render an adult vulnerable to the stressor and place him/her at risk for negative outcomes. However, on the gains side of the ledger, the neonates would not have perceived the event to be threatening or harmful, and would not have responded to the event in such a way that would have resulted in the depletion of their physiological and psychological resources. In fact, when rescuers reached the babies, they found some of them asleep! Such resource conserving activity no doubt contributed in a significant way to their survival. Resource conserving behaviours have been observed in most stages of the lifespan; for example, in pre-school children following reunion with mothers from whom they had been separated. Following their mothers' return, children demonstrated decreased positive affect, activity, heart rate, and active sleep, features which are also present in adult depression. This pattern is hypothesised to be homeostatic or resource-conserving, following as it does, a period of increased arousal during the period of separation (Field, 1996; Field & Reite, 1984).

Human development unfolds simultaneously on multiple levels and in multiple domains of human functioning (physical, cognitive, and psychosocial), all mutually influencing the developmental trajectories that children follow to adulthood. For example, there is a complex relationship between the onset of puberty in girls and the emergence of dieting and eating disorders. Puberty results, among other changes, in the accumulation of fat around the hips and thighs, which can be disturbing to some adolescent females. Attitudes to their changing body shape may be mediated by prevailing community attitudes and media influences, as well as by a range of factors associated with individual cognitive and social development (Rutter, 1994). Although puberty may trigger abnormal eating behaviours and poor body image, other factors related to intra-and interpersonal difficulties are more strongly related to maintenance and severity of eating disorders (Attie & Brooks-Gunn, 1989; Kenny & Adams, 1995).

Changes in the ability to cope are linked to major maturational changes throughout the lifespan, such as the development of language, the capacity to walk, and the onset of puberty. The younger the child, the greater the need for external structures to reduce the child's vulnerability to maladaptive coping behaviours in stressful situations (Maccoby, 1983). As the child matures and develops internal structures for self-regulation of affect arousal, the need for environmental control diminishes. Very young children have a limited bank of prepared reactions to stressful situations. The over-arching strategy is to retreat to the attachment figure. This pattern of coping in very young children was elegantly demonstrated in the strange situation experiments conducted by Mary Ainsworth (1973). As children grow, they develop situationally specific coping strategies and learn to seek support from other important figures, such as peers, siblings, and teachers, and to rely less on the attachment figure. If the initial attachments were faulty, this creates potential vulnerabilities at each stage of the lifespan. In a later section, the central role of secure attachment in healthy development will be discussed. For now, let us turn our attention to life events research and its contribution to our understanding of stress and coping in childhood and adolescence.

LIFE EVENTS IN CHILDHOOD AND ADOLESCENCE

Current conceptualisations of life-span development are underpinned by transactional models in which genes, persons, and environments are thought to influence each other in reciprocal ways (Compas, 1987; Rutter, 1997; Scarr, 1992; Scarr & McCartney, 1983). Plomin, DeFries, McClearn & Rutter (1997) have described three such interactions.

> ... passive correlations that arise because parental genes, insofar as they influence parental behaviour, also influence the child's experiences ... evocative correlations that derive from the effect of one person's characteristics in eliciting particular responses in other people ... [and] active correlations that arise from the processes by which individuals shape and select their environments (Rutter, 1997, p. 393).

In contrast, life events research has remained rooted in a linear model in which life events are seen as causal factors in the development of coping and psychopathology (Compas, 1987). As with many linear models, the direction of causality in the observed associations between life events and psychopathology or illness is problematic. Do stressful life events cause physical or mental illness or are vulnerable individuals more likely to experience life events as stressful? Life events research has also suffered from problems in classification, definition, and measurement (Boekaerts, 1996). Various classificatory systems have been developed to describe different life events, but most have proven unsatisfactory (Goodyer, 1988). Brim and Ryff (1980) argue for a central role for life events within lifespan developmental theory, conceptualising them as states of disequilibrium that make further development possible. Rutter (1994) on the other hand, argued that life events are more likely to exacerbate or accentuate pre-existing psychological characteristics, rather than to change them or to deflect development along another trajectory.

The majority of life event studies have employed a checklist or questionnaire format, asking participants to indicate which of the listed life events they have experienced in a given time frame (Goodyer, 1990; Program for Prevention Research, 1992; Sandler, Ramirez & Reynolds, 1986). One of the problems in life events research with children and adolescents is the failure to obtain subjective appraisals of particular life events to permit the variance in individual perception of events to be accounted for (Monroe, 1982). Westen (1995) and Shedler, Mayman & Manis (1995) also caution against reliance on self-report (i.e. checklist or questionnaire) data, because at best, they can only reveal aspects of an individual's functioning of which s/he is aware. The existence of both explicit (conscious) and implicit (unconscious) knowledge of oneself has been demonstrated in many domains of human functioning, including memory (Schacter, 1992), cognitions (Holyoak & Spellman, 1993), and affect and motivation (Westen, 1990). Moreover, reliance on self-report may result in misclassification of people as psychologically healthy, when expert clinical judgment and physiological measures indicate that some of these individuals are psychologically distressed (Shedler, Mayman & Manis, 1995). Defensive denial of psychological distress has been reported in both adults and adolescents (Weinberger, 1990). Methods for assessing implicit or unconscious knowledge need to be developed in stress research, particularly with children and adolescents.

A large number of life events have been implicated in the psychological and physical well-being of children and adolescents. These include hospital admission (Rudolph, Dennig & Weisz, 1995), birth of a sibling (Rutter, 1983), parental conflict and/or divorce (Sandler, Tein & West, 1994), and loss of a parent (Brown, 1988). Specific illnesses, such as asthma, recurrent abdominal pain, headaches, and juvenile rheumatoid arthritis have also been linked to stressful life events (Forman, 1993). Reporting long lists of observed associations between particular life events and particular physical and psychological outcomes does not advance knowledge about the causal chain in these associations. Rather, a shift in focus from enumerating discrete events to a search for underlying mechanisms, such as parental reflective self-function, quality of attachment, social support, self-concept, and adaptability that link multiple variables is likely to be a more fruitful methodology in the study of the impact of stressful life events on children and adolescents, and of the outcome of such experiences in terms of vulnerability and resilience.

A life event is a rather crude measure of life experience or life change. Life events do not provide information about the desirability or frequency of the occurrence, the duration of impact, controllability, or personal meaning to the individual. Timing (in terms of development) of onset of the event, experience with similar previous events, and the intensity of the event will also have an impact on the effect of the event on individuals.

Life events research will only advance our understanding of human stress and coping if causal models are developed and tested. The field of developmental psychopathology has taken up this challenge, shifting from a conceptualisation of aetiology based on linear models of causality involving discrete factors, such as gender, birth order, family size, and socioeconomic status; specific life events such as death of a significant other; and acute stressors, such as separation from a caregiver or the birth of a sibling, to a view that is transactional and based on interacting processes. More complex interactive models that examine the combined and potentiating effects of specific life events or adversities have been proposed to overcome the shortcomings of earlier methodologies (Chess & Thomas, 1983; Goodyer, 1990).

A hierarchical model has been proposed by Rutter and his colleagues (Brown & Harris, 1986; Rutter, 1985, 1986, 1987) in which factors either contribute a direct effect to subsequent pathology or indirect or modifier effects of risk. If a particular factor intensifies the risk, the variable is described as a vulnerability factor; if the risk is diminished, the factor exerts a protective effect against risk. In many cases, vulnerability and protection may indicate the presence or absence of the same factor. These factors can also exert catalytic effects as they may change the mechanisms and effects of other variables.

Although this line of investigation has contributed major insights into our understanding of the putative factors in the development of resilience and psychopathology, Lyons-Ruth (1996) has argued that such models still do not resolve the methodological problem of focusing on variables rather than individuals. Like Westen (1995), she questions

> whether the current analytic models that ... use variables as units of analysis rather than individuals and which emphasise causal, linear relations among variables, are well suited to identifying and describing organisational coherence in individual behaviour (p. 71).

Compas, Hinden, and Gerhardt (1995) also call for a shift from the search for 'static markers' (p. 273) of risk to a ' ... search for processes and mechanisms that account for negative outcomes during adolescence' (p. 273).

THEORIES OF ATTACHMENT

Empirical theories of attachment which brought the significance of the maternal-child relationship into sharp focus had their origins in the work of John Bowlby (1951, 1969, 1973, 1980), Ainsworth (1973), and White & Watts (1973), among others. Subsequently, many researchers have emphasised the importance of the empathic capacity of a primary caregiver as a protective factor against chronic family discord and other ongoing adverse social experiences (Rutter, 1985), and the development of child, adolescent, and adult psychopathology (Bowlby, 1980; Cantwell & Rutter, 1994; Hinde, 1987; Hinde & Stevenson-Hinde, 1988; Kenny & Waters, 1995; Rutter, 1985, 1986, 1987; Sroufe & Fleeson, 1988). Parallel work reported in the literature of psychology and psychoanalysis, particularly object relations theory and self-psychology, over the past 20 years, have drawn similar conclusions (Garmezy & Rutter, 1985; Kohut, 1977; Ornstein, 1981).

Recent conceptualisations of attachment have described a process that may occur across the lifespan (Field, 1985), is almost certainly a universal occurrence (Petrovich & Gewirtz, 1985), and that may involve multiple caregivers (Tronick, Winn & Morelli, 1985). Field (1996) has suggested a need for alternative methods to the strange situation paradigm (Ainsworth, 1967) for studying attachment, to include the study of how mothers and infants interact in everyday situations, and that the list of attachment behaviours be expanded to include those that occur with attachment figures other than the mother, for example, fathers, siblings, and peers. Field proposes the following definition. 'Attachment is viewed as a relationship that develops between two or more organisms as they become attuned to each other, each providing the other meaningful stimulation and arousal modulation' (Field, 1996, p. 545). The critical features of recent definitions of attachment include its capacity for arousal reduction through the caregiver's prompt response to distress and negative affect, the reinstatement of a sense of security following arousal, and the open and synchronous responsiveness to infant communications (Lyons-Ruth, 1996).

The path from attachment to resilience is complex, and a number of theories have been proposed to account for the relationship. Fonagy, Steele, Steele, Higgit & Target (1994), for example, argue that the key factor is the capacity for reflective-self function in at least one primary caregiver that is most associated with secure attachment in the infant. In a series of studies, Fonagy and his colleagues demonstrated that attachment quality is based on the inter-generational transmission of internal working models of relationships, that is, their object relations. Object relations are defined as the internalised, cognitive representations of relationships experienced with the primary attachment figures. These representations provide a secure base for cognitive development and the development of social cognition (Revelle, 1995). Parents at risk of transmitting insecurity to their children, by virtue of rejection, abuse, neglect, deprivation, or other risk factors in their own childhoods, but who do not do so, can be differentiated from at risk parents who have insecurely attached children by the complexity of their internal working models of relationships. Parents demonstrating such complexity differ from parents who do not in their capacity for reflective self-function. Differences in reflective-self function account for individual differences in parental sensitivity or empathy. Each parent transmits his/her working model independently of the other parent. Belonging to a two parent family can therefore be a protective factor against the development of insecurity of attachment and/or later psychopathology if one of the parents is depressed, alcoholic, violent, or in some way emotionally unavailable to their child. The independence of the transmission of each parent's internal working model can account for resilient maltreated children, and other resilient children who have developed normally under conditions of risk.

Garmezy & Masten (1986) argue that attachment influences resilience through the child's capacity to develop cognitive and social competence. A resilient child is defined as one who remains competent despite exposure to adverse events or experiences. The terms competence and coping have sometimes been used interchangeably, with some researchers claiming that the advantage of assessing competence rather than coping or coping style is that competence can be operationalised and has a measurable outcome while coping is a process that lends itself less well to operational definition and measurement (Garmezy, Masten & Tellegen, 1984). Others (e.g. Zeidner & Endler, 1996) describe coping as a multi-component process, incorporating perception of the stressor, coping repertoire, and coping goals. Unlike competence, which implies successful coping, coping per se may include all attempts, whether adaptive or maladaptive, to deal with taxing situations. The term competence, as it is used here, refers to the adaptive coping repertoire available to an individual, and its appropriate application in given situations.

How does attachment influence the development of competence? A number of sources of evidence is available to make such a link. Firstly, attachment quality has consistently been related to the degree to which infants use their primary caregiver as a secure base to explore the environment. The maintenance of a strong sense of security in the infant supports optimal interaction with the environment, which in turn provides many opportunities for the infant to develop cognitive competence through a process of exploration, problem-solving, and the development of mastery over both the social and non-social environments (Basic Behavioural Science Task Force of the National Advisory Mental Health Council, 1996; Field, 1996; Jacobson, Edelstein & Hofmann, 1994; Lyons-Ruth, 1996; Maccoby, 1983).

Secondly, there is evidence for a link between attachment quality and later cognitive development, suggesting that early experiences related to cognitive challenges may have an enduring impact on subsequent cognitive development. In one study, infants displaying disorganised attachments in infancy were found to have lower infant mental development scores at 18 months, compared to securely attached children (Lyons-Ruth, 1996). Other studies (Cox, Puckering, Pound & Mills, 1987; Mills, Puckering, Pound & Cox, 1985) have identified direct pathways from maternal depression, to impaired attachment and subsequent cognitive and social deficits in children.

Thirdly, there is a strong association between secure attachment and the development of social competence. For example, securely attached infants exhibited more prosocial behaviours towards parents and peers in the preschool years (Bretherton, 1985), compared to children displaying either avoidant or disorganised attachment patterns, whose behaviour was characterised by a range of maladaptive responses including aggression, hyperactivity, passive withdrawal, helplessness, and depression (Main & Solomon, 1990; Renken, Egeland, Marvinney, Mangelsdorf & Sroufe, 1989). Longitudinal studies of insecurely attached infants found that at ages 10–14 years, these children were more dependent, less socially competent, and demonstrated lower self-esteem and resilience compared to children of the same ages who had been securely attached infants. Goodyer (1990) summed up from this research that:

> ... early secure attachments provide a learning experience through which individuals internalise or represent relationships. This representation of relations seems to be carried forward to influence expectations and attitudes towards the self and others. Thus early parenting experiences exert a significant influence on relations in later social interactions (p. 25).

Once adequate mental representations ie object relations of significant relationships have been established, they constitute a protective factor against potentially adverse experiences such as separation from a caregiver (Fonagy et al., 1994; Goodyer, 1990; Quinton & Rutter, 1988; Wolkind & Rutter, 1985). Conversely, the absence of a confiding, empathic relationship with one's mother (or primary caregiver), that results in one of the several forms of impaired attachment (see Lyons-Ruth, 1996), is one of the most powerful and most frequently cited vulnerability factors for a range of adverse outcomes, including deficits in social and cognitive competence and the development of psychopathology (Zeanah, 1996). Such representations form the basis of the capacity to perceive social support as helpful, thereby facilitating the individual's willingness to seek and receive it in times of need. This ability is resource conserving and is critical to coping.

Object relations theory has been theoretically useful in linking affective and cognitive development. The theoretical formulations of object relations theory have now found experimental validation in the work of Fonagy et al. (1994) and others. Westen (1995), for example, has proposed a 'clinical-empirical model of personality' (p. 495) that integrates theories of coping and attachment, and is based on three central questions: (a) What psychological resources—cognitive, affective, and behavioural dispositions—does the individual have at his or her disposal? Westen describes four major classes of psychological resources, assessment of which are necessary to describe personality, as follows: (1) cognitive functioning, expectancies, and belief systems, (2) capacity for, and awareness of affective experience, (3) affect regulation, including coping strategies, and (4) behavioural skills, including physical and motor skills, and other procedural skills that translate thought into action. Most personality theories neglect the role of objective or external resources, and how their presence or absence impacts on an individual's personality development or capacity to cope. Lazarus and Folkman (1984) and Hobfoll (1989) have correctly included such resources in their models of stress, in a manner similar to the incorporation of social, historical, and cohort effects in theories of lifespan development (Baltes, 1987).

The second and third questions posed by Westen—What does the person wish for, fear, and value, and how do these motives combine and conflict?); and How does the person experience the self and others and to what extent can the individual enter into intimate relationships? (p. 495)—pertain to the nature of the individual's attachment experiences and how these have impacted upon the development of the self-concept, self-awareness, and the capacity to seek, obtain, and provide social support. Westen's theory, in accord with the attachment theories described above, demonstrates the relationships between secure and insecure attachment and later abilities to express and fulfil needs, to resolve intrapsychic conflict, and to develop a coherent set of values that guide behaviour and contribute to identity formation. Westen (1995) emphasises the roles of observation, clinical judgment, and the case study in providing dynamic explanations as opposed to static descriptions of personality, methodologies that also have a strong tradition in developmental psychology (Garmezy & Masten, 1986; Piaget, 1951, 1952, 1954).

STRESS AND HEALTH

Biopsychosocial models link stress, coping, and psychological adjustment with health and illness. (Ader & Cohen, 1984; Andersen, Kiecolt-Glaser & Glaser, 1994). Essentially, such models propose that stressors, whether of maximum (e.g. negative life events, chronic psychological distress, natural disasters, wars, poverty) or minimum (e.g. choices, challenges, daily hassles, or irritations) magnitude, are consistently associated with autonomic and neuroendocrine responses, which in some cases result in down regulation of the immune system, thereby rendering the organism more vulnerable to illness (Cacioppo, 1996).

Stress serves a somewhat paradoxical function for humans, since it is both necessary for survival and strongly associated with susceptibility to disease, disease severity, and prognosis (Cacioppo, 1996). For example, caregiver stress has been associated with longer episodes of respiratory and viral illnesses, and poorer wound healing (Kiecolt-Glaser, Glaser, Gravenstein, Malarkey & Sheridan, 1996). Marital conflict (Kiecolt-Glaser et al., 1987), examination stress (Kiecolt-Glaser et al., 1984), clinical depression (Herbert & Cohen, 1993a), and psychological distress (Herbert & Cohen, 1993b) have all been associated with down regulation of the immune system. Stressful life events per se appear to be more strongly associated with subsequent disease onset than either the perception of stress, the negative affect generated, or the degree to which the person coped adequately with the stressor (Cohen, Tyrell & Smith, 1991, 1993). However, studies of the relationship between stressful life events and immune function have generally reported small effects. Life events per se can only provide a crude measure of both the quantity or the quality of stress experienced by individuals. Moreover, life event studies often fail to consider either the intra-personal or inter-personal context in which the stressful event is occurring (Brown & Harris, 1989). Measuring stress reactivity, that is, the physiological, autonomic, and endocrine changes that result from identified stressors as a means for understanding individual differences in responding to stress that occur in individuals under certain conditions, may overcome some of the problems associated with life event approaches. Stress reactivity has been shown to vary between individuals whose life circumstances, self-report of stress, coping behaviour, and performance have been found to be similar (Cacioppo et al., 1992; Shedler, Mayman & Manis, 1995).

A similar relationship between stress and illness has been found in infants and young children (Forman, 1993). For example, significant changes in salivary cortisol and behavioural response to the pain of immunisation injections during the first six months of life have been reported (Lewis, 1988; Lewis & Thomas, 1990; Worobey & Lewis, 1989). This decrease suggests that as the infant matures, it becomes more able to cope with stressors, such as pain. Response to pain stimuli has been proposed as a possible benchmark for assessing an individual's stress reactivity, since many pain stimuli, particularly those induced by medical procedures, have some uniformity from one individual to another in terms of the physiological impact of the pain stimulus (Haggerty, Sherrod, Garmezy & Rutter, 1994). There appear to be individual differences over and above those explained by maturation, that are demonstrable from about two months of age in infants' responses to pain stress. During follow-up at 18 months of age, infants who quieted more quickly following immunisation at two months of age had significantly fewer atopic disorders and infections than infants who were slow to quiet. In an interesting and innovative study, Lewis, Thomas, and Worobey (1990) demonstrated a developmental trend in newborns' ability to cope with stressful situations and subsequent illness. They found that although reactivity at two days of age was inversely related to subsequent frequencies of illnesses at 18 months, reactivity at two months of age strongly predicted this association. Healthier neonates, defined by Apgar and birth weight scores, were more reactive at birth, but rapidly became less reactive at two months of age, suggesting that they were developing effective coping strategies to control their reactivity to painful stimuli (i.e. immunisation). Generally, coping with pain improves with age, although decreases in overt signs of distress are not always followed by similar decreases in self-reports of pain or anxiety. Further, there are qualitative differences in the way that younger and older children express their distress. Younger children tend to cry and thrash about, while older children will flinch and groan (Le Baron & Zeltzer, 1984). Older children are more likely to employ cognitive coping i.e. secondary control strategies when confronted with uncontrollable medical procedures. Younger children may be able to generate such strategies but are less able to implement them in the stressful setting (Rudolph, Dennig & Weisz, 1995). A number of other factors affect a child's response to the stress of pain, including gender and prior experience with the stressor. Boys tend to display less overt signs of distress when experiencing pain than girls, a difference attributed to different socialisation experiences (McGrath, 1993). Conflicting evidence regarding the effect of prior experience with painful medical procedures exists, since both habituation and sensitisation experiences may co-occur in the one experience (Rudolph, Dennig & Weisz, 1995). There has been recent interest in the role that temperament plays in moderating stress and coping responses of children and adolescents. Individuals vary on both biological and psychological dimensions such as physiological reactivity and behavioural adaptability, dimensions which impact directly on responsiveness to stressors (Boyce, Barr & Zeltzer, 1992).

In a review of available studies of the stress-illness association in children and adolescents, Barr, Boyce and Zeltzer (1994) concluded that modest, significant relationships exist between psychosocial stressors and onset, duration, and severity of both physical and mental illnesses in children and adolescents. Individual variation in stress reactivity was hypothesised to underlie the modest associations found, and a case was made for the role of mediator and moderator variables to enhance our understanding of the role of individual differences in responsiveness to stressors. For example, in one study, children displaying high laboratory induced cardiac stress reactivity had significantly more injuries than children displaying low cardiac stress reactivity under high but not under low stress conditions. Cardiovascular reactivity therefore functioned as a moderator variable, elucidating the relationship between reactivity and injury proneness (Boyce, Chesney, Kaiser, Alkon-Leonard & Tschann, 1992). Recent evidence indicates that the cluster of characteristics described as Type A personality in adults can be observed in children, and that such a biobehavioural pattern involving both greater heart rate and blood pressure reactivity and increased competitiveness, aggression, impatience, and anger demonstrates modest stability throughout the lifespan (Haggerty et al., 1994). Measures of autonomic and neuroendocrine reactivity have utility in further clarifying the direction and strength of associations between stressors and morbidity (Barr, Boyce & Zeltzer, 1994).

Further support for the link between biology and behaviour is provided by studies that demonstrate improved immune function and prognosis of disease outcome following psychological interventions (Eysenck & Grossarth-Maticek, 1991; Fawzy, Fawzy, Hyun, Gutherie, Fahey & Morton, 1993; Gruber et al., 1993). There has been little parallel work in this area with children and adolescents (Rutter, 1994), although there have been some recent attempts to develop programs that promote the development of social competence as a stress buffering strategy (The Consortium on the School-based Promotion of Social Competence, 1994; Pless & Stein, 1994).

COPING

Freud's theory of the defences (Freud, 1938) is arguably the first theory of coping, although current formulations ignore this work in favour of a social-cognitive perspective that is predicated on the (implicit) assumption that the cognitive appraisal that underlies coping behaviours is conscious and that it can be reliably accessed through self-report (Auerbach & Gramling, 1998). However, some forms of coping become habitual and automatic (i.e. unconscious) such that we engage in coping behaviour without being aware of any cognitive appraisal occurring prior to the event, and without being able to articulate our reasons for acting in the way that we did (Boekearts, 1996; Kihlstrom, 1987; Loftus & Klinger, 1992). Westen (1995) argues that the unconscious components of coping are the expectancies and belief systems around self-efficacy and behaviour-outcome expectancies that impact upon the motivation to perform and the performance itself. These unconscious expectancies are akin to Freudian defences, which are activated in certain circumstances to regulate affect (Eisenberg & Fabes, 1992; Westen, 1994). Another feature of dynamic formulations which are missing from social-cognitive perspectives of stress and coping is the possible existence of conflicting motives, goals, and behaviours and the unique solutions that individuals find to compromise among these (Brenner, 1982).

Numerous attempts abound to identify, classify and categorise both the types of stressors experienced and the coping strategies used by children and adolescents. For example, some of the commonest family stressors identified by adolescents include arguments with parents and siblings, not having enough money, and being treated like a child (Thomas & Groer, 1986). School based stressors have been divided into academic (i.e. mastery of subject matter, academic performance, evaluation, and meeting the high expectations of others); and social stressors (i.e. relationships with teachers and peers, fear of rejection) (Matheny, Aycock & McCarthy, 1993). Elkind (1986) identified three categories of stressors faced by students: (1) forseeable and avoidable stress (e.g. drug use and breaking the law); (2) unforseeable and unavoidable (e.g. illness and death); and (3) forseeable but unavoidable (e.g. examinations).

Using *The Ways of Coping Checklist*, Folkman & Lazarus (1985) identified two main types of coping—problem-focused and emotion-focused—that could be broken down into eight subcategories, three that are problem-focused (confrontive coping, planful problem-solving, and seeking social support to solve the problem); and five that are emotion-focused (distancing, self-control, accepting responsibility, escape-avoidance, positive re-appraisal, and seeking emotional support). A number of other typologies of coping styles and dispositions have been proposed. These usually take the form of uni-dimensional scales, and include behavioural versus cognitive coping (Curry & Russ, 1985); primary control, secondary control, and relinquished control (Weisz, McCabe & Dennig, 1994); approach versus avoidance (Ebata & Moos, 1991; Hubert, Jay, Saltoun & Hayes, 1988; Suls & Fletcher, 1986); avoidant versus transformational coping (Maddi, 1981); repression-sensitization (Byrne, 1961); internal-external locus of control (Rotter, 1966); coper-avoider (DeLong, 1970); and monitoring-blunting (Miller, 1987). A number of comprehensive reviews on coping styles are available (see Rudolph, Dennig & Weisz, 1995; Sandler, Tein & West, 1994; Zeidner & Endler, 1996).

There appears to be considerable variability in the dimensions derived from different studies to aid our understanding of the ways in which children and adolescents cope with stress. Moreover, the dimensions derived from factor analysis, cluster analysis, or other exploratory statistical techniques often lack a clear theoretical underpinning and therefore have limited explanatory power (Sandler, Tein & West, 1994). These conceptualisations of coping are oversimplifications of a complex phenomenon, and therefore leave much of the variance in coping behaviours unexplained. It seems unlikely that individuals would respond to stressors in a unilateral way, that is, with either a problem-focused or an emotion-focused coping response, and there is some evidence that all coping involves both problem-focused and emotion- focused strategies (Patterson & McCubbin, 1987). A number of researchers have pointed to the primacy of affect in directing behaviour; good moods induce optimism which in turn increases the probability of positive coping rather than a retreat into defensive responding (Maccoby, 1983). Current mood not only influences behaviour, but also biases later recall. People who are currently depressed are more likely to recall depressing events, while other more optimistic individuals are more likely to recall positive experiences (Bower, 1981). Westen (1995) suggests that actions, including coping attempts, are motivated by wishes, fears, and values, each of which involves both cognitive and affective components: that is, the cognitive representation has affect inextricably attached to it. Similarly, MacDonald (1995) argues that personality itself is a series of motivational systems with an affective core, and that the attainment or avoidance of certain affective states is at the core of what motivates people to act.

From a very early age, infants engage in combinations of problem- and emotion-focused coping. The quintessential coping strategy, crying, elicits both problem-solving behaviour (e.g. offer of milk) and emotional comfort from the care-giver. Indeed, most of the infant's other early attempts at mastery of the environment, for example, self-exploration, such as sucking on lips, hands, fingers and toes, serves a problem-solving function while simultaneously providing emotional comfort through self-soothing. Many of the infant's early self-directed behaviours appear to have affect regulation as their primary goal. These prototypical coping attempts are tested within the relationship with primary attachment figures. If the response is sufficiently attuned to the infant, such that the interaction results in affect arousal reduction and a growing sense of mastery over one's reactions and the environment, a sufficient basis is laid for later coping (Bandura, 1990; Rutter, 1990; Suomi, 1991). Future research on coping may benefit from the adoption of a clinical-empirical methodology described by Westen (1995).

In this chapter, I have argued that attachment is a key resource upon which other resources are built, which in turn influence coping. Temperament and intelligence are two such resources. Intelligence has consistently been associated with resilience (Cohler, 1987; Egeland, Jacobvitz & Sroufe, 1988; Felsman & Vaillant, 1987; Garmezy & Rutter, 1985; Werner, 1995), but intelligence, in the absence of a secure attachment, does not, by itself, enhance coping. Recent attempts to identify other predictors of coping have led to the description of a number of personality traits, such as hardiness (Kobasa, 1982), locus of control orientation (Rotter, 1966; Strentz & Auerbach, 1988), learned resourcefulness (Rosenbaum, 1990), self-efficacy (Bandura, 1990), and learned helplessness/optimism (Seligman, 1991), among others. Successful personal mastery experiences form the basis for the development of such characteristics (Aldwin, Sutton & Lachman, 1996). These begin in infancy, as described above, in the presence of a secure attachment with a primary caregiver, who is both attuned to the child's needs and responds appropriately by providing the child with a safe environment in which to explore and solve problems. The attributions that we make about why we coped, our ability to generalise these coping strategies appropriately, and our capacity to modify ineffective coping behaviours are also important factors in later adjustment (Auerbach & Gramling, 1998).

Coping models have been variously described as 'stress resistance', 'invulnerability', 'resilience', 'protective factors', 'hardiness', or 'learned resourcefulness' (see for example, Anthony & Cohler, 1987; Garmezy, 1987; Kobasa & Pucetti, 1983; Rutter, 1989). Longitudinal studies that have examined the interplay of risk and protective factors in developmental psychopathology and resilience (see, for example, Magnusson & Bergman, 1988; Sameroff, Seifer, Zax & Barocas, 1987; Werner & Smith, 1982) concluded that

> resilience is associated with two groups of protective factors (1) personal resources or dispositional characteristics of the individual and (2) social resources or characteristics of the relationships and support within or outside the family (Bliesener & Losel, 1990, p. 300–301).

Protective factors within the individual include a coping pattern that combines an easy temperament, autonomy together with the willingness to seek assistance and ask for help when one's own resources are not sufficient; intelligence and academic achievement; internal locus of control, and a positive self-concept (Egeland, Jacobvitz & Sroufe, 1988; Werner, 1995). The primary protective factor within the family is the presence of at least one competent, emotionally stable and empathic caregiver who is attuned to the needs of the child (Anthony, 1987; Wallerstein & Blakeslee, 1989). Other factors interact with gender to produce resilient boys and girls. For example, resilient boys have usually experienced a positive male role model, and have grown up in an environment that has clear structures and rules. Resilient girls, on the other hand, have experienced encouragement to take risks and to develop independence in the context of reliable support from a female caregiver (Block & Gjerde, 1986, in Werner, 1995). Protective factors within the community include adult (e.g. teacher, coach) and peer support that is available in times of crisis, and structures such as school, church and youth groups (Werner, 1995).

Using this framework, psychopathology can be understood in terms of inadequate resources, in particular, impaired attachments, competencies, temperament, and self-esteem, and the subsequent problems arising as a consequence, that form the basis of impaired capacities to seek, obtain, and give social support. These impaired capacities in turn impair the individual's capacity to conserve resources and to cope adequately with stress. The group of resources proposed by Hobfoll (1988) may interact in additive or synergistic ways to enhance or deplete the overall reservoir of resources available to the individual. For example, economic hardship may exert a direct negative effect on the quality of the marital relationship, which in turn may impact upon the couple's capacity or energy for parenting. Poor quality parenting may result in impaired attachments in their children which may lead to psychological distress, psychopathology, or illness during childhood or adolescence. Impaired attachments and psychological distress negatively influence cognitive functioning, which in turn may lead to poor school grades, lowered self-esteem, reduced capacity to deal effectively with stressors, fewer vocational opportunities, and so on. Such a model suggests a range of possible interventions to break this negative cycle of resource depletion, since it suggests many possibilities to decrease stress by enhancing resources via the most accessible route. Relieving the economic hardship would constitute a sensible and fundamental intervention, but this may not be possible. Providing compensatory attachment figures and academic support to the children through the school may constitute an effective intervention to prevent educational disadvantage.

CONCLUSION

In this paper I have attempted to provide a synthesis of the literature in key but discrete areas of investigation and to propose a heuristic model that links each of these bodies of knowledge in such a way that multiple interventions are suggested at different levels of complexity. I have attempted to argue that theorising about stress and coping without providing a developmental and social context in which the stress and coping occurs, is to provide an incomplete picture of individual differences that remains rooted in description rather than explanation. The proper starting point for an investigation of how and why people experience stress in the way that they do and cope with it in idiosyncratic ways must begin with an examination of the social and relational context of the first attempts to interact with the world. This includes an elucidation of parental internal working models of relationships, their reflective self-function, and how these interact with child characteristics, including temperament, intelligence, physical characteristics, and early life experiences to determine the quality of attachment, the development of object relations and other resources, and how these combine to determine coping.

Future research will need to elucidate the relationships between parental internal working models, attachment, and coping; the relationships between attachment quality, immune function, and health; the relationships between quality of attachment and learned helplessness/resourcefulness; and importantly, since prevention is the best cure, how we can ensure the development of adequate attachment and object relations in the majority of children, so that resilience is the major outcome of exposure to risk.

References

Abouserie, R. (1994) Sources and levels of stress in relation to locus of control and self esteem in university students. *Educational Psychology*, **14**(3), 323–330.
Ader, R. & Cohen, N. (1984) Behavior and the immune system. In *Handbook of Behavioral Medicine*, edited by W. D. Gentry, pp. 117–173. New York: Guilford Press.

Ainsworth, M. D. S. (1967) *Infancy in Uganda: Infant Care and the Growth of Love*. Baltimore: John-Hopkins Press.

Ainsworth, M. D. S. (1973) The development of infant-mother attachment. In *Review of Child Development Research*, edited by B. M. Caldwell & H. N. Ricciuti, vol III. Chicago: University of Chicago Press.

Aldwin, C. M., Sutton, K. J. & Lachman, M. (1996) The development of coping resources in adulthood. *Journal of Personality*, **64**, 837–872.

Andersen, B. L., Kiecolt-Glaser, J. K. & Glaser, R. (1994) A biobehavioural model of cancer stress and disease course. *American Psychologist*, **49**(5), 389–404.

Anthony, E. J. (1987) Children at high risk for psychosis growing up successfully. In *The Invulnerable Child*, edited by E. J. Anthony & B. J. Cohler, pp. 147–184. New York: Guilford Press.

Anthony, E. J. & Cohler, B. J. (eds.) (1987) *The Invulnerable Child*, pp. 147–184. New York: Guilford Press.

Antonovsky, A. (1979) *Health, Stress and Coping*. San Francisco, CA: Jossey-Bass.

Antonucci, T. C. (1985) Social support: Theoretical advances, recent findings and pressing issues. In *Social Support: Theory, Research and Application*, edited by I. G. Sarason & B. R. Sarason, pp. 391–414. The Hague, The Netherlands: Nijhoff.

Attie, I. & Brooks-Gunn, J. (1989) Development of eating problems in adolescent girls: A longitudinal study. *Developmental Psychology*, **25**, 70–79.

Auerbach, S. M. & Gramling, S. E. (1998) *Stress Management: Psychological Foundations*. Sydney: Prentice-Hall.

Baltes, P. B. (1987) Theoretical propositions of life-span developmental psychology: On the dynamics between growth and decline. *Developmental Psychology*, **23**(5), 611–626.

Baltes, P. B. (1997) On the incomplete architecture of human ontogeny: Selection, optimization, and compensation as foundation of developmental theory. *American Psychologist*, **52**(4), 366–380.

Bandura, A. (1990) Conclusion: Reflections on nonability determinants of competence. In *Competence Considered*, edited by R. J. Sternberg & J. Kolligan, pp. 315–362. New Haven: Yale University Press.

Bandura, A. (ed.) (1995) *Self-efficacy in Changing Societies*. New York: Cambridge University Press.

Barr, R. G., Boyce, W. T. & Zeltzer, L. K. (1994) The stress-illness association in children: A perspective from the biobehavioral interface. In *Stress, Risk and Resilience in Children and Adolescents: Processes, Mechanisms and Interventions*, edited by R. J. Haggerty, L. R. Sherrod, N. Garmezy & M. Rutter, (pp. 182–224). Cambridge: Cambridge University Press.

Basic Behavioral Sciences Task Force of the National Advisory Mental Health Council (1996) Basic Behavioral Science Research for Mental Health: Vulnerability and resilience. *American Psychologist*, **51**(1), 22–28.

Berkman, L. F., Leo-Summers, L. & Horwitz, R. I. (1992) Emotional support and survival following myocardial infarction: A prospective population-based study of the elderly. *Annals of International Medicine*, **117**, 1003–1009.

Bliesener, T. & Losel, F. (1990) Resilience in adolescence: A study on the generalizability of protective factors. In *Health Hazards in Adolescence*, edited by K. Hurrelmann & F. Losel, pp. 299–320. Berlin: Aldine de Gruyter.

Block, J. & Gjerde, P. F. (1986) *Early Antecedents of Ego Resilience in Late Adolescence*, Paper presented at the annual meeting of the American Psychological Association, Washington, DC, August, 1986.

Boekaerts, M. (1996) Coping with stress in childhood and adolescents. In *Handbook of Coping: Theory, Research, Applications*, edited by M. Zeidner & N. S. Endler, pp. 452–484. Brisbane: John Wiley and Sons.

Bower, G. H. (1981) Mood and memory. *American Psychologist*, **36**, 129–148.

Bowlby, J. (1951) *Maternal Care and Mental Health*. Geneva: World Health Organization.

Bowlby, J. (1969) *Attachment and Loss. vol. 1: Attachment.* London: Hogarth Press.

Bowlby, J. (1973) *Attachment and Loss. vol. 2: Separation.* New York: Basic Books.

Bowlby, J. (1980) *Attachment and Loss. vol. 3: Loss, Sadness and Depression.* New York: Basic Books.

Boyce, W. T., Barr, R. G. & Zeltzer, L. K. (1992) Temperament and the psychology of childhood stress. *Pediatrics,* **90**(suppl.), 483–486.

Boyce, W. T., Chesney, M., Kaiser, P., Alkon-Leonard, A. & Tschann, J. (1992) Childcare stressors, cardiovascular reactivity, and injury incidence in preschool children (abstract). *Pediatric Research,* **31**, 9A.

Brenner, C. (1982) *The Mind in Conflict.* New York: International Universities Press.

Bretherton, I. (1985) Attachment theory: Retrospect and prospect. In I. Bretherton & E. Waters (eds.), Growing points of attachment theory and research. *Monographs of the Society for Research in Child Development,* **50**(1–2, Serial No. 209), 66–104.

Brim, O. G., Jr. & Ryff, C. D. (1980) On the properties of life events. In *Life-span Development and Behavior,* vol. 3, edited by P. Baltes & O. G. Brim, Jr., pp. 368–388. New York: Academic Press.

Brown, G. W. (1988) Early loss of parent and depression in adult life. In *Handbook of Life Stress, Cognition and Health,* edited by S. Fisher & J. Reason, pp. 441–465. John Wiley & Sons: Chichester, England.

Brown, G. W. & Harris, T. (1986) Stressor, vulnerability and depression—a question of replication. *Psychological Medicine,* **16**, 739–744.

Brown, G. W. & Harris, T. O. (1989) *Life Events and Illness.* New York: Guilford Press.

Burnham, D. K. (1986) Developmental loss of speech perception: Exposure to and experience with a first language. Special issue: Language loss. *Applied Psycholinguistics,* **7**(3), 207–239.

Burnham, D. K., Earnshaw, L. J. & Clark, J. E. (1991) Development of categorical identification of native and non-native bilabial stops: Infants, children and adolescents. *Journal of Child Language,* **18**(2), 231–260.

Byrne, D. (1961) The repression-sensitisation scale: Rationale, reliability and validity. *Journal of Personality,* **29**, 334–349.

Cacioppo, J. T. (1996) Somatic Responses to Psychological Stress: The reactivity hypothesis. *Invited Address Presented at the XXVI International Congress of Psychology, Montreal, Canada, August, 1996.*

Cacioppo, J. T., Uchino, B. N., Crites, S. L., Jr., Snydersmith, M. A., Smith, G., Berntson, G. G. & Lang, P. J. (1992) Relationship between facial expressiveness and sympathetic activation in emotion: A critical review, with emphasis on modelling underlying mechanisms and individual differences. *Journal of Personality and Social Psychology,* **62**, 110–128.

Cantwell, D. & Rutter, M. (1994) Classification: Conceptual issues and substantive findings. In *Child and Adolescent Psychiatry: Modern Approaches,* edited by M. Rutter, E. Taylor & L. Hersov, (pp. 3–21). London: Blackwell Scientific Publications.

Chess, S. & Thomas, A. (1983) *Origins and Evolution of Behavior Disorders: From Infancy to Adult Life.* New York: Brunner Mazel.

Cohen, S. & Syme, S. L. (1985) *Social Support and Health.* London, New York: Academic Press.

Cohen, S., Tyrrell, D. A. J. & Smith, A. P. (1991) Psychological stress and susceptibility to the common cold. *New England Journal of Medicine,* **325**, 606–612.

Cohen, S., Tyrrell, D. A. J. & Smith, A. P. (1993) Life events, perceived stress, negative affect, and susceptibility to the common cold. *Journal of Personality and Social Psychology,* **64**, 131–140.

Cohen, S. & Wills, T. A. (1985) Stress, social support, and the buffering hypothesis. *Psychological Bulletin,* **98**, 310–357.

Cohler, B. J. (1987) Adversity, resilience, and the study of lives. In *The Invulnerable Child,* edited by E. J. Anthony & B. J. Cohler, (pp. 363–424). New York: Guilford.

Compas, B. E. (1987) Coping with stress during childhood and adolescence. *Psychological Bulletin,* **101**, 393–403.

Compas, B. E., Hinden, B. R. & Gerhardt, C. A. (1995) Adolescent development: Pathways and processes of risk and resilience. *Annual Review of Psychology*, **46**, 265–293.

Cox, A. D., Puckering, C., Pound, A. & Mills, M. (1987) The impact of maternal depression in young children. *Journal of Child Psychology and Psychiatry*, **28**, 917–928.

Curry, S. L. & Russ, S. W. (1985) Identifying coping strategies in children. *Journal of Clinical Child Psychology*, **14**, 61–69.

De la Fuente, R. (1990) Las consecuencias del desastre en la salud mental. (Disaster consequences in regard to mental health.) Symposium: The September 1985 earthquakes in Mexico City: Medical aspects (1986, Mexico City, Mexico). *Salud Mental*, **9**(3), 3–8.

DeLong, R. D. (1970) Individual differences in patterns of anxiety arousal, stress-relevant information and recovery from surgery. *Doctoral Dissertation*. University of California, Los Angeles.

Dohrenwend, B. P. & Dohrenwend, B. S. (1981) Socioenvironmental factors, stress, and psychopathology. *American Journal of Community Psychology*, **9**(2), 128–164.

Dufka, C. L. (1988) The Mexico City earthquake disaster. *Social Casework*, **69**(3), 162–170.

Ebata, A. T. & Moos, R. H. (1991) Coping and adjustment in distressed and healthy adolescents. *Journal of Applied and Developmental Psychology*, **12**, 33–54.

Egeland, B., Jacobvitz, D. & Sroufe, L. A. (1988) Breaking the cycle of child abuse. *Child Development*, **59**, 1080–1088.

Eisenberg, N. & Fabes, R. A. (eds.) (1992) *Emotion and Regulation in Early Development: New Directions for Child Development* (Vol. 55). San Francisco: Jossey-Bass.

Elkind, D. (1967) Egocentrism in adolescence. *Child Development*, **38**, 1025–1034.

Elkind, D. (1986) Stress and the middle grader. *School Counseling*, 196–206.

Eysenck, H. J. & Grossarth-Maticek, R. (1991) Creative novation behaviour therapy as a prophylactic treatment for cancer and coronary heart disease: II. Effects of treatment. *Behaviour Research & Therapy*, **29**(1), 17–31.

Fawzy, F. I., Fawzy, N. W., Hyun, C. S., Gutherie, D., Fahey, J. L. & Morton, D. (1993) Malignant melanoma: Effects of an early structured psychiatric intervention, coping, and affective state on recurrence and survival six years later. *Archives of General Psychiatry*, **50**, 681–689.

Felsman, J. K. & Vaillant, G. E. (1987) Resilient children as adults: A 40 year study. In *The Invulnerable Child*, edited by E. J. Anthony & B. J. Cohler. New York: Guilford Press.

Felston, G. (1991) Influences of situation-specific mastery beliefs and satisfaction with social support on appraisal of stress. *Psychological Reports*, **69**(2), 483–495.

Field, T. (1985) Attachment as psychobiological attunement: Being on the same wavelength. In *Psychobiology of Attachment and Separation*, edited by M. Reite & T. Field, (pp. 455–480). New York: Academic.

Field, T. (1996) Attachment and separation in young children. *Annual Review of Psychology*, **47**, 541–561.

Field, T. & Reite, M. (1984) Children's responses to separation from mother during the birth of another child. *Child Development*, **55**, 1308–1316.

Flavell, J. H. (1979) Metacognition and cognitive monitoring. *American Psychologist*, **34**, 906–911.

Folkman, S. & Lazarus, R. S. (1985) If it changes it must be a process: Study of emotion and coping during three stages of a college examination. *Journal of Personality and Social Psychology*, **48**, 150–170.

Fonagy, P., Steele, M., Steele, H., Higgitt, A. & Target, M. (1994) The Emanuel Miller memorial lecture 1992: The theory and practice of resilience. *Journal of Child Psychology and Psychiatry*, **35**(2), 231–257.

Forman, S. (1993) *Coping Skills Interventions for Children and Adolescents*. San Francisco: Jossey-Bass.

Freud, S. (1938) In A. A. Brill (ed. & translation), *The Basic Writings of Sigmund Freud*. New York: Modern Library.

Garmezy, N. (1983) Stressors of childhood. In *Stress, Coping and Development in Children*, edited by N. Garmezy & M. Rutter, pp. 43–84. Baltimore, MD: Johns Hopkins University Press.

Garmezy, N. (1987) Stress, competence, and development: Continuities in the study of schizophrenic adults, children vulnerable to psychopathology, and the search for stress-resistant children. *American Journal of Orthopsychiatry*, **57**, 159–174.

Garmezy, N. & Masten, A. S. (1986) Stress, competence, and resilience: Common frontiers for therapist and psychopathologist. *Behavior Therapy*, **17**, 500–521.

Garmezy, N., Masten, A. S. & Tellegen, A. (1984) The study of stress and competence in children: A building block for developmental psychopathology. *Child Development*, **55**, 97–111.

Garmezy, N. & Rutter, M. (1985) Acute reactions to stress. In *Child Psychiatry: Modern Approaches*, edited by M. Rutter & L. Hersov. Oxford: Blackwell.

Gentry, W. D. & Kobasa, S. C. (1984) Social and psychological resources mediating stress-illness relationships in humans. In *Handbook of Behavioral Medicine*, edited by W. D. Gentry, pp. 87–113. New York: Guilford Press.

Goodyer, I. M. (1988) Stress in childhood and adolescence. In *Handbook of Life Stress, Cognition and Health*, edited by S. Fisher & J. Reason, (pp. 23–40). England: John Wiley & Sons.

Goodyer, I. M. (1990) *Life Experiences, Development and Childhood Psychopathology*. England: John Wiley & Sons Ltd.

Gruber, B. L., Hersh, S. P., Hall, N. R., Waletzky, L. R., Kunz, J. F., Carpenter, J. K., Kverno, K. S. & Weiss, S. M. (1993). Immunological responses of breast cancer patients to behavioral interventions. *Biofeedback and Self-Regulation*, **18**, 1–22.

Haggerty, R. J., Sherrod, L. R., Garmezy, N. & Rutter, M. (eds.) (1994) *Stress, Risk and Resilience in Children and Adolescents: Processes, Mechanisms and Interventions*. Cambridge: Cambridge University Press.

Hansson, R. O., Jones, W. H. & Carpenter, B. N. (1984) Relational competence and social support. *Review of Personality and Social Psychology*, **5**, 265–284.

Herbert, T. B. & Cohen, S. (1993a) Depression and immunity: A meta-analytic review. *Psychological Bulletin*, **113**, 472–486.

Herbert, T. B. & Cohen, S. (1993b) Stress and immunity in humans: A meta-analytic review. *Psychosomatic Medicine*, **55**, 364–379.

Hinde, R. A. (1987) *Individuals, Relationships and Culture*. Cambridge: Cambridge University Press.

Hinde, R. A. & Stevenson-Hinde, J. (eds.) (1988) *Relationships within Families*. Oxford: Clarendon Press.

Hobfoll, S. E. (1985) Personal and social resources and the ecology of stress resistance. In *Review of Personality and Social Psychology*, vol. 6, edited by P. Shaver, pp. 265–290. Beverly Hills, CA: Sage.

Hobfoll, S. E. (1988) *The Ecology of Stress*. Washington, D. C.: Hemisphere.

Hobfoll, S. E. (1989) Conservation of resources: A new attempt at conceptualising stress. *The American Psychologist*, **44**, 513–524.

Hobfoll, S. E. & Lerman, M. (1988) Personal relationships, personal attributes, and stress resistance: Mothers' reactions to their child's illness. *American Journal of Community Psychology*, **16**(4), 565–589.

Hobfoll, S. E., Schwarzer, R. & Chon, K. K. (1996) Disentangling the stress labyrinth: Interpreting the meaning of the term stress as it is studied. Paper presented for the First Meeting of the International Society of Health Psychology, Montreal Quebec, Canada, August 1996.

Holahan, C. J. & Moos, R. H. (1986) Personality, coping and family resources in stress resistance. A longitudinal analysis. *Journal of Personality and Social Psychology*, **51**, 389–395.

Holahan, C. J. & Moos, R. H. (1987) Risk, resistance and psychological distress: A longitudinal analysis with adults and children. *Journal of Abnormal Psychology*, **96**, 3–13.

Holyoak, K. & Spellman, B. (1993) Thinking. *Annual Review of Psychology*, **44**, 265–315.

House, J. S. (1981) *Work Stress and Social Support*. Reading, MA.: Addison-Wesley.

Hubert, N. C., Jay, S. M., Saltoun, M. & Hayes, M. (1988) Approach-avoidance and distress in children undergoing preparation for painful medical procedures. *Journal of Clinical Child Psychology*, **17**, 194–202.

Inhelder, B. & Piaget, J. (1958) *The Growth of Logical Thinking from Childhood to Adolescence*. New York: Basic Books.

Jacobson, T., Edelstein, W. & Hofmann, V. (1994) A longitudinal study of the relation between representations of attachment in childhood and cognitive functioning in childhood and adolescence. *Developmental Psychology*, **30**, 112–124.

Jalajas, D. S. (1994) The role of self-esteem in the stress process: Empirical results from job hunting. *Journal of Applied Social Psychology*, **24**(22), 1984–2001.

Kellerman, E. & Smith, M. S. (1986) *Crosslinguistic Influence in Second Language Acquisition*. Oxford, England: Permagon Press.

Kessler, R. C. (1992) Perceived support and adjustment to stress: Methodological considerations. In *The Meaning and Measurement of Social Support*, edited by H. O. F. Veiel & U. Baumann, (pp. 259–271). New York: Hemisphere.

Kenny, D. T. & Adams, R. (1995) Body shape, gender, age and adolescent eating attitudes. In *Australia's Adolescents: A Health Psychology Perspective*, edited by D. T. Kenny & R. F. S. Job, (pp. 45–52). Armidale, NSW: University of New England Press.

Kenny, D. T. & Waters, B. (1995) Current issues in adolescent mental health. In *Australia's Adolescents: A Health Psychology Perspective*, edited by D. T. Kenny & R. F. S. Job, (pp. 68–88). Armidale, NSW: University of New England Press.

Kiecolt-Glaser, J. K., Fisher, L., Ogrocki, P., Stout, J. C., Speicher, C. E. & Glaser, R. (1987) Marital quality, marital disruption and immune function. *Psychosomatic Medicine*, **49**, 13–34.

Kiecolt-Glaser, J. K., Garner, W., Speicher, C. E., Penn, G. M., Holliday, J. & Glaser, R. (1984) Psychosocial modifiers of immunocompetence in medical students. *Psychosomatic Medicine*, **46**, 7–14.

Kiecolt-Glaser, J. K., Glaser, R., Gravenstein, S., Malarkey, W. B. & Sheridan, J. (1996) Chronic stress alters the immune response to influenza virus vaccine in older adults. *Proceedings of the National Academy of Sciences*, **93**, 3043–3047.

Kihlstrom, J. F. (1987) The cognitive unconscious. *Science*, **237**, 1445–1452.

Kliewer, W. & Sandler, I. N. (1992) Locus of control and self-esteem as moderators of stressor-symptom relations in children and adolescents. *Journal of Abnormal Child Psychology*, **20**(4), 393–413.

Kobasa, S. C. (1982) The hardy personality: Toward a social psychology of stress and health. In *Social Psychology of Health and Illness*, edited by G. Sanders & J. Suls, pp. 3–32. Hillsdale, N. J. : Erlbaum.

Kobasa, S. C. & Puccetti, M. C. (1983) Personality and social resources in stress resistance. *Journal of Personality and Social Psychology*, **45**, 839–850.

Kohut, H. (1977) *The Restoration of the Self*. New York: International Universities Press Inc.

Kreger, D. W. (1995) Self-esteem, stress, and depression among graduate students. *Psychological Reports*, **76**(1), 345–346.

Lane, C. & Hobfoll, S. E. (1992) How loss affects anger and alienates potential supporters. *Journal of Consulting and Clinical Psychology*, **60**(6), 935–942.

Lazarus, R. S. & Folkman, S. (1984) *Stress, Appraisal and Coping*. New York: Springer Publishing Co.

LeBaron, S. & Zeltzer, L. (1984) Assessment of acute pain and anxiety in children and adolescents by self-reports, observer reports, and a behavior checklist. *Journal of Consulting and Clinical Psychology*, **52**, 729–738.

Lewis, M. (1988) Psychology of Stress: Infants Behavioral and Salivary Cortisol Responses to Stress. Paper presented at the Sixth Biennial International Conference on Infant Studies, Washington, DC.

Lewis, M. & Thomas, D. (1990) Cortisol release in response to inoculation. *Child Development*, **61**, 50–59.

Lewis, M., Thomas, D. & Worobey, J. (1990) Developmental organization, stress and illness. *Psychological Science*, **1**(5), 316–318.

Loftus, E. F. & Klinger, M. R. (1992) Is the unconscious smart or dumb? *American Psychologist*, **47**, 761–765.

Lopez, M. I. & Leon, N. A. (1989) Babies of the Earthquake: Follow-up study of their first 15 months. *Hillside Journal of Clinical Psychiatry*, **11**(2), 147–168.

Lyons-Ruth, K. (1996) Attachment relationships among children with aggressive behavior problems: The role of disorganized early attachment patterns. *Journal of Consulting and Clinical Psychology*, **64**(1), 64–73.

Maccoby, E. E. (1983) Social-emotional development and response to stressors. In *Stress, Coping and Development in Children*, edited by N. Garmezy & M. Rutter. New York: McGraw-Hill.

MacDonald, K. (1995) Evolution, the Five Factor Model, and levels of personality. *Journal of Personality*, **63**(3), 525–567.

Maddi, S. (1981) Individual development: Its significance for stress responsivity and stress adaptation. Personality development. In *Adolescence and Stress*, edited by C. Moore, (DHHS Publication No. ADM 81-10098). Washington, DC.: US Government Printing Office, 15–33.

Magnusson, D. & Bergman, L. R. (1988) Individual and variable-based approaches to longitudinal research no early risk factors. In *Studies of Psychosocial Risk: The Power of Longitudinal Data*, edited by M. Rutter, pp. 45–61. Cambridge: Cambridge University Press.

Main, M. & Solomon, J. (1990) Procedures for identifying infants as disorganized/ disoriented during the Ainsworth Strange Situation. In *Attachment in the Preschool Years: Theory, Research and Intervention*, edited by M. Greenberg, D. Cicchetti & E. M. Cummings, pp. 121–160. Chicago: University of Chicago Press.

Matheny, K. B., Aycock, D. W. & McCarthy, C. J. (1993) Stress in school-aged children and youth. *Educational Psychology Review*, **5**(2), 109–133.

McGrath, P. (1993) Psychological aspects of pain perception. In *Pain in Infants, Children and Adolescents*, edited by N. Schecter, C. Berde & M. Yaster, pp. 39–63. Baltimore: Williams & Wilkins.

Medvedova, L. (1995) Personal resources of adaptive coping with stress in adolescents. *Studia Psychologica*, **37**(3), 177–179.

Meyerowitz, B. (1996) Cited in Azur, B., Scientists examine cancer patients fears. *APA Monitor*, **27**(9), 32.

Miller, S. M. (1987) Monitoring and blunting: Validation of a questionnaire to assess styles of information seeking under threat. *Journal of Personality and Social Psychology*, **52**, 345–353.

Mills, M., Puckering, C., Pound, A. & Cox, A. (1985) What is it about depressed mothers that influences their children's functioning. In *Recent Advances in Developmental Psychopathology*, edited by J. Stevenson. Permagon Press: Oxford.

Monroe, S. M. (1982) Life events assessment: Current practices, emerging trends. *Clinical Psychology Review*, **2**, 435–453.

Ornstein, A. (1981) Self-pathology in childhood: Developmental and clinical considerations. *Psychiatric Clinics of North America*, **4**(3), 435–453.

Patterson, J. M. & McCubbin, H. I. (1987) Adolescent coping style and behaviours: Conceptualisation and measurement. *Journal of Adolescence*, **10**, 163–186.

Petrovich, S. B. & Gewirtz, J. L. (1985) The attachment learning process and its relation to cultural and biological evolution: Proximate and ultimate consideration. In *Psychobiology of Attachment and Separation*, edited by M. Reite & T. Field, pp. 51–92. New York: Academic.

Piaget, J. (1951) *Play, Dreams and Imitation in Childhood*. New York: Norton.

Piaget, J. (1952) *The Origins of Intelligence in Children*. New York: International Universities Press.

Piaget, J. (1954) *The Construction of Reality in the Child*. New York: Basic Books.

Piaget, J. (1970) Piaget's theory, In *Carmichael's Manual of Child Psychology*, edited by P. H. Mussen. New York: Wiley.

Piaget, J. (1972) Intellectual evolution from adolescence to adulthood. *Human Development*, **15**, 1–12.

Pless, I. B. & Stein, R. E. K. (1994) Intervention research: Lessons from research on children with chronic disorders. In *Stress, Risk and Resilience in Children and Adolescents: Processes, Mechanisms and Interventions (Chapter 9)*, edited by R. J. Haggerty. Cambridge: Cambridge University Press.

Plomin, R., DeFries, J. C., McClearn, G. & Rutter, M. (1997) *Behavioral Genetics* (3rd ed). New York: W. H. Freeman.

Program for Prevention Research (1992) *Divorce Adjustment Project Documentation*. (Available from the Program for Prevention Research, Arizona State University, Tempe, AZ).

Quinton, D. & Rutter, M. (1988) *Parenting Breakdown: The Making and Breaking of Intergenerational Links*. Aldershot: Averbury.

Renken, B., Egeland, B., Marvinney, D., Mangelsdorf, S. & Stroufe, L. A. (1989) Early childhood antecedents of aggression and passive-withdrawal in early elementary school. *Journal of Personality*, **57**, 257–281.

Revelle, W. (1995) Personality processes. *Annual Review of Psychology*, **46**, 295–328.

Rook, K. S. (1984) The negative side of social interaction: Impact on psychological well-being. *Journal of Personality and Social Psychology*, **46**, 1097–1108.

Rosenbaum, M. (1990) Role of learned resourcefulness in self-control of health behavior. In *Learned Resourcefulness: On Coping Skills, Self-control and Adaptive Behavior*, edited by M. Rosenbaum , pp. 3–30. New York: Springer.

Rotter, J. B. (1966) Generalized expectancies for internal versus external control of reinforcement. *Psychological Monographs*, **80** (1, Whole No. 609).

Rudolph, K. D., Dennig, M. D. & Weisz, J. R. (1995) Determinants and consequences of children's coping in the medical setting: Conceptualization, review and critique. *Psychological Bulletin*, **118**(3), 328–357.

Rutter, M. (1983) Stress, Coping, and Development: Some issues and some questions. In *Stress, Coping and Development in Children*, edited by N. Garmezy & M. Rutter, pp. 1–41. New York: McGraw-Hill.

Rutter, M. (1985) Family and school influences on cognitive development. In *Social Relationships and Cognitive Development*, edited by R. A. Hinde, A. N. Perret-Clermont & J. Stevenson-Hinde. Oxford: Clarendon Press.

Rutter, M. (1986) Psychosocial resilience and protective mechanisms. In *Risk and Protective Factors in the Development of Psychopathology*, edited by D. Cicchetti, K. Neuchterlein & S. Weintraub. Cambridge: Cambridge University Press.

Rutter, M. (1987) Temperament, personality and personality disorder. *British Journal of Psychiatry*, **150**, 443–458.

Rutter, M. (1989) Psychosocial resilience and protective mechanisms. In *Risk and Protective Factors in the Development of Psychopathology*, edited by J. Rolf, A. Master, D. Chichetti, K. Nuecherlein & S. Weintraub. New York: Cambridge University Press.

Rutter, M. (1990) Psychosocial resilience and protective mechanisms. In *Risk and Protective Factors in the Development of Psychopathology*, edited by J. Rolf, A. S. Masten, D. Chicchetti, K. H. Neuchterlein & S. Weintraub, pp. 181–214. New York: Cambridge University Press.

Rutter, M. L. (1994) Stress research: Accomplishments and tasks ahead. In *Stress, Risk and Resilience in Children and Adolescents: Processes, Mechanisms and Interventions*, edited by R. J. Haggerty, pp. 354–385. Cambridge: Cambridge University Press.

Rutter, M. L. (1997) Nature-nurture integration: The example of antisocial behavior. *American Psychologist*, **52**(4), 390–398.

Sameroff, A. J., Seifer, R., Zax, M. & Barocas, R. (1987) Early indicators of developmental risk: Rochester Longitudinal Study. *Schizophrenia Bulletin*, **13**, 383–394.

Sandler, I. N., Ramirez, R. & Reynolds, K. (1986) *Life Stress for Children of Divorce, Bereaved and Asthmatic Children*. Poster presented at the American Psychological Association Convention, Washington, DC.

Sandler, I. N., Tein, J. Y. & West, S. G. (1994) Coping, stress, and the psychological symptoms of children of divorce: A cross-sectional and longitudinal study. *Child Development*, **65**(6), 1744–1763.

Sarason, I. G. & Sarason, B. R. (1985) Social support: Insights from assessment and experimentation. In *Social Support: Theory, Research and Application*, edited by I. G. Sarason & B. R. Sarason, pp. 391–414. The Hague, The Netherlands: Nijhoff.

Sarason, B. R., Sarason, I. G. & Pierce, G. R. (1990) Traditional views of social support and their impact on assessment. In *Social Support: An Interactional View*, edited by B. R. Sarason & G. R. Pierce, pp. 9–25. New York: Wiley.

Scarr, S. (1992) Developmental theories for the 1990s: Developmental and individual differences. *Child Development*, **63**, 1–19.

Scarr, S. & McCartney, K. (1983) How people make their own environments: A theory of genotype—environment effects. *Child Development*, **54**, 424–435.

Schacter, D. L. (1992) Understanding implicit memory: A cognitive neuroscience approach. *American Psychologist*, **47**, 559–569.

Scheier, M. F. & Carver, C. S. (1992) Effects of optimism on psychological and physical well-being: Theoretical overview and empirical update. *Cognitive Therapy and Research*, **16**, 201–228.

Scheier, M. F. & Carver, C. S. (1993) On the power of positive thinking: The benefits of being optimistic. *Current Directions in Psychological Science*, **2**, 26–30.

Schwarzer, R. (1994) Optimism, vulnerability, and self-beliefs as health-related cognitions: A systematic overview. *Psychology and Health*, **9**, 161–180.

Seligman, M. E. P. (1991) *Learned Pptimism*. New York: Alfred A. Knopf.

Shedler, J., Mayman, M. & Manis, M. (1995) The illusion of mental health. *American Psychologist*, **48**(11), 1117–1131.

Shumaker, S. A. & Brownell, A. (1984) Toward a theory of social support: Closing conceptual gaps. *Journal of Social Issues*, **40**, 11–36.

Strentz, T. & Auerbach, S. M. (1988) Adjustment to the stress of simulated captivity: Effects of emotion-focused vs. problem-focused preparation on hostages differing in locus of control. *Journal of Personality and Social Psychology*, **55**, 652–660.

Suls, J. & Fletcher, B. (1986) The relative efficacy of avoidant and nonavoidant coping strategies: A meta-analysis. *Health Psychology*, **4**, 249–288.

Suomi, S. J. (1991) Early stress and adult emotional reactivity in rhesus monkeys. In *The Childhood Environment and Adult Disease*, edited by G. R. Bock & J. Whelan, pp. 171–188. Chichester: Wiley.

The Consortium on the School-Based Promotion of Social Competence (1994) The school-based promotion of social competence: Theory, research, practice and policy. In *Stress, Risk and Resilience in Children and Adolescents: Processes, Mechanisms and Interventions* (Chapter 8), edited by R. J. Haggerty, L. R. Sherrod, N. Garmezy & M. Rutter. Cambridge: Cambridge University Press.

Thoits, P. A. (1985) Social support and psychological wellbeing: Theoretical possibilities. In *Social Support: Theory, Research and Applications*, edited by I. G. Sarason & B. R. Sarason. The Hague, The Netherlands: Nijhoff.

Thoits, P. A. (1986) Social support as coping assistance. *Journal of Consulting and Clinical Psychology*, **54**(4), 416–423.

Thomas, S. P. & Groer, M. W. (1986) Relationship of demographic, life-style and stress variables to blood pressure in adolescents. *Nursing Research*, **35**(3), 169–172.

Tronick, E. Z., Winn, S. & Morelli, G. A. (1985) Multiple caretaking in the context of human evolution: Why don't the Efe know the western prescription for child care? In *Psychobiology of Attachment and Separation*, edited by M. Reite & T. Field, pp. 292–322. New York: Academic.

Turner, R. J. (1992) Measuring social support: Issues of concept and method. In *The Meaning and Measurement of Social Support*, edited by H. O. F. Veiel & U. Baumann, pp. 217–233. New York: Hemisphere.

Vaux, L. (1992) Assessment of social support. In *The Meaning and Measurement of Social Support*, edited by H. O. F. Veiel & U. Baumann, pp. 193–216. New York: Hemisphere.

Vega, L., Ollinger, E., Zimmerman, R., Figueroa, J. et al (1987) Children's representation of earthquakes. *Salud Mental*, **10**(1), 66–71.

Veiel, H. O. F. & Baumann, U. (1992) The many meanings of social support. In *The Meaning and Measurement of Social Support*, edited by H. O. F. Veiel & U. Baumann, pp. 1–12. New York: Hemisphere Publications.

Wallerstein, J. S. & Blakeslee, S. (1989) *Second Chances: Men, Women, and Children a Decade After Divorce*. New York: Ticknor & Fields.

Weinberger, D. (1990) The construct validity of the repressive coping style. In *Repression and Dissociation: Implications for Personality Theory, Psychopathology and Health*, edited by J. L. Singer, pp. 337–385. Chicago: University of Chicago Press.

Weisz, J. R., McCabe, M. & Dennig, M. D. (1994) Primary and secondary control among children undergoing medical procedures: Adjustment as a function of coping style. *Journal of Consulting and Clinical Psychology*, **62**, 324–332.

Werner, E. E. (1995) Resilience in development. *Current Directions in Psychological Science*, **4**(3), 81–85.

Werner, E. E. & Smith, R. S. (1982) *Vulnerable But Invincible: A Study of Resilient Children*. New York: McGraw-Hill.

Westen, D. (1990) Psychoanalytic approaches to personality. In *Handbook of Personality: Theory and Research*, edited by L. Pervin, pp. 21–65. New York: Guilford.

Westen, D. (1994) Toward an integrative model of affect regulation: Applications to social-psychological research. *Journal of Personality*, **62**, 641–667.

Westen, D. (1995) A Clinical-Empirical Model of Personality: Life after the Mischelian Ice Age and the MEO-Lithic Era. *Journal of Personality*, **63**(3), 495–524.

White, B. L. & Watts, J. C. (1973) *Experience and Environment: Major Influences on the Development of the Young Child*. Englewood Cliffs, N.J.: Prentice-Hall.

Williams, R. B., Barefoot, J. C., Califf, R. M., et al. (1992) Prognostic importance of social and economic resources among medically treated patients with angiographically documented coronary artery disease. *Journal of the American Medical Association*, **267**, 520–524.

Winnubst, J. A. M., Buunk, B. P. & Marcelissen, F. H. G. (1988) Social support and stress: Perspectives and processes. In *Handbook of Life Stress, Cognition and Health*, edited by S. Fisher & J. Reason, pp. 511–528. Chichester, England: John Wiley and Sons.

Wolkind, S. & Rutter, M. (1985) Separation, loss and family relationships. In *Chid Psychiatry-Modern Approaches*, edited by M. Rutter & L. Hersov. Blackwell: Oxford.

Worobey, J. & Lewis, M. (1989) Individual differences in the reactivity of young infants. *Developmental Psychology*, **25**, 663–667.

Younger, J. B. (1991) A theory of mastery. *Advances in Nursing Science*, **14**(1), 76–89.

Chapter 5

CHRONIC PAIN—NEURAL BASIS AND INTERACTIONS WITH STRESS

David. J. Tracey, PhD Judith S. Walker, PhD and John J. Carmody, PhD

INTRODUCTION

When tissue is injured, nociceptors are activated by strong mechanical, thermal or chemical stimuli. These anatomically unspecialised sensory receptors are preferentially sensitive to such noxious stimuli and when acute pain results it serves as a useful signal of tissue damage, either actual or potential. Pain has therefore been defined as 'an unpleasant sensory and emotional experience associated with actual or potential tissue damage, or described in terms of such damage' (Merskey, 1979, p. 250). The nociceptors have 'free' nerve endings in skin, joints, muscles and viscera (Cervero & Belmonte, 1996). These free endings have unmyelinated axons (C-fibres) or thinly myelinated axons (Aδ-fibres) which are slowly conducting. Activation of the free nerve endings of nociceptors generates action potentials which are conducted towards the central nervous system along the axons, whose central endings make synaptic contacts with neurons in the dorsal horn of the spinal cord (or the trigeminal nuclei for facial sensation). Activation of these second order neurons will have two main results: reflex actions such as withdrawal of the injured limb to prevent further tissue damage, and in human at least, a conscious sensation of pain. Under normal circumstances, once the painful stimulus is removed and any tissue damage has been repaired, the nociceptors will no longer be activated, and pain sensation will cease. This kind of acute pain, which does not outlast painful stimuli or tissue injury, is easy to understand and comparatively easy to treat.

Unfortunately, this simple mechanism which is normally beneficial can go seriously wrong, so that pain continues well past any useful role in warning us of tissue damage or helping us to recuperate. This is chronic pain, and may be caused by damage to peripheral nerves or by a continuing inflammatory process. It is often spontaneous, in other words it outlasts the duration of painful stimuli and may not even depend on the activation of nociceptors. It is generally accompanied by hyperalgesia, where the patient shows greater sensitivity than usual to a painful stimulus, and by allodynia, where normally innocuous stimuli are perceived as painful. The mechanisms underlying chronic pain are complex, and it is difficult to treat. In this chapter, we will look at how plasticity of the nervous system contributes to chronic pain. Firstly, we will consider the peripheral nervous system and mechanisms which could sensitise the nociceptors. We will then examine some of the ways in which changes in neurons in the spinal cord and supraspinal centres can result in chronic pain. Finally, to give these mechanisms a functional context, we will deal briefly with interactions between stress and chronic pain.

THEORY AND RESEARCH

Peripheral Mechanisms

By peripheral mechanisms we mean those which involve sensory receptors, particularly nociceptors and mechanoreceptors. These mechanisms include sensitisation of nociceptors by the actions of inflammatory mediators and by upregulation of ion channels, the effects of neuromodulators and neurotrophins on the nociceptor, the sprouting of the central endings of mechanoreceptors into abnormal regions of the spinal cord, and the controversial role of the sympathetic nervous system.

Sensitisation of Nociceptors by Inflammatory Mediators
One of the notable features of pain is that the relation between stimulus and response is not fixed (Figure 5.1). The increase in slope and leftward shift are due in part to sensitisation of nociceptors. This sensitisation may be produced by nerve injury or by inflammation. At first glance, one might think that nerve injury and inflammation have little in common. However, injury to any tissue will result in the recruitment or proliferation of immune cells such as macrophages and mast cells which release inflammatory mediators. These mediators include bradykinin (Bk, a peptide derived from high molecular weight precursors in damaged tissue), eicosanoids such as prostaglandins E_2 and I_2 (PGE_2 & PGI_2, released by macrophages, sympathetic nerve terminals and possibly Schwann cells as well), cytokines such as interleukin-1 and interleukin-6 (IL-1 & IL-6, produced by macrophages and other immune cells), serotonin (5-HT, released from blood platelets and mast cells) and even nitric oxide (NO, a short-lived gaseous neurotransmitter produced by several cell types). All of these are known to sensitise nociceptive afferents or to produce hyperalgesia (Rang, Bevan & Dray, 1991). Some of these effects are shown in Figure 5.2. The Schwann cell is not normally thought of as an immune cell (it was believed

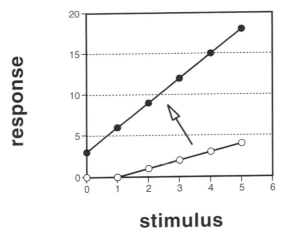

Figure 5.1 Normal relationship between stimulus and response (open circles) is altered in chronic pain (closed circles). The slope of the relationship in the schematic graph becomes steeper and the plot is shifted to the left. In chronic pain, a given stimulus results in a greater response than it normally would (hyperalgesia), and there may even be a response without a stimulus (spontaneous pain).

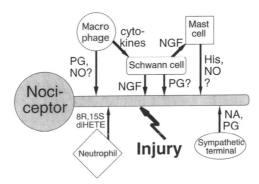

Figure 5.2 Actions of inflammatory mediators on the nociceptor in the periphery. Several cell types (mainly immune cells) release inflammatory mediators, some of which act on the nociceptor to sensitise or activate it. Cytokines include interleukin-1 and interleukin-6. Abbreviations—His: histamine; NA: noradrenaline; NGF: nerve growth factor; NO: nitric oxide; PG: prostaglandins (primarily PGE_2 and PGI_2); 8R,15S-diHETE: (8R,15S)-dihydroxyicosa (5E-9,11,13Z) tetraenoic acid.

for many years to play a rather passive role in the support, maintenance and insulation of peripheral axons) but recent work suggests that it too could release algesic agents such as prostaglandins under conditions of damage or inflammation (Constable, Armati, Toyka & Hartung, 1994; Heywood, Ansselin & Tracey, 1996). Inflammatory mediators not only sensitise regular nociceptors, they also sensitise a group of 'silent nociceptors' which do not respond to any kind of mechanical stimulus in normal tissue (Michaelis, Habler & Jänig, 1996) (Figure 5.6). When tissue such as skin or joint capsule is inflamed, this population of 'silent nociceptors' is sensitised by the inflammatory mediators mentioned above, so that the silent nociceptors now respond to innocuous as well as noxious mechanical stimuli (Schaible & Grubb, 1993). This finding helps to explain the everyday experience that inflamed tissue is sensitive to quite mild mechanical stimuli which would not ordinarily be painful—the phenomenon referred to as allodynia.

How do inflammatory mediators sensitise nociceptors? The mechanism will depend on the particular mediator, but in most cases the mediator will bind to a specific receptor on the nerve membrane—for example, serotonin may bind to a 5-HT_3 receptor, bradykinin may bind to a B1 or B2 receptor. With some mediators (e.g. serotonin) the receptor is directly linked to an ion channel which is permeable to sodium or calcium ions, so that activation of the receptor causes influx of these ions into the neuron. This results in depolarisation, making it easier to activate the nociceptor. With other mediators (e.g. bradykinin) the receptor is linked to second messenger systems (such as adenylate cyclase) which in turn regulate the permeability of ion channels and produce a longer term increase in the excitability of the nociceptor (Figure 5.3) (Rang, Bevan & Dray, 1994). Sensitisation of nociceptors also gives rise to allodynia by a central mechanism, described below. Recent work on how nociceptors are sensitised by inflammatory mediators may lead to new treatments for neuropathic pain as well as inflammatory pain in man (Dray, 1995).

Sensitisation of Nociceptors by Upregulation of Ion Channels
Release of inflammatory mediators is by no means the only mechanism which is likely to contribute to sensitisation of nociceptive afferents. Activation of nociceptors is a result of depolarisation of the neuronal cell membrane at the sensory terminal, and this depends in turn on the influx of cations such as sodium (Na^+) ions and calcium (Ca^{2+}) ions into the terminal. It is this depolarisation which elicits action potentials, which are conducted along the axon of the nociceptor towards its central terminations. There is now evidence that sodium channels and calcium channels are present at greater densities in the cell membrane of axons in injured nerves (Matzner & Devor, 1994; Xie & Xiao, 1993). This increased density will sensitise nociceptive axons by reducing the strength of stimulus needed to elicit action potentials. In fact some algesic mediators (including PGE_2 and serotonin) appear to act on a specific type of sodium channel found in the cell membrane of nociceptors (Gold, Reichling, Shuster & Levine, 1996). Recent work also suggests that the hyperalgesia produced by nerve injury can be relieved using calcium channel blockers (Xiao & Bennett, 1995) suggesting that they could be developed as a treatment for chronic pain.

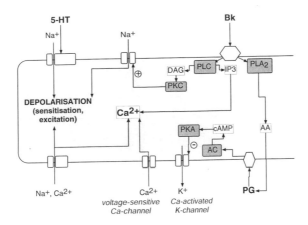

Figure 5.3 Cellular mechanisms of sensitisation of nociceptors. Nociceptors are sensitised in the periphery by the action of agents such as inflammatory mediators on specific receptors in the cell membrane. Some of these receptors, e.g. receptors for serotonin are coupled directly to ion channels (ionotropic receptors, left side of diagram) while others, e.g receptors for bradykinin or prostaglandins are coupled to second messengers such as phospholipase or adenylate cyclase (metabotropic receptors, right side of diagram). The result is either depolarisation of the nociceptor, which sensitises the cell by making it easier to generate action potentials, or an increase in the internal concentration of Ca^{2+} ions, which leads to longer term changes in the metabolism of the cell which also result in sensitisation. Abbreviations: 5-HT: 5-hydroxytryptamine (serotonin); AA: arachidonic acid; AC: adenylate cyclase; Bk: bradykinin; cAMP: cyclic adenosine monophosphate; DAG: diacylglycerol; IP3: inositol-1,4,5-trisphosphate; PLA_2: phospholipase A_2; PLC: phospholipase C; PKA: cAMP-dependent protein kinase A; PKC: protein kinase C. Diagram modified from Rang et al. (1991).

Upregulation of Neuromodulators

In the last few years, it has been found that nerve damage or experimental arthritis induce changes in the neuropeptide content of nociceptive neurons. Neuropeptides include substance P, neurokinin A and calcitonin gene-related peptide (CGRP). They are stored in dense-cored vesicles in the central terminals of nociceptive afferents, and some are known to produce a slow and relatively long-lasting depolarisation of nociceptive neurons in the spinal cord. When a peripheral nerve is cut (the sciatic nerve in most experiments), neuropeptides such as substance P and CGRP are depleted from nociceptive neurons. At the same time, other neuropeptides such as galanin and vasoactive intestinal peptide (VIP) are apparently upregulated—they are found in greater quantities and in a larger number of sensory neurons. Because neuropeptides are known to modulate the responsiveness of spinal neurons which respond to noxious stimuli, it has been suggested that the upregulation of neuropeptides such as VIP may play a role in the increased sensitivity of spinal neurons following nerve damage (Hökfelt, Zhang & Wiesenfeld-Hallin, 1994).

However, the importance of this role is not yet clear. In adjuvant arthritis, an animal model of chronic joint inflammation where the hindpaws are affected, substance P and CGRP are both found in increased quantities in the sciatic nerve as well as the dorsal root ganglia and the dorsal horn of the spinal cord (Donnerer, Schuligoi & Stein, 1992). These neuropeptides probably play a dual role in chronic pain due to inflammation; when released from the peripheral endings of the nociceptors, they contribute to the inflammatory process, and when released from the central endings of the nociceptor, they enhance synaptic transmission between the nociceptor and the spinal neurons which it contacts (Urban, Thompson, Fox, Jeftinija & Dray, 1995).

Contribution of Sensory Nerves to Inflammatory Pain
Chronic pain is symptomatic of a number of diseases including neuropathic pain, cancer and rheumatoid arthritis. It is likely that in such conditions a variety of chemical mediators like SP are able to alter the functions of peripheral nerves. Changes in local blood flow and vascular permeability, activation and migration of immune cells, and changes in the release of trophic and growth factors are also likely to be involved. Enormous potential thus exists for interactions between neural (sensory and autonomic nerves) and non neural (vascular and immune cells) systems. In particular, several studies have suggested a contribution of afferent fibres and neuropeptides to the expression of arthritis. For example, the development of adjuvant arthritis is less severe when sensory function has been impaired by pre-treatment with the neurotoxin capsaicin, while infusion of the neuropeptide SP into the knee increased the severity of experimental arthritis. Involvement of the nervous system in arthritis is also supported by the clinical observation that patients who have experienced a stroke and later develop arthritis experience a less severe form of the disease on the side affected by the stroke (the paretic limb) (Glick, 1967). In animals more severe arthritis develops in joints that are densely innervated by SP-containing neurons (Levine et al., 1984). In support of this, high-risk joints contain higher amounts of SP than low-risk joints. However, despite strong evidence linking neuropeptides to the pain and inflammation of arthritis, further work is required to determine the precise stage at which neuropeptides are involved and how interfering with their actions might alter the course of arthritis and chronic pain.

Modulation by Neurotrophins
Recently it has been suggested that neurotrophic factors such as nerve growth factor (NGF) play a key role in inflammatory hyperalgesia (Lewin, 1995) since peripheral injection of NGF causes hyperalgesia, and administration of agents which sequester NGF prevents development of the hyperalgesia which normally accompanies inflammation (Lewin, Rueff & Mendell, 1994; McMahon, Bennett, Priestley & Shelton, 1995). Furthermore,

NGF expression is upregulated in adjuvant arthritis and other inflammatory conditions (Donnerer et al., 1992; McMahon et al., 1995). It is not yet clear how NGF elicits hyperalgesia, although one intriguing possibility is that NGF somehow acts on sympathetic axons which normally innervate blood vessels in the neighbourhood of the dorsal root ganglia, inducing these axons to sprout and invade the dorsal root ganglion and make abnormal terminations on the cell bodies of sensory neurons in the ganglia (Davis, Albers, Seroogy & Katz, 1994). Autonomic activity which would normally be directed to controlling the diameter of blood vessels could then cause abnormal firing of sensory neurons, which would in turn lead to chronic pain. The sensory neurons themselves may also form abnormal connections within the spinal cord, and this will be discussed in more detail in the next section.

Abnormal Central Terminations of Nociceptors and Mechanoreceptors
The central terminals of nociceptive afferent fibres mostly terminate in the two most superficial layers of the dorsal horn in the spinal cord—the marginal layer, (lamina 1) and the substantia gelatinosa (lamina 2). Some of the neurons in lamina 1 are referred to as 'nociceptive specific' because they are activated only by noxious stimuli. By contrast, the central terminals of mechanoreceptors (e.g. touch and pressure receptors in the skin, spindles and tendon organs of muscle) terminate in the deeper layers of the dorsal horn (laminae 3 to 6). Here they activate neurons which may be 'low threshold' (LT neurons, activated only by mechanoreceptors) or 'wide dynamic range' (WDR neurons). The WDR neurons receive inputs from mechanoreceptors as well as from nociceptors, with the input from nociceptors mediated by interneurons. Following nerve injury, the terminals of mechanoreceptors change their configuration and wander out of their allotted space in the deeper dorsal horn, and into the superficial layers as seen in Figure 5.4 (Lekan, Carlton & Coggeshall, 1996; Shortland & Woolf, 1993). This means that after nerve injury, low-threshold mechanoreceptors may be able to activate nociceptive neurons in the superficial laminae, and offers an anatomical explanation for allodynia—the perception of innocuous stimuli as painful.

Role of the Sympathetic Nervous System
Since the work of Leriche in the First World War, it has been known that sympathectomy of the affected area may relieve naropathic pain and return sensation to normal; this has been well documented in human (Jänig & Schmidt, 1992) although doubts have recently been expressed over the importance of the sympathetic nervous system in chronic pain (Verdugo & Ochoa, 1994). Certainly the mechanism by which the sympathetic nervous system generates or maintains pain is not clear (Jänig & Koltzenburg, 1991; Koltzenburg & McMahon, 1991). One suggestion is that α-1 adrenoreceptors on the peripheral terminals of nociceptive fibres are

RAT DORSAL HORN - Aβ Hair Follicle Afferents

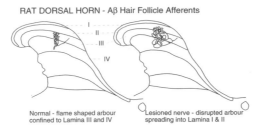

Normal - flame shaped arbour
confined to Lamina III and IV

Lesioned nerve - disrupted arbour
spreading into Lamina I & II

Figure 5.4 Nerve injury results in abnormal terminations of mechanoreceptors in the spinal cord. Injury to the sciatic nerve results in sprouting and reorganisation of the central terminals of mechanoreceptors, such as afferents from hair follicles. These endings are normally confined to lamina III and deeper layers of the dorsal horn (left panel), but after nerve damage they penetrate into lamina II and even lamina I (right panel), where nociceptive neurons are located. Diagram modified from Shortland and Woolf (1993).

upregulated by increased activity in the nociceptors themselves; these adrenoreceptors would then be activated by noradrenaline released by sympathetic terminals in the periphery (Campbell, Meyer, Davis & Raja, 1992). An alternative suggestion, originally put forward by Levine, is that noradrenaline does not act directly on nociceptors, but rather on α-2 adrenoreceptors on the sympathetic terminals themselves. Activation of the adrenoreceptors leads to synthesis and release of PGE_2 or PGI_2 by the sympathetic terminals, and the prostaglandins then sensitise the nociceptor (Levine, Taiwo, Collins & Tam, 1986; Tracey, Cunningham & Romm, 1995). A third possibility is the formation of abnormal connections between sympathetic axons and the cell bodies of afferents in the dorsal root ganglia, mentioned above in the section dealing with neurotrophins (McLachlan, Jänig, Devor & Michaelis, 1993). Activity in sympathetic axons could then lead to abnormal activity in sensory fibres, giving rise to pain. While the sympathetic nervous system may contribute to pain resulting from nerve damage, there is little evidence that it contributes to acute or chronic pain resulting from inflammation (Kidd, Cruwys, Mapp & Blake, 1992; Raja, 1995).

Central Mechanisms

In the previous section, we have outlined how nociceptors may be sensitised to external stimuli such as mechanical pressure, temperature changes and increased concentration of chemical agents. Similarly, spinal neurons may be sensitised to synaptic inputs from nociceptors or even mechanoreceptors. In this case, the relation between stimulus and response would be changed for the spinal neuron as shown in Figure 5.1; here the stimulus is synaptic input while the response is the number of action potentials generated. A good example of this is the phenomenon referred to as 'wind-up'. If a nociceptive neuron in the dorsal horn is activated by electrical stimulation of a peripheral nerve at a strength above threshold for C-fibres, the response to the first few stimuli is relatively low, but it then increases markedly and stabilises at a level much greater than the original response (Dickenson, 1990) (Figure 5.5). Nociceptive neurons can therefore be sensitised by repeated bursts of activity in C-fibres. In fact there are two main classes of nociceptive neuron: the WDR neuron, referred to above, and the nociceptive specific ('NS') neuron, which is activated only by noxious stimuli. It appears that the WDR neuron, which responds to inputs from innocuous as well as noxious stimuli, is the one most likely to be responsible for the conscious awareness of painful stimuli (Dubner, Kenshalo, Maixner, Bushnell & Oliveras. Furthermore, sensitisation of the WDR neuron by a barrage of activity in C-fibres makes it respond more vigorously not only to noxious stimuli, but also to innocuous stimuli-resulting in allodynia as well as hyperalgesia (Cervero & Laird, 1996; Roberts, 1986). This means that both forms of hypersensitivity found in chronic pain can be alleviated by blocking C-fibres (Koltzenburg, Lundberg & Torebjörk, 1992). Chronic pain may therefore start with sensitisation of nociceptors in the periphery, and be reinforced by sensitisation of WDR neurons in the dorsal horn of the spinal cord. The chronic pain state will continue so long as it is maintained by excessive activity in C-fibres, but is usually relieved when this activity ceases.

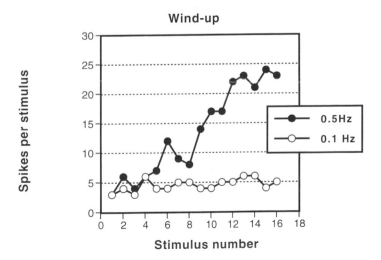

Wind-up

Figure 5.5   Wind-up in nociceptive neurons of the dorsal horn. When a nociceptive neuron in the dorsal horn is repeatedly activated by stimulating a peripheral nerve electrically at a strength above threshold for C-fibres, the response to each stimulus remains small at a low stimulus frequency (0.1 Hz). However, at a higher stimulus frequency, the response to each stimulus tends to be greater than the previous one. This is a form of sensitisation. Diagram modified from Dickenson (1990).

Sensitisation of WDR Neurons by Glutamate

Some hints about the mechanisms which underlie sensitisation of WDR neurons are given by the actions of neurotransmitters and neuromodulators on neurons in the dorsal horn. The central terminals of nociceptors contain the excitatory amino acids glutamate and aspartate (De Biasi & Rustioni, 1988; Tracey, De Biasi, Phend & Rustioni, 1991). These are neurotransmitters which excite nociceptive neurons in the dorsal horn. They are contained in synaptic vesicles, the contents of which are released into the synaptic cleft between the synaptic terminal and the spinal neuron. Glutamate then binds to receptors on the postsynaptic membrane, leading to activation of the spinal neuron (Figure 5.7). There are at least four types of glutamate receptor—three ionotropic receptors (linked to ion channels), namely the NMDA receptor and two non-NMDA receptors (kainate and AMPA receptors). In addition there is a metabotropic glutamate receptor, which is linked to a second messenger system rather than to an ion channel. All of these receptors are found on neurons in the dorsal horn which receive nociceptive inputs. Under normal circumstances, the non-NMDA receptors are activated by glutamate release, and mediate a rapid, short-latency

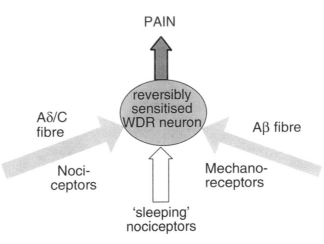

Figure 5.6   Sensitisation of nociceptive neuron in the dorsal horn of the spinal cord. The neuron shown is a wide dynamic range neuron (WDR neuron), so called because it responds in a graded fashion to low-intensity stimuli (signalled by mechanoreceptors with myelinated axons, e.g. Aβ axons) as well as to high-intensity stimulil (signalled by nociceptors with unmyelinated axons—C fibres, or by thinly myelinated axons—Aδ fibres). Increased activity in nociceptors sensitises the neuron, which now responds more vigorously to nociceptive inputs as well as to inputs from mechanoreceptors. The increased responsiveness to nociceptive inputs contributes to hyperalgesia; the increased responsiveness to mechanoreceptive inputs contributes to allodynia. Activation of 'sleeping' nociceptors by inflammatory mediators will also contribute to sensitisation of the WDR neuron. Interactions between nociceptors and mechanoreceptors may also contribute to allodynia (Cervero & Laird, 1996) but are not shown in the diagram.

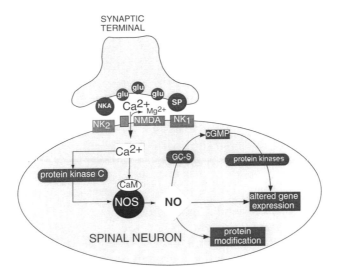

Figure 5.7 Cellular mechanisms of sensitisation of nociceptive spinal neurons. The synaptic terminal of a nociceptor carries synaptic vesicles containing neurotransmitters, the most important of which is glutamate (an excitatory amino acid). Glutamate acts on several receptor types, only one of which (the NMDA receptor) is shown. Glutamate has relatively little effect on the NMDA receptor unless the cell membrane is depolarised by the action of glutamate on non-NMDA receptors (not shown) or the action of neuromodulators such as NKA or SP on their respective receptors (NK2 and NK1 receptors). This depolarisation removes Mg^{2+} ions from the ion channel associated with the NMDA receptor, allowing Ca^{2+} ions to enter the cell. As in the nociceptor, increased levels of Ca^{2+} have several long-term effects, including activation of NOS, leading to the production of NO, which leads in turn to altered gene expression and protein modification. These factors can modulate the ion channels responsible for depolarisation of the cell, so that the neuron is sensitised to synaptic inputs from nociceptors and mechanoreceptors outlined in the previous figure. Abbreviations: CaM: calmodulin; cGMP: cyclic GMP; GC-S: soluble guanylate cyclase; glu:glutamate; NKA: neurokinin A; NK1: NK1 receptor; NK2: NK2 receptor; NMDA: NMDA receptor; NO: nitric oxide; NOS: nitric oxide synthase. Diagram modified from Meller and Gebhart (1993).

depolarisation of the spinal neuron. Activation of these non-NMDA receptors by C-fibres appears to mediate responses to acute painful stimuli. By contrast, the NMDA receptor is partially inactivated by physiological concentrations of Mg^{2+} ion, and mediates a slow, long-latency depolarisation which is relatively weak and does not contribute to responses to acute painful stimuli. With repetitive stimulation, the NMDA component becomes more pronounced (Urban et al., 1995) and contributes to wind-up (Chapman & Dickenson, 1992; Ren, 1994). Depolarisation reverses the inactivation of NMDA produced by Mg^{2+} ions and increases the conductivity of the ion channel associated with the NMDA receptor. As the spinal neuron is depolarised, the conductivity of the NMDA channel increases, leading to further depolarisation and so on. A voltage-dependent increase in the permeability of the NMDA receptor therefore contributes to sensitisation of the spinal nociceptive neuron. This increase in permeability leads to an influx of Ca^{2+} ions into the neuron, which makes a further contribution to sensitisation (see below). One would therefore expect that NMDA receptor blockers should prevent or relieve hyperalgesia, and this has been shown in animal models of inflammation and neuropathic pain (Neugebauer, Lücke & Schaible, 1993; Qian, Brown & Carlton, 1996). NMDA receptor blockers hold some promise for pain treatment in humans as well (Gordh, Karlsten & Kristensen, 1995). Most of the evidence for involvement of the NMDA receptor in hyperalgesia relates to an increased sensitivity to thermal stimuli (Meller, Dykstra & Gebhart, 1996). However, recent evidence implicates non-NMDA receptors in the generation and maintenance of increased sensitivity to mechanical stimuli. This work suggests that mechanical hyperalgesia is produced not by activation of NMDA receptors, but rather by the combined activation of ionotropic AMPA receptors and metabotropic glutamate receptors (Meller, Dykstra & Gebhart, 1993).

Sensitisation of WDR Neurons by Neuropeptides
It was mentioned earlier that the synaptic terminals of nociceptors contain neuropeptides. In fact neuropeptides such as substance P and neurokinin A are co-localised in some synaptic vesicles with glutamate (De Biasi & Rustioni, 1988) so that neuropeptides are released into the synaptic cleft at the same time as excitatory amino acids. Once released, these two neuropeptides act on neurokinin (NK) receptors (substance P acts primarily on NK_1 receptors, while neurokinin A acts primarily on NK_2 receptors). Neurokinin A normally contributes to the synaptic potential, but substance P does not. However, after continued activity in C-fibres as a result of inflammation or nerve damage, substance P starts to contribute to the synaptic potential. At the same time, activation of both NK_1 and NK_2 receptors appears to activate NMDA receptors via intracellular second messengers (Chen & Huang, 1992). This activation of NMDA receptors happens even at normal concentrations of Mg^{2+} and at resting membrane potential, and will contribute to sensitisation as described in the previous paragraph. These results, obtained in slice preparations of the spinal cord *in vitro*, are consistent with findings of recent *in vivo* experiments. These showed that during experimental inflammation of the knee joint, neurokinin A mediates both the development and maintenance of hyperexcitability of dorsal horn neurons (Neugebauer, Rumenapp & Schaible, 1996), while substance P is involved in maintenance rather than development of central sensitisation (Neugebauer, Weiretter & Schaible, 1995). As yet, intrathecal application of neurokinin antagonists has not been used clinically to relieve chronic pain.

Sensitisation of Nociceptive Dorsal Horn Neurons by Second Messengers
It can be seen from the above outline that excitatory amino acids and neuropeptides act on dorsal horn neurons, resulting in sensitisation of the neurons to innocuous as well as noxious stimuli. What are the intracellular mechanisms underlying this sensitisation? There is some evidence that these mechanisms may be different for mechanical and thermal hyperalgesia (Meller et al., 1993; Meller et al., 1996). In thermal hyperalgesia, activation of NMDA receptors is involved, and this leads to influx of Ca^{2+} ions. The increased Ca^{2+} concentration activates nitric oxide synthase, which generates nitric oxide (NO). This gas forms an important link in the chain of events between the activation of receptors on the surface of the neuron and long-term changes in the neuron, such as gene expression. Nitric oxide activates soluble guanylate cyclase, leading to an increased concentration of cyclic GMP in the neuron (Figure 5.7). This in turn activates protein kinases and leads to altered gene expression (Coderre, 1993; Meller et al., 1996; Meller & Gebhart, 1993). In mechanical hyperalgesia, it has been suggested that co-activation of AMPA receptors and metabotropic glutamate receptors is required. Activation of these receptors also leads to Ca^{2+} influx, as described for the NMDA receptor. If activation of NMDA receptors leads to thermal hyperalgesia while activation of AMPA and metabotropic receptors leads to mechanical hyperalgesia, there must be some difference in the intracellular messengers evoked by these distinct glutamate receptors.

Involvement of Supraspinal Structures in Chronic Pain
Since nociceptive neurons in the dorsal horn of the spinal cord are sensitised in chronic pain conditions, it is not surprising that neurons in higher centres such as the thalamus also become more active. The evidence for this is much less extensive than at the spinal level. However, such changes have been shown in a rat model of peripheral mononeuropathy. Rats with a chronic constriction injury of the sciatic nerve showed increased metabolic activity in a number of brain regions including the thalamus (posterior thalamic nucleus and ventral posterolateral thalamus), amygdala, somatosensory cortex and cingulate cortex. Extensive activation of many brain regions related to processing of sensory-discriminative aspects of pain was reported. In addition, limbic structures such as the amygdala and cingulate cortex, which have been implicated in affective-motivational aspects of pain, were also activated in this rat model of chronic pain (Mao, Mayer & Price, 1993). Electrophysiogical data from patients with chronic pain confirms that the activity of some thalamic neurons is increased. 'Hyperactive' neurons (neurons showing a high frequency of discharge) were found in the ventral posterolateral thalamic nucleus of rats with sectioned dorsal roots, as well as in thalamic nuclei of patients with chronic pain (Yamashiro et al., 1994). Patients with chronic

neuropathic pain show activation of several cortical areas, including the anterior cingulate cortex, on the basis of positron emission tomography (Hsieh, Belfrage, Stone-Elander, Hansson & Ingvar, 1995). It has also been reported that somatosensory cortex shows evidence of reorganization in patients with chronic back pain (Flor, Braun, Elbert & Birbaumer, 1997).

Stress and Pain

Animal Studies
Pain of any kind—especially chronic pain—provides a major therapeutic challenge for clinicians. Despite their many advantages it is clear that morphine and the anti-inflammatory drugs leave much to be desired in the treatment of chronic pain conditions. It is important, therefore, that improvements in our understanding be constantly evaluated from a therapeutic perspective: there is some promise, for example, that the dynamic properties of the nervous system may also be exploited to assist with clinical analgesia. If, for example, clinically acceptable ways were found to activate the phenomenon that is currently known as stress-analgesia or auto-analgesia, it would represent a great advance. This analgesia has been evoked in experimental animals by diverse stimuli, one of the most popular of which has been swimming with rats or mice. Classical stress leads to increased secretion of CRH (corticotrophin-releasing hormone) by hypothalamic neurons and hence release of both ACTH and β-endorphin from the anterior pituitary (Guillemin et al., 1977). This is clearly one factor in auto-analgesia: mice that cannot produce β-endorphin do not have the capacity for this opioid-analgesia, although they have a normal sensitivity to exogenous opiates (Rubinstein et al., 1996). Stress doubtless has effects elsewhere in the CNS too, probably in the brainstem where electrical stimulation (especially involving the periaqueductal gray (PAG) has potent effects on nociception, most likely through inhibition of the transmission of nociceptive afferents within the dorsal horn of the spinal cord. Some brainstem stimulation evokes opioid-based inhibition and may lead to opioid independent analgesia (Cannon, Prieto, Lee & Liebeskind, 1982).

Depending on the details, this stress-induced analgesia also proves to have both opioid and non-opioid components. One study (Tierney, Carmody & Jamieson, 1991) reported that extremely short swims (e.g. 15 s) in water at room temperature produce an early non-opioid analgesia (i.e. its properties were not affected by opiate antagonist drugs) whereas longer swims (3 min) induce analgesia that is wholly opioid in nature (blocked completely by naloxone). Furthermore, these two analgesic systems interact: as the more severer stress activates the opioid system, the non-opioid analgesia is suppressed. Other workers have found a comparable duality of the analgesia but reported that milder stress evoked the opioid analgesia while more severe stress was required to evoke the non-opioid form of analgesia (Mogil, Sternberg, Balian, Liebeskind & Sadowski, 1996). It seems likely that the ups-and-downs of everyday living act to keep the opioid system partially activated (Carmody, Carroll & Morgans, 1979). It is noteworthy that in some circumstances, stress can increase pain sensitivity (Vidal & Jacob, 1986). Clearly the systems involved with nociception are extremely labile, acutely as well as chronically.

Finally, it is worth mentioning the co-operative action of peripheral and central factors in pain modulation. Not only is hypothalamic CRH involved in the release of β-endorphin but CRH may also be released from cells in non-neural peripheral tissues, thereby triggering opioid release from certain immune cells (Schafer, Mousa, Zhang, Carter & Stein, 1996). This implies that the immune system plays a role in pain control. It also raises the issue of the role of the concomitant release of β-endorphin and ACTH from the anterior pituitary and then of the corticosteroids which the ACTH will release from the adrenal. ACTH activates the adrenal cortex to release cortisol, which acts on the immune system and the endogenous opioid system. It has recently been suggested that, 'If the output of cortisol is prolonged, or excessive, or of abnormal patterning, it may produce destruction of muscle, bone and neural tissue and produce the conditions for many kinds of chronic pain' (Melzack, 1997). There is thus the possibility of an integrated operation such as is seen in aspects of endocrine function. In other words, central and peripheral CRH may have complementary functions. It has been argued that the opioid analgesia is only part of an opioid-based recuperative phenomenon involving numerous body systems (Carmody, 1992); likewise there may be integrative neuro-immune interactions in pain control which may be amenable to clinical exploitation.

CLINICAL APPLICATIONS AND EVALUATIONS

As might be expected, human studies have sought to confirm the idea that there is a relationship between stress and pain sensitivity. In fact the interaction between stress and pain works both ways—stress may enhance chronic pain, while chronic pain in turn leads to stress.

Stress Enhances Chronic Pain

Stressful events may enhance chronic pain (Craig, 1994; Weisenberg, 1977). Thus day-to-day stresses were reported to be strongly associated with increased pain (Sternbach, 1986) and recurrent painful episodes may be triggered by perceived stress in children (Kain & Rimar, 1995). Greater stress-related lability of the back muscles was reported in patients with chronic, painful lower-back conditions than in normal, pain-free subjects (Flor, Turk & Birbaumer, 1985). Headache sufferers were reported to experience greater life stress ('daily hassles') than headache-free controls

(De Benedittis & Lorenzetti, 1992), while patients scoring high in hospital stress tended to report more pain during hospitalisation and less improvement after discharge than patients scoring low in hospital stress (Volicer, 1978). However, on the basis of a study on the relation between pain and stress in patients with rheumatoid arthritis, Radanov, Frost, Schwarz and Augustiny (1996) suggest that the importance of psychosocial stress as a factor in chronic intractable pain needs to be reassessed, and some authors believe that the relationship between stress and pain is not a strong one (Merskey, 1994). Such work is at odds with the animal experiments which demonstrated stress analgesia. However, stress-induced analgesia has been shown in human subjects, using anticipation of a noxious footshock as a stress and a flexion reflex as the nociceptive test (Willer, Dehen & Cambier, 1981). Recent work on painful intracutaneous stimuli to the hand has shown that stress-induced analgesia can be classically conditioned in humans (Flor & Birbaumer, 1994). In both of these studies, stress-induced analgesia was found to be opioid-mediated. This work points to clear plasticity of nociceptive mechanisms; an important clinical challenge is to find ethical and reliable means to activate those systems which will induce analgesia, especially in patients with chronic pain.

Chronic Pain Produces Stress

It is hardly surprising that chronic pain gives rise to stress. In fact chronic pain may result in several types of emotional and behavioural disturbance, in particular depression (Barkin et al., 1996; Craig, 1994). Recent work on stress as a result of pain has focused on post-traumatic stress disorder (PTSD). This disorder may be initiated by the acute pain of childbirth (Fones, 1996; Reynolds, 1997) or other forms of uncontrolled acute pain (Schreiber & Galai-Gat, 1993). PTSD also has a high prevalence in individuals with chronic pain (Geisser, Roth, Bachman & Eckert, 1996), although much of the work on the relationship between PTSD and chronic pain has been based on case studies. There is some agreement that targeting PTSD symptoms may be a useful approach to enhance treatment outcomes for chronic pain and PTSD (Eisendrath, 1995; Geisser et al., 1996).

Treatment of Chronic Pain

Geisser et al. (1996) observed that behavioural treatments such as cognitive behavioural therapy, systematic desensitization and relaxation training have often been employed to treat chronic pain (Holzman, Turk & Kerns, 1986) as well as PTSD (Ebbinghaus, Bauer & Priebe, 1996; Foy, Donahoe, Carrol, Gallers & Reno, 1987). It has been suggested that these treatments may share a common physiological mechanism relying in part on activation of endogenous opioids (Egan, Carr, Hunt & Adamson, 1988). In some forms of chronic pain, (cancer pain) opioids are the mainstay of pain relief. However, other forms of chronic pain (e.g. neuropathic pain) may be unresponsive to opioids. This disparity highlights the question of effective pharmacological treatment for chonic pain. Current evidence from randomised controlled trials supports the use of tricyclic antidepressants as first choice medication for chronic pain (Rowbotham, 1995) except where pain is associated with peripheral nervous system injury or trigeminal neuralgia, in which case anti-convulsants and anti-arrhythmics may be more appropriate. Antidepressants have also been shown to be effective in pharmacological intervention for PTSD (Ebbinghaus et al., 1996; Katz, Fleisher, Kjernisted & Milanese, 1996; Sutherland & Davidson, 1994). Most clinicians would agree that a multifaceted approach is useful for syndromes as complex as chronic pain. It would appear that a combination of some form of behavioural therapy such as cognitive therapy and one of the antidepressants is most likely to help relieve symptoms of chronic pain combined with PTSD, particularly in view of the interaction between stress and chronic pain discussed above.

CONCLUSION

In this brief outline of the neural mechanisms of chronic pain, we have shown that chronic pain and its modulation by stress are based on demonstrable changes in the anatomy, physiology and pharmacology of the nervous system. While psychological changes inevitably take place as a result of the unpleasantness of chronic pain, the doctor should not give the patient the additional burden of believing that chronic pain is 'all in the mind'.

Acknowledgments

We would like to thank Dr Aihua Song and Professor R.F. Schmidt for constructive criticism of of the manuscript.

References

Barkin, R. L., Lubenow, T. R., Bruehl, S., Husfeldt, B., Ivankovich, O. & Barkin, S. J. (1996) Management of chronic pain. Part II. *Disease-A-Month*, **42**(8), 457–507.

Campbell, J. N., Meyer, R. A., Davis, K. D. & Raja, S. N. (1992) Sympathetically maintained pain: a unifying hypothesis. In *Hyperalgesia and Allodynia*, edited by W. D. Willis, Jr., pp. 141–149. New York: Raven.

Cannon, J. T., Prieto, G. J., Lee, A. & Liebeskind, J. C. (1982) Evidence for opioid and non-opioid forms of stimulation-produced analgesia in the rat. *Brain Research*, **243**(2), 315–321.

Carmody, J. J. (1992) Stress-induced analgesia: is it a protective phenomenon? In *Animal Pain: Ethical and Scientific Perspectives*, edited by T. Kuchel, M. Rose & J. Burrell. Adelaide: ACCART.

Carmody, J. J., Carroll, P. R. & Morgans, D. (1979) Naloxone increases pain perception in rats and mice. *Life Sciences*, **24**(13), 1149–1152.

Cervero, F. & Belmonte, C. (eds.) (1996) *Neurobiology of Nociceptors*. Oxford: Oxford Univ. Press.

Cervero, F. & Laird, J. M. A. (1996) Mechanisms of touch-evoked pain (allodynia): a new model. *Pain*, **68**, 13–23.

Chapman, V. & Dickenson, A. H. (1992) The combination of NMDA antagonism and morphine produces profound antinociception in the rat dorsal horn. *Brain Research*, 573(2), 321–323.

Chen, L. & Huang, L. Y. (1992) Protein kinase C reduces Mg^{2+} block of NMDA-receptor channels as a mechanism of modulation. *Nature*, 356(6369), 521–523.

Coderre, T. J. (1993) The role of excitatory amino acid receptors and intracellular messengers in persistent nociception after tissue injury in rats. *Molecular Neurobiology*, 7(3–4), 229–246.

Constable, A. L., Armati, P. J., Toyka, K. V. & Hartung, H. P. (1994) Production of prostanoids by Lewis rat Schwann cells *in vitro*. *Brain Research*, 635(1–2), 75–80.

Craig, K. D. (1994) Emotional aspects of pain. In *Textbook of Pain*, 3rd ed., edited by P. D. Wall & R. Melzack, pp. 261–274. Edinburgh: Churchill Livingstone.

Davis, B. M., Albers, K. M., Seroogy, K. B. & Katz, D. M. (1994) Overexpression of nerve growth factor in transgenic mice induces novel sympathetic projections to primary sensory neurons. *Journal of Comparative Neurology*, 349(3), 464–474.

De Benedittis, G. & Lorenzetti, A. (1992) The role of stressful life events in the persistence of primary headache: major events vs. daily hassles. *Pain*, 51(1), 35–42.

De Biasi, S. & Rustioni, A. (1988) Glutamate and substance P coexist in primary afferent terminals in the superficial laminae of spinal cord. *Proceedings of the National Academy of Sciences of the United States of America*, 85(20), 7820–7824.

Dickenson, A. H. (1990) A cure for wind up: NMDA receptor antagonists as potential analgesics. *Trends in Pharmacological Sciences*, 11(8), 307–309.

Donnerer, J., Schuligoi, R. & Stein, C. (1992) Increased content and transport of substance P and calcitonin gene-related peptide in sensory nerves innervating inflamed tissue: evidence for a regulatory function of nerve growth factor *in vivo*. *Neuroscience*, 49(3), 693–698.

Dray, A. (1995) Inflammatory mediators of pain. *British Journal of Anaesthesia*, 75(2), 125–131.

Dubner, R., Kenshalo, D. R., Jr., Maixner, W., Bushnell, M. C. & Oliveras, J. L. (1989) The correlation of monkey medullary dorsal horn neuronal activity and the perceived intensity of noxious heat stimuli. *Journal of Neurophysiology*, 62(2), 450–457.

Ebbinghaus, R., Bauer, M. & Priebe, S. (1996) Behandlung der posttraumatischen Belastungsstörung. *Fortschritte der Neurologie-Psychiatrie*, 64(11), 433–443.

Egan, K. J., Carr, J. E., Hunt, D. D. & Adamson, R. (1988) Endogenous opiate system and systematic desensitization. *Journal of Consulting & Clinical Psychology*, 56(2), 287–291.

Eisendrath, S. J. (1995) Psychiatric aspects of chronic pain. *Neurology*, 45(12 Suppl. 9), S26–34.

Flor, H. & Birbaumer, N. (1994) Basic issues in the psychobiology of pain. In *Progress in Pain Research and Management*, Vol. 2, edited by G. F. Gebhart, D. L. Hammond, & T. S. Jensen, pp. 113–125. Seattle: IASP Press.

Flor, H., Braun, C., Elbert, T. & Birbaumer, N. (1997) Extensive reorganization of primary somatosensory cortex in chronic back pain patients. *Neuroscience Letters*, 224(1), 5–8.

Flor, H., Turk, D. C. & Birbaumer, N. (1985) Assessment of stress-related psychophysiological reactions in chronic back pain patients. *Journal of Consulting and Clinical Psychology*, 53(3), 354–364.

Fones, C. (1996) Posttraumatic stress disorder occurring after painful childbirth. *Journal of Nervous and Mental Disease*, 184(3), 195–196.

Foy, D. W., Donahoe, C. P. J., Carrol, E. M., Gallers, J. & Reno, R. (1987) Posttraumatic stress disorder. In *Anxiety and Stress Disorders: Cognitive-Behavioral Assessment and Treatment*, edited by L. Michelson & L. M. Ascher, pp. 361–378. New York: Guilford Press.

Geisser, M. E., Roth, R. S., Bachman, J. E. & Eckert, T. A. (1996) The relationship between symptoms of post-traumatic stress disorder and pain, affective disturbance and disability among patients with accident and non-accident related pain. *Pain*, 66(2–3), 207–214.

Glick, E. N. (1967) Asymmetrical rheumatoid arthritis after poliomyelitis. *British Medical Journal*, 3(556), 26–28.

Gold, M. S., Reichling, D. B., Shuster, M. J. & Levine, J. D. (1996) Hyperalgesic agents increase a tetrodotoxin-resistant Na+ current in nociceptors. *Proceedings of the National Academy of Sciences of the United States of America*, 93(3), 1108–1112.

Gordh, T., Karlsten, R. & Kristensen, J. (1995) Intervention with spinal NMDA, adenosine, and NO systems for pain modulation. *Annals of Medicine*, **27**(2), 229–234.

Guillemin, R., Vargo, T., Rossier, J., Minick, S., Ling, N., Rivier, C., Vale, W. & Bloom, F. (1977) beta-Endorphin and adrenocorticotropin are secreted concomitantly by the pituitary gland. *Science*, **197**(4311), 1367–1369.

Heywood, G., Ansselin, A. & Tracey, D. J. (1996) Adult Schwann cells release prostaglandins *in vitro*. *Proc. Aust. Neurosci. Soc.*, **7**, 233.

Hökfelt, T., Zhang, X. & Wiesenfeld-Hallin, Z. (1994) Messenger plasticity in primary sensory neurons following axotomy and its functional implications. *Trends in Neurosciences*, **17**(1), 22–30.

Holzman, A. D., Turk, D. C. & Kerns, R. D. (1986) The cognitive-behavioral approach to the management of chronic pain. In *Pain Management: A Handbook of Psychological Treatment Approaches*, edited by A. D. Holzman & D. C. Turk, pp. 31–50. New York: Pergamon Press.

Hsieh, J. C., Belfrage, M., Stone-Elander, S., Hansson, P. & Ingvar, M. (1995) Central representation of chronic ongoing neuropathic pain studied by positron emission tomography. *Pain*, **63**(2), 225–236.

Jänig, W. & Koltzenburg, M. (1991) What is the interaction between the sympathetic terminal and the primary afferent fiber? In *Towards a New Pharmacotherapy of Pain*, edited by A. I. Basbaum & J.-M. Besson, pp. 331–352. New York: John Wiley.

Jänig, W. & Schmidt, R. F. (eds.) (1992) *Reflex Sympathetic Dystrophy*. Weinheim: VCH.

Kain, Z. N. & Rimar, S. (1995) Management of chronic pain in children. *Pediatrics in Review*, **16**(6), 218–222.

Katz, L., Fleisher, W., Kjernisted, K. & Milanese, P. (1996) A review of the psychobiology and pharmacotherapy of posttraumatic stress disorder. *Canadian Journal of Psychiatry —Revue Canadienne de Psychiatrie*, **41**(4), 233–238.

Kidd, B. L., Cruwys, S., Mapp, P. I. & Blake, D. R. (1992) Role of the sympathetic nervous system in chronic joint pain and inflammation. *Annals of the Rheumatic Diseases*, **51**(11), 1188–1191.

Koltzenburg, M., Lundberg, L. E. & Torebjörk, H. E. (1992) Dynamic and static components of mechanical hyperalgesia in human hairy skin. *Pain*, **51**(2), 207–219.

Koltzenburg, M. & McMahon, S. B. (1991) The enigmatic role of the sympathetic nervous system in chronic pain. *Trends Pharmacol. Sci.*, **12**, 399–402.

Kuraishi, Y., Nanayama, T., Ohno, H., Fujii, N., Otaka, A., Yajima, H. & Satoh, M. (1989) Calcitonin gene-related peptide increases in the dorsal root ganglia of adjuvant arthritic rat. *Peptides*, **10**(2), 447–452.

Lekan, H. A., Carlton, S. M. & Coggeshall, R. E. (1996) Sprouting of A-beta fibers into Lamina II of the rat dorsal horn in peripheral neuropathy. *Neuroscience Letters*, **208**(3), 147–150.

Levine, J. D., Clark, R., Devor, M., Helms, C., Moskowitz, M. A. & Basbaum, A. I. (1984) Intraneuronal substance P contributes to the severity of experimental arthritis. *Science*, **226**(4674), 547–549.

Levine, J. D., Taiwo, Y. O., Collins, S. D. & Tam, J. K. (1986) Noradrenaline hyperalgesia is mediated through interaction with sympathetic postganglionic neurone terminals rather than activation of primary afferent nociceptors. *Nature*, **323**(6084), 158–160.

Lewin, G. R. (1995) Neurotrophic factors and pain. *Seminars in the Neurosciences*, **7**, 227–232.

Lewin, G. R., Rueff, A. & Mendell, L. M. (1994) Peripheral and central mechanisms of NGF-induced hyperalgesia. *Europ. J. Neurosci.*, **6**, 1903–1912.

Mao, J., Mayer, D. J. & Price, D. D. (1993) Patterns of increased brain activity indicative of pain in a rat model of peripheral mononeuropathy. *Journal of Neuroscience*, **13**(6), 2689–2702.

Matzner, O. & Devor, M. (1994) Hyperexcitability at sites of nerve injury depends on voltage-sensitive Na$^+$ channels. *Journal of Neurophysiology*, **72**(1), 349–359.

McLachlan, E. M., Jänig, W., Devor, M. & Michaelis, M. (1993) Peripheral nerve injury triggers noradrenergic sprouting within dorsal root ganglia. *Nature*, **363**(6429), 543–546.

McMahon, S. B., Bennett, D. L. H., Priestley, J. V. & Shelton, D. L. (1995) The biological effects of endogenous nerve growth factor on adult sensory neurons revealed by a trkA-IgG fusion molecule. *Nature Medicine*, **1**(8), 774–780.

Meller, S. T., Dykstra, C. & Gebhart, G. F. (1996) Acute thermal hyperalgesia in the rat is produced by activation of N-methyl-D-aspartate receptors and protein kinase C and production of nitric oxide. *Neuroscience*, **71**(2), 327–335.

Meller, S. T., Dykstra, C. L. & Gebhart, G. F. (1993) Acute mechanical hyperalgesia is produced by coactivation of AMPA and metabotropic glutamate receptors. *Neuroreport*, **4**(7), 879–882.

Meller, S. T. & Gebhart, G. F. (1993) Nitric oxide (NO) and nociceptive processing in the spinal cord. *Pain*, **52**(2), 127–136.

Melzack, R. (1993) Pain: past, present and future. *Candadian Journal of Experimental Psychology*, **47**, 615–629.

Merskey, H. (1979) Pain terms: a list with definitions and notes on usage. *Pain*, **6**, 249–252.

Merskey, H. (1994) Pain and psychological medicine. In *Textbook of Pain*, edited by P. D. Wall & R. Melzack, (3rd ed., pp. 903–920). Edinburgh: Churchill Livingstone.

Michaelis, M., Habler, H. J. & Jaenig, W. (1996) Silent afferents: a separate class of primary afferents? *Clinical and Experimental Pharmacology and Physiology*, **23**(2), 99–105.

Mogil, J. S., Sternberg, W. F., Balian, H., Liebeskind, J. C. & Sadowski, B. (1996) Opioid and nonopioid swim stress-induced analgesia: a parametric analysis in mice. *Physiology and Behavior*, **59**(1), 123–132.

Neugebauer, V., Lücke, T. & Schaible, H. G. (1993) N-methyl-D-aspartate (NMDA) and non-NMDA receptor antagonists block the hyperexcitability of dorsal horn neurons during development of acute arthritis in rat's knee joint. *Journal of Neurophysiology*, **70**(4), 1365–1377.

Neugebauer, V., Rumenapp, P. & Schaible, H. G. (1996) The role of spinal neurokinin-2 receptors in the processing of nociceptive information from the joint and in the generation and maintenance of inflammation-evoked hyperexcitability of dorsal horn neurons in the rat. *European Journal of Neuroscience*, **8**(2), 249–260.

Neugebauer, V., Weiretter, F. & Schaible, H. G. (1995) Involvement of substance P and neurokinin-1 receptors in the hyperexcitability of dorsal horn neurons during development of acute arthritis in rat's knee joint. *Journal of Neurophysiology*, **73**(4), 1574–1583.

Qian, J., Brown, S. D. & Carlton, S. M. (1996) Systemic ketamine attenuates nociceptive behaviors in a rat model of peripheral neuropathy. *Brain Research*, **715**(1–2), 51–62.

Radanov, B. P., Frost, S. A., Schwarz, H. A. & Augustiny, K. F. (1996) Experience of pain in rheumatoid arthritis—an empirical evaluation of the contribution of developmental psychosocial stress. *Acta Psychiatrica Scandinavica*, **93**(6), 482–488.

Raja, S. N. (1995) Role of the sympathetic nervous system in acute pain and inflammation. *Annals of Medicine*, **27**(2), 241–246.

Rang, H. P., Bevan, S. & Dray, A. (1991) Chemical activation of nociceptive peripheral neurones. *British Medical Bulletin*, **47**(3), 534–548.

Rang, H. P., Bevan, S. & Dray, A. (1994) Nociceptive peripheral neurons: cellular properties. In *Textbook of Pain*, edited by P. D. Wall & R. Melzack, 3rd edn., pp. 57–78. Edinburgh: Churchill Livingstone.

Ren, K. (1994) Wind-up and the NMDA receptor: from animal studies to humans. *Pain*, **59**(2), 157–158.

Reynolds, J. L. (1997) Post-traumatic stress disorder after childbirth: the phenomenon of traumatic birth. *Canadian Medical Association Journal*, **156**(6), 831–835.

Roberts, W. J. (1986) A hypothesis on the physiological basis for causalgia and related pains. *Pain*, **24**(3), 297–311.

Rowbotham, M. C. (1995) Chronic pain: from theory to practical management. *Neurology*, **45**(12 Suppl. 9), S5–10; discussion S35–36.

Rubinstein, M., Mogil, J. S., Japon, M., Chan, E. C., Allen, R. G. & Low, M. J. (1996) Absence of opioid stress-induced analgesia in mice lacking beta-endorphin by site-directed mutagenesis. *Proceedings of the National Academy of Sciences of the United States of America*, **93**(9), 3995–4000.

Schafer, M., Mousa, S. A., Zhang, Q., Carter, L. & Stein, C. (1996) Expression of corticotropin-releasing factor in inflamed tissue is required for intrinsic peripheral opioid analgesia. *Proceedings of the National Academy of Sciences of the United States of America*, **93**(12), 6096–6100.

Schaible, H. G. & Grubb, B. D. (1993) Afferent and spinal mechanisms of joint pain. *Pain*, **55**(1), 5–54.

Schreiber, S. & Galai-Gat, T. (1993) Uncontrolled pain following physical injury as the core-trauma in post-traumatic stress disorder. *Pain*, **54**(1), 107–110.

Shortland, P. & Woolf, C. J. (1993) Chronic peripheral nerve section results in a rearrangement of the central axonal arborizations of axotomized A beta primary afferent neurons in the rat spinal cord. *Journal of Comparative Neurology*, **330**(1), 65–82.

Sternbach, R. A. (1986) Pain and 'hassles' in the United States: findings of the Nuprin pain report. *Pain*, **27**(1), 69–80.

Sutherland, S. M. & Davidson, J. R. (1994) Pharmacotherapy for post-traumatic stress disorder. *Psychiatric Clinics of North America*, **17**(2), 409–423.

Tierney, G., Carmody, J. & Jamieson, D. (1991) Stress analgesia: the opioid analgesia of long swims suppresses the non-opioid analgesia induced by short swims in mice. *Pain*, **46**(1), 89–95.

Tracey, D. J., Cunningham, J. E. & Romm, M. A. (1995) Peripheral hyperalgesia in experimental neuropathy: mediation by alpha 2-adrenoreceptors on post-ganglionic sympathetic terminals. *Pain*, **60**(3), 317–327.

Tracey, D. J., De Biasi, S., Phend, K. & Rustioni, A. (1991) Aspartate-like immunoreactivity in primary afferent neurons. *Neuroscience*, **40**(3), 673–686.

Urban, L., Thompson, S. W., Fox, A. J., Jeftinija, S. & Dray, A. (1995) Peptidergic afferents: physiological aspects. *Progress in Brain Research*, **104**, 255–269.

Verdugo, R. J. & Ochoa, J. L. (1994) 'Sympathetically maintained pain.' I. Phentolamine block questions the concept. *Neurology*, **44**(6), 1003–1010.

Vidal, C. & Jacob, J. (1986) Hyperalgesia induced by emotional stress in the rat: an experimental animal model of human anxiogenic hyperalgesia. *Annals of the New York Academy of Sciences*, **467**, 73–81.

Volicer, B. J. (1978) Hospital stress and patient reports of pain and physical status. *Journal of Human Stress*, **4**(2), 28–37.

Weisenberg, M. (1977) Pain and pain control. *Psychological Bulletin*, **84**, 1008–1044.

Willer, J. C., Dehen, H. & Cambier, J. (1981) Stress-induced analgesia in humans: endogenous opioids and naloxone-reversible depression of pain reflexes. *Science*, **212**(4495), 689–691.

Xiao, W. H. & Bennett, G. J. (1995) Synthetic omega-conopeptides applied to the site of nerve injury suppress neuropathic pains in rats. *Journal of Pharmacology and Experimental Therapeutics*, **274**(2), 666–672.

Xie, Y. K. & Xiao, W. H. (1993) Inhibitory effect of anisodamine on the neuropathic hyperalgesia following peripheral nerve injury .2. *Science in China Series B—Chemistry Life Sciences and Earth Sciences*, **36**(7), 824–834.

Yamashiro, K., Mukawa, J., Terada, Y., Tomiyama, N., Ishida, A., Mori, K., Tasker, R. R. & Albe-Fessard, D. (1994) Neurons with high-frequency discharge in the central nervous system in chronic pain. *Stereotactic and Functional Neurosurgery*, **62**(1–4), 290–294.

Chapter 6

STRESS, SENESCENCE AND LONGEVITY: How Are They Connected?

Paul J. Rosch, MD

Stress, aging, and death are inescapable, inevitable consequences of life on earth. It should not be surprising, therefore, to find that they are often interrelated and interwoven into a fabric with intriguing motifs and patterns. Longevity, biological aging, and senescence frequently follow some sort of sequential pattern that suggests a cause-effect relationship. As Shakespeare noted, the end stage is 'mere oblivion, sans teeth, sans eyes, sans taste, sans everything'. On the other hand, not everyone suffers this inevitable fate. Some individuals well into their eighties and even nineties continue to be almost as physically active, mentally alert, and spry as they were a decade or two earlier. Others may have all their mental faculties, but their bodies show the ravages of time, or conversely, they may be physically fit, but mentally senile.

What determines the considerable variation that is seen in different individuals? Longevity and hardiness do seem to run in certain families, and it seems obvious that there are certain heritable factors over which we have little control. However, there are also modulating environmental and lifestyle influences. Smoking can hasten the development of certain characteristics of biologic aging, but regular aerobic exercise can retard others. Similarly, since there is good evidence that stress can accelerate the aging process, it would seem plausible that stress reduction strategies might have a reverse effect. However, proving such a hypothesis is hazardous, since both biologic aging and stress are so difficult to define.

WHAT IS BIOLOGIC AGING?

There are numerous physical and physiologic changes associated with biologic aging, as noted in Table 6.1. Mental and emotional alterations that also increase after we become senior citizens are listed in Table 6.2.

Table 6.1   Physical and physiologic changes associated with biologic aging

- Increased atherosclerosis
- Decreased cardiac output and blood flow
- Increased blood pressure
- Decreased kidney, liver and pulmonary function
- Decreased elasticity of blood vessels
- Loss of muscle mass and strength
- Increased osteoporosis
- Increased osteoarthritis
- Diminished hearing, especially for higher frequencies
- Diminished sense of taste and smell
- Cataracts, macular degeneration, arcus senilis
- Slower reaction time
- Progressive graying and loss of hair
- Drier, rougher, more wrinkled, and keratotic skin changes
- Declining levels of estrogen, testosterone, melatonin, DHEA
- Impaired immune system responses
- Atrophy or hyperplasia of cells
- Increased intracellular pigments associated with degeneration
- Increased amyloid, calcium, and immune complex deposits

TABLE 6.2   Cognitive and emotional changes associated with biologic aging.

- Progressive inability to remember recent events
- Surprisingly improved memory for things well in the past
- Poorer personal hygiene habits and sanitary standards
- Lack of attention to appearance and cleanliness
- Progressive loss of a sense of independence and control
- Easy fatiguability, lack of pep, energy, or 'get up and go'
- A more conservative attitude about events and people
- Feelings of loss of attractiveness
- Increased feelings of loneliness, and social isolation
- Tendency to paranoia, depression, and emotional instability
- Increased concerns and anxiety about possible future health problems, financial insecurity, and having fewer friends

All of the alterations associated with aging differ for each of us with respect to when or whether they will occur, with no predictable pattern or order of appearance. As indicated, some individuals develop gray hair or cataracts in their twenties or thirties, and yet retain almost all of their teeth well into their seventies and eighties. Certain centenarians remain bright and alert although crippled with the physical infirmities of old age, while senile dementia can strike healthy individuals in superb physical condition in their forties. Some of these benchmarks of aging are inherited, others may be affected more by post natal factors, and in many instances, it is likely that a combination of the two is responsible. In addition, both genetic and environmental factors can have positive or negative influences. Such variable and unknown contributions to the protean manifestations of aging obviously makes it quite difficult to determine the efficacy of any intervention.

WHAT IS STRESS?

Trying to define or measure stress is even more arduous. Hans Selye, who coined the term as it is presently used, originally defined it as 'the non-specific response of the body to any demand for change' (Selye, 1946). This was based on the observation that when experimental animals were subjected to severe but very different physical and emotional challenges, they all showed the same pathologic changes in the stomach, adrenal glands and lymphoid tissues. Exposure to scorching heat could cause a burn and dilatation of blood vessels, while freezing produced frostbite and vasoconstriction. However, both these temperature extremes produced the identical picture of gastric ulcerations, adrenal cortical hypertrophy, and dissolution of the thymus and lymphatic tissues at autopsy. Persistent physical exertion to the point of exhaustion, exposure to bright lights, loud noises, and extended emotional and mental stress also resulted in this same, non-specific pathological picture.

He chose the word 'stress' to describe this phenomenon, which turned out to be an unhappy decision that would haunt him the rest of his life. The term originally came from the Latin *strictus* (tight, narrow) and *stringere* (to draw tight). This became *estrece* (narrowness, oppression) in Old French, and *stresse* (hardship, oppression) in Middle English. From a practical standpoint, stress is generally viewed as a contraction or variant of distress. Unfortunately, Selye was not aware that stress had been used for centuries in physics in an attempt to explain elasticity, the property of a material that allows it to resume its original size and shape after having been compressed or stretched by an external force. As expressed in Hooke's Law (1658), the magnitude of an external force, or stress, produces a proportional amount of deformation or strain. The maximum amount of stress a material could withstand before becoming permanently deformed was referred to as its elastic limit. This ratio of stress to strain, called the modulus of elasticity, is a characteristic property of each material; its value is high for rigid things like steel, and much lower for flexible metals like tin. Selye once complained to me that had his knowledge of English been more precise, he would have gone down in history as the father of the 'strain' concept.

This created considerable confusion when his research had to be translated into foreign languages. There was no suitable word or phrase that could convey what stress meant, since he was really describing strain. In 1946, when he was asked to give an address at the prestigious Collège de

France, the academicians responsible for maintaining the purity of the French language struggled with this problem for several days, and subsequently decided that a new word would have to be created. Apparently, the male chauvinists prevailed, and *le stress* was born, quickly followed by *el stress*, *il stress*, *lo stress*, *der stress* in other European languages, and similar neologisms in Russian, Japanese, Chinese and Arabic. Stress is one of the very few words you will see preserved in English in these latter languages. Twenty-four centuries previously, Hippocrates wrote that disease was not only *pathos* (suffering), but also *ponos* (toil), as the body fought to restore normalcy. While these might have sufficed, the Greeks also settled on stress.

Selye's concept of stress and its relationship to illness quickly spread from the research laboratory to all branches of medicine, and stress ultimately became a 'buzz' word in vernacular speech. However, the term was used interchangeably to describe both physical and emotional challenges, the body's response to such stimuli, as well as the ultimate result of this interaction. Thus, an unreasonable and over demanding boss might give you heartburn or stomach pain, which eventually resulted in an ulcer. For some people, stress was the bad boss, while others used stress to describe either their 'agita' or their ulcer. Because it was clear that most people viewed stress as some unpleasant threat, he had to create a new word, stressor, to refer to this, in order to distinguish between stimulus and response. Even Selye had difficulties, and in helping to prepare the *First Annual Report On Stress* in 1951, I included the comments of one critic, who, using verbatim citations from Selye's own writings, concluded that 'Stress, in addition to being itself, was also the cause of itself, and the result of itself'. Stress is an ambiguous term in colloquial use, since it is still used indiscriminately to refer to noxious stimuli, the response of the body to such challenges, as well as their physical and emotional consequences.

Stress is also difficult to define, because our individual responses can be so markedly different. Some people blush, or experience palpitations and anxiety, while others become pale, depressed, or develop hives. In addition, situations that are terrifyingly distressful for some, can be an enjoyable delight for others, or seemingly produce little emotional response. As can be readily illustrated by observing passengers on a steep roller coaster ride, stress can be one man's meat and another's poison, the spice of life, or the kiss of death. It can be good or bad, acute and severe, or a chronic annoyance. Winning a race or election can be just as stressful as losing, or more so. A passionate kiss and contemplating what might ensue might be stressful, but is hardly the same feeling you have when undergoing extensive root canal reparation. While heart rate and blood pressure reactions to varied stressors may be similar, neuroendocrine responses are likely to be quite different. Acute, life threatening stress elicits 'fight or flight' autonomic nervous system and hormonal reactions that can have profound effects on the cardiovascular system, including sudden death.

However, the insidious and more subtle stress of loneliness and chronic frustration impact more on the immune system, resulting in lowered resistance to infections and malignancies.

As Selye was fond of pointing out, everyone knows what stress is, but in actuality, nobody really knows. He recognized that his original definition was inappropriate and useless, and struggled all his life to come up with something more meaningful. Many others have also tried, and after more than 45 years in the field, I can attest to the fact that trying to define stress to a scientist's satisfaction, is like trying to nail a piece of jelly to a tree. However, in his later years, in attempting to explain the significance of his research to a lay audience, Selye redefined stress as 'the rate of wear and tear on the body' (Selye, 1956, pp.273–274). I find this description particularly pertinent to this presentation since 'the rate of wear and tear on the body' is also a fairly accurate description of biologic aging. To support his premise, Selye cited various anecdotal reports demonstrating that stress could accelerate certain aspects of aging, such as someone's hair turning gray overnight following a severe shock. In addition, he was able to convincingly demonstrate the ability of stress to accelerate various hallmarks of aging in his experimental animals, including graying of the hair, wrinkled skin, premature atherosclerosis, and microscopic evidence of malignant changes and intracellular pigment accumulation which were usually not seen in litter mates until they were much older. Since then, additional supportive experimental and clinical data have accumulated. More importantly, there is evidence that stress reduction strategies may be effective in delaying the appearance and progression of certain manifestations of aging.

PREMATURE AND DELAYED BIOLOGICAL AGING

Some individuals age much faster biologically than they do chronologically. This is vividly illustrated in progeria, or the Hutchinson-Guilford Syndrome, a rare condition characterized by premature senility and dwarfism. Afflicted individuals generally appear normal at birth, but by three years, and occasionally within six months, growth slows down dramatically, and eventually ceases due to early epiphyseal fusion. Various changes associated with advanced age are seen, such as loss of scalp hair and severe arteriosclerosis. Complete baldness is common, the skin becomes taut, dry and scaly, and the face assumes a peculiar birdlike look, because of narrow sunken features that cause the nose to resemble a beak. Bone age is usually advanced, the joints are enlarged, thickened and stiff, and there is muscle and soft tissue wasting, which makes superficial veins appear unusually prominent. Death usually occurs during the second decade due to infection or advanced arteriosclerosis, and coronary occlusion may occur before the age of eight. There is usually severe mental deficiency, not unlike that seen in senile elderly individuals. Although there is no history of a familial occurrence, the reported patients look so similar that they most likely share some common genetic defect.

Other conditions are also characterized by premature aging. Patients with Werner's syndrome have short stature, a peculiar habitus with thin extremities, cataracts, premature graying and loss of hair, a high pitched voice, severe arteriosclerosis and skin atrophy, especially below the knees, which often leads to persistent ulcerations of the feet and ankles. Many develop adult onset diabetes in the first decade and there are other associated endocrine defects. Females tend to have irregular menses, poor breast development, and very early menopause, and testicular atrophy is not uncommon in young males.

Conversely, there are numerous accounts of individuals with amazing longevity coupled with vitality. The Old Testament states that Adam had Seth at the age of 130, and additional children over the next 800 years. His progeny, Kenan, Mahalalel, Jared, Enoch, and Methuselah, had similar fertility and longevity records; Methuselah lived to be 969, had Noah at the age of 182, and lived another 595 years, during which he sired additional children. Noah was allegedly over 500 years old when Shem, Ham and Japheth were born. 'Moses was an hundred and twenty years old when he died: his eye was not dim, nor his natural force abated'. The oldest existing written record of medicine, *The Yellow Emperor's Canon Of Internal Medicine* (circa 2000 B.C.) (Veith, 1972), indicates that in still earlier times, people regularly lived to be over 100, and attributed this to the absence of stress in their lives.

Although such anecdotal reports appear grossly exaggerated and hard to swallow, there is evidence that some individuals have occasionally lived to very advanced ages without significant reduction of physical abilities or mental faculties. Among the 5th and 6th century B.C. Greeks, Isocrates, an Athenian orator, lived to be 98, and the philosopher Heraclitus, as well as the great mathematician, Pythagoras, continued to teach and be productive well past the age of ninety. In 1799, Easton identified some 1,712 individuals who had lived at least 100 years since the onset of the Christian era, including Thomas Parr, who died in 1635 at the age of 152, and was buried in Westminster Abbey. Parr had been brought to London from Shropshire by the Earl of Arundel, to be presented to Charles I because of his remarkable age and vigor. He was subsequently retained as a domestic by the Earl, but died due to the increased stress of city life, and exposure to 'the foul London air', according to Sir William Harvey, who performed his autopsy (cited in Pelletier, 1981, p.1).

The Guinness Book Of World Records has allegedly authenticated the records of individuals from all over the globe who lived to be well over 100, including one who reportedly died at the age of 254. There also appear to be some scattered communities around the world, where an unusual number of inhabitants remain active and well into their nineties and beyond, including:

- The Vilcabamba Indians in the valleys of the Ecuadorian Andes
- The Abkhazians in the Caucasus Mountains of Georgia
- The Tarahumara Indians of the Sierra Madre
- The Hunza of the Karakoram Range of the Himalayas

Most scientists question the authenticity of these claims, and believe that the upper limit of chronological age that can be achieved is less than 130 years. However, there is well documented evidence that elderly people can still be productive and creative in their eighth and ninth decades, including: Titian – 99, Pablo Picasso – 92, Grandma Moses – 101 (started at age 76), Santayana – 88, Bertrand Russel – 91, numerous statesmen (Churchill, De Gaulle), musicians and symphony conductors (Sir Adrian Boult – 104), and entertainers, like George Burns and Bob Hope. Goya entitled a drawing done in his eighties, *'I Am Still Learning'*. A common factor in these and other individuals appears to be that they are engaged in pursuits that provide pride of accomplishment, social support, and doing something enjoyable that benefits others, which Selye referred to as 'altruistic egotism'. All of these attributes have been shown to have powerful stress buffering activities.

THE ROLE OF PSYCHOSOCIAL STRESS IN AGING

While exceptional longevity is quite likely determined largely by genetic factors, the relative absence of certain stigmata of biologic aging in very old individuals may also be related to lifestyle influences. In the very elderly but healthy populations noted above, many are engaged in daily physical activities at high altitudes, which increases their aerobic conditioning and cardiovascular fitness. Dietary factors could also play a role because of an increased intake of yogurt and fibrous fruits and vegetables, that are rich in vitamins, phytosterols, and other antioxidants. The relative absence of stress may also be crucial. As noted previously, *The Yellow Emperor's Canon Of Internal Medicine*, written more than 40 centuries ago, referred to the unusual longevity that was apparently common in earlier times, noting:

> ... I have heard that in early times, the people lived to be over 100 years old. But these days people reach only half that age, and must curtail their activities. Does the world change from generation to generation—or does man become negligent of the laws of nature?

> ... Today, people do not know how to find contentment within. They are not skilled in the control of their spirits. For these reasons, they reach only half of their 100 years, and then they disintegrate (Veith, 1972, p.67).

The relative absence of stress was also considered to be responsible for the unusual longevity seen in certain populations. One of the best documented groups are the Hunza natives in the Kashmir, who were studied intensively by Sir Robert McCarrison during the early part of this century. He had been assigned by the British Army to establish a hospital and health care delivery system in the region. He was astounded by the magnificent physical and mental status of the very elderly, and being a very alert and perceptive physician, searched for some explanation. He traced family records, conducted detailed interviews, performed careful physical examinations, and kept meticulous records for almost a decade. After reviewing all the information he had gathered, McCarrison concluded that the unusual longevity and extraordinarily good health of the Hunzas well into the eighth and ninth decades was due to the absence of the stresses of contemporary civilization, noting:

> ... and they are far removed from the refinements of civilization. Certain of these races are of magnificent physique, preserving until late in life, the character of their youth; they are unusually fertile and long-lived, and endowed with nervous systems of notable stability ... Cancer is unknown (cited in Stefansson, 1960, p.135).

Similar comments were made by Vilhalmur Stefansson concerning the Eskimos on his first expedition to the Arctic Circle, and by Albert Schweitzer about African natives, on his initial visit to the Congo. Both attributed the complete absence of cancer to the absence of stressful Western lifestyles. Both also lived to witness its appearance and steady increase, as these aboriginal, primitive peoples became progressively 'civilized'.

WHAT CAUSES BIOLOGIC AGING?

Numerous factors can influence different aspects of the aging process. However, the preponderance of evidence suggests that almost all the common manifestations of old age, including an increase in atherosclerosis, malignancies, gray hair, cataracts, and wrinkled skin, are caused by the cumulative effects of oxidative stress. In respiration, oxygen attaches to the hemoglobin molecule, and is transported to cells throughout the body, where it is exchanged for their waste products, which are then eliminated in the form of carbon dioxide and water. During this process, hundreds of thousands of molecular and chemical changes take place. Some oxygen molecules are not completely utilized, and are unstable, since they lack one or more electrons in their outer shell, and are known as free radicals. Of these, the (–OH), or hydroxyl radical, which has an unpaired electron in its outer shell, appears to cause the most destruction. Hydroxyl radicals are highly charged and extremely unstable, and must instantly find some way to correct this deficiency. As a result, they race around the body, latching on to and destroying cell membranes, and oxidizing cholesterol,

DNA, and anything else they come in contact with. It has been estimated that each cell in the body is bombarded by free radicals 10,000 times every day. This disrupts and distorts normal functions, resulting in the formation of other free radicals, and precipitating a chain reaction which produces further damage and destruction.

For example, cholesterol is a vital constituent of all cell membranes, and since this large molecule is relatively inert, it has always been difficult for scientists to understand how it could cause atherosclerotic plaque, which has inflammatory characteristics. Most now believe that the real culprit is oxidized cholesterol, caused by free radical activity. Once cholesterol becomes oxidized, it acts as a magnet to attract other cells, which cumulatively form an atherosclerotic plaque that eventually clogs up arteries.

Low density lipoproteins (LDL), which are smaller molecules that can more readily infiltrate tissue, seem to be the worst offenders. Oxidized LDL resulting from free radical bombardment also attracts white cells, which release chemicals that cause proliferation of smooth muscle cells in the arterial wall, causing further vessel constriction. It is generally not appreciated that emotional stress has a far more powerful effect on cholesterol than diet. Increased fat intake has surprisingly little influence on serum cholesterol. In contrast, the stress of an important examination can cause dramatic rises in a few hours. Tax accountants also show a progressive increase as the end of the financial year approaches, despite little dietary changes.

Oxygen free radicals are a regular byproduct of routine metabolic activities. Anything that increases the rate of metabolism, including exercise and eating, increases free radical production. Flies housed in quarters that allowed them only enough room to walk, lived twice as long as those given room to fly. Researchers were able to correlate this increased longevity with a corresponding lower degree of free radical oxidative damage. In another study, flies who were periodically exposed to lower levels of oxygen lived longer than those breathing regular air, because they also suffered less oxygen free radical injury. Honey bees born in the summer live an average of 35 days. Those born in the cooler days of fall and winter expend less energy during daily activities, and can live for 8 months. The more you exercise, the more free radicals you generate.

This seems to fly in the face of conventional advice urging people to exercise more. There is little doubt that moderate regular aerobic exercise confers cardiovascular and other health benefits that can outweigh adverse free radical effects. However, it is widely believed that the more you exercise, the greater the rewards. This 'no pain, no gain' philosophy is erroneous. Several reports have shown that accomplished marathoners have higher mortality rates from heart attacks and malignancies. This is attributed to their regular and excessive production of free radicals. Jim Fixx, George Sheehan, and other popular exercise gurus have died from heart attacks and malignancies at relatively early ages, and Kenneth

Cooper, who coined the term 'aerobics', has warned about this in his latest books.

The grueling Hawaii Ironman Triathlon requires swimming 2.4 miles in the ocean, bicycling for 112 miles, and then running 26.2 miles, all in immediate succession. A recent study of elite athletes competing in this event revealed that more than one in four had elevated blood levels of troponins immediately after the race. These are proteins produced by injured heart cells, and in some instances, concentrations in participants were as high as those seen in acute heart attack patients. None of them had evidence of any heart disease or abnormal troponin concentrations prior to the competition. Most of the cardiovascular benefits associated with jogging three or four miles daily can be achieved by just taking a brisk 20–30 minute walk three times a week. Some authorities believe that the reduction in coronary morbidity and mortality associated with regular jogging and walking may result in part from their ability to lower stress levels and associated catecholamines known to cause myocardial damage.

The more you eat, the greater your rate of metabolism and production of free radicals. Sharply restricting caloric intake significantly prolongs the life of experimental animals. A variety of anti-aging effects have also been shown in humans, as shown in Table 6.3.

There are numerous other factors that can increase free radical production, including exposure to toxic emissions, ultraviolet rays, cigarette smoke, and a high intake of iron and other oxidative metals. Not surprisingly, these are also associated with higher rates of malignancies and heart disease.

ANTIOXIDANTS, STRESS REDUCTION AND AGING

Antioxidants help prevent the devastating damage due to free radicals by supplying electrons that make them stable. Superoxide dismutase and glutathione are among the natural antioxidants normally manufactured in the body. In addition, estrogen, testosterone, DHEA and melatonin also

TABLE 6.3   Anti-aging effect associated with low caloric intake

- Slower connective tissue degeneration
- Slower development of osteoporosis and atherosclerosis
- Delayed loss of fertility
- Decreased loss of brain dopamine receptors
- Less crystalline loss from the lens of the eye
- Diminished decline in immune system function
- Reduction in age related decline in muscle mass and strength
- Reduction in age related increase in serum cholesterol
- A lower incidence of malignancies and infections

have antioxidant properties, and some have been shown to have certain anti-aging effects. Melatonin, which is secreted by the pineal gland during darkness, is the most powerful scavenger for the deadly hydroxyl free radical. Under normal circumstances, these naturally produced substances are able to block free radical damage, but our ability to manufacture them declines sharply as we grow older. Vitamins C, E, and beta carotene are also powerful antioxidants, as are a variety of herbal preparations such as *Panax ginseng* and *Ginkgo biloba*, and numerous nutrients found in fruits, vegetables and fresh dairy products, red wine and green tea.

Most of the support for their use comes from large scale studies showing that populations consuming diets rich in these vitamins have lower rates of heart disease and cancer, and also live longer. Whether these supplements are as effective as the antioxidants found in fibrous fruits, vegetables, yogurt, red wine, and other foods is still not clear. There may be some synergistic effect of the combinations of different antioxidants found in foods. It is also conceivable that taking massive doses of antioxidants may suppress the body's ability to manufacture its own free radical scavengers. In some studies, beta carotene supplements have been linked with an increased incidence of cancer, especially in smokers. Taking large amounts of antioxidants in combination with other supplements, as is often done, can also cause problems. For example, when megadoses of Vitamin C are taken along with the iron found in many multivitamin-mineral preparations, the combination has a deleterious result that promotes oxidation. Taking large amounts of vitamin E appears to reduce the efficacy of other antioxidants.

Thus, although all living cells and tissues become injured and eventually die when deprived of oxygen, an excess of oxygen also damages cells. Under normal conditions, the body maintains equilibrium by producing antioxidants as needed to offset free radical production resulting from exercise, eating, and stress. These antioxidants safeguard and sustain cellular integrity, much like other antioxidants that are used to prevent foods from spoiling, or rubber and other compounds from deteriorating. Similarly, metals are preserved, as long as they are protected from excess exposure to oxygen, which causes them to oxidize or rust. Thus, in a very real sense, we do not wear out, but rather rust out. Strategies to prevent this include finding the appropriate amount of exercise for your age, reducing caloric intake, avoiding environmental pollutants, increasing dietary intake of foods rich in natural antioxidants, and sensible antioxidant supplementation. However, much more attention should be devoted to the role of emotional stress in facilitating free radical damage. Studies show that within 15 minutes after the onset of provoked mental stress, there is a significant rise in free radical production, and oxidized LDL levels. Stress induced increased cortisol secretion causes atrophy of the hippocampus and loss of memory and cognitive skills identical to those seen in aging. Such changes have been demonstrated in patients suffering from posttraumatic stress disorder and depression, both of which may be associated with chronic high cortisol levels. Hippocampal shrinkage is due to free radical damage, and can be prevented or reversed by administering certain antioxidants, especially those found in ginkgolides. It would seem logical that reducing stress also offers the potential for preventing and minimizing such damage. Apoptosis, or programmed cell death, and telomerase activity may also be important factors in the aging process, and stress may possibly influence these genetic traits.

Everyone wants to live long, but nobody wants to grow old. Learning how to reduce stress and minimize its harmful effects may be the best way to achieve this goal. It will not only add years to your life, but also provide a better quality of life to those years, which is even more important.

References

Pelletier, K. R. (1981) in *Longevity: Finding Our Biological Potential,* p. 1. New York: Delacorte Press.

Selye, H. (1946) The general adaptation syndrome and the diseases of adaptation. *Journal of Clinical Endocrinology,* **6**, 117–230.

Selye, H. (1956) *The Stress Of Life,* pp. 273–274. New York: McGraw-Hill.

Stefansson, V. (1960) *Cancer: Disease of Civilization?* p. 135. New York: Hill and Wang

Veith, I., (Trans.) (1972) *Nei Ching: The Yellow Emperor's Canon of Internal Medicine,* p.67. Berkely: University of California Press.

Chapter 7

STRESS AND SEXUAL FUNCTION

Marita P. McCabe, PhD

OVERVIEW

Stress has been associated with a wide range of physical and psychological problems. However, the difficulty with the stress concept is that it may be defined as either a stimulus or a response. For example, attending a job interview may be a stressful event, but the effect of this event, and whether it generates a stress reaction, may depend on a number of moderating factors (Lazarus & Folkman, 1984). The way in which the individual appraises the event, the importance of the event for the person, and the individual's perceived competence to deal with the event are all factors which influence the magnitude of the response. Other chapters within this book will examine various general aspects of the stress reaction. This chapter will be confined to an evaluation of the effect of stress on sexual function.

The nature of the stress reaction in terms of sexual functioning may depend in part on the type of stressor. Stress which results from daily hassles and major life events is likely to have a different impact from social stress which develops from problems in personal relationships. It has been demonstrated that stress from events in everyday life leads to lowered levels of testosterone and elevated blood levels of corticoids (Herbert, 1996). Other results suggest that socially dominant men have higher levels of testosterone (Zumoff et al., 1984). However, these results do not directly inform us on the association between stress and sexual function. Although there has been much theorising about this relationship, as yet there has been no adequate exploration of the direct effects of either general stress or social stress on sexual behaviour in human males. There is an even greater dearth of information on the effect of stress on sexual function in human females. This poor state of understanding stems partly from the lack of knowledge about the physiological changes associated with stress which influence sexual functioning. The available literature on the effect of stress on the sexual function of men and women is discussed below.

EFFECTS OF STRESS ON THE SEXUAL RESPONSE OF MEN

Studies with primates indicate that the subordinate males in a group of monkeys show lower levels of testosterone than higher ranking males, and also lower levels of sexual activity with female monkeys (Yodyengyuad, Eberhart & Keverne, 1982). There seem to be strong interrelationships between levels of testosterone, social stress and sexual activity. Stress is associated with lowered levels of testosterone, which is associated with less social dominance and, in turn, lower levels of sexual activity. It is difficult to ascertain the direction of these influences: does stress lead to lower social position, which lowers sexual activity, or does lower social position increase stress, as well as decreasing sexual activity?

The situation with human males is even less clearly defined. Much of the literature which has investigated the effect of testosterone on sexual behaviour is compromised by the interchangeable use of such terms as sexual desire, sexual behaviour and sexual capacity. Although the study was not directly evaluating the relationship between stress and sexual behaviour, Schiari, White, Mandeli and Levine (1997) found that testosterone injections administered to males with erectile dysfunction led to an increase in the frequency of ejaculation among respondents. However, there was no change in the level of sexual desire, masturbation, frequency of sex with partner, erections or sexual satisfaction. These findings highlight the importance of clearly specifying the nature of the sexual responses that are being explored, and the initial sexual functioning of the participants in the study; sexually functional males administered additional testosterone may respond quite differently from sexually dysfunctional males. There may be a critical level of testosterone below which a man may experience problems in sexual functioning. However, there is evidence to suggest that this critical level may vary from one individual to another. Further, sexually dysfunctional males may also experience psychological factors which impede sexual function, even when their testosterone is restored to normal levels.

Physical stress in men, such as when in battle or after strenuous exercise, is known to lower levels of testosterone. Given the intense levels of stress inherent in major life events, one could predict that these would also lead to lowered levels of testosterone. But the effect of daily hassles, where there is constant low level stress, has not been explored.

Although there is anecdotal evidence that social stress may have a detrimental effect on sexual function in human males, the evidence is far from clear, and the pathway is unlikely to be as direct as that for monkeys. Social stress may stem from an evaluation by the male that he does not possess the attributes which make him attractive to females. This stress may have a physiological effect, as for monkeys, of lowering levels of free testosterone, or it may lead to a psychological response of feelings of inadequacy, which leads, in turn, to a decrement in sexual functioning quite independent of testosterone levels.

There is some evidence that social support has a moderating effect on the relationship between stress and sexual functioning. Social support may be provided by a partner, family, friend or co-worker. Within the context of a sexual relationship, it is likely that it would be provided by the person's partner. Morokoff and Gillilland (1993) found that the stress associated with unemployment among males in a relationship led to erectile difficulties. Unemployed men were more likely to experience erectile problems, after allowing for age and health problems. This finding was apparent for both self reported erectile capacity and, as indicated by an earlier study (Morokoff, Baum, McKinnon & Gillilland, 1987), physiological responses of the unemployed men to an erotic videotape. The sexual response of unemployed men after an acute stressor was more likely to be impaired when they viewed an erotic videotape than was the case for employed men. Although there was no assessment of levels of testosterone, these results demonstrate that the stress associated with unemployment led to an increase in erectile problems. It is unclear whether levels of sexual desire or other aspects of sexual functioning and behaviour were also reduced.

An interesting finding by Morokoff and Gillilland (1993) was that the stress associated with unemployment was mediated by the social support provided by their partner. For men who were unemployed, there was a strong relationship between the marital satisfaction of the wife and the sexual functioning of the male. Unemployed men in a poor quality relationship (as defined by the wife) were more likely to experience greater erectile difficulties. Similar relationships between erectile functioning and marital satisfaction were not found for employed men. A possible explanation for these findings is that wives who were involved in a satisfying marital relationship provided support for their husbands when they were unemployed. This support reduced the level of stress experienced by the unemployed men, which led, in turn, to less impairment in their sexual functioning. It is interesting to note that the level of marital satisfaction experienced by the unemployed men themselves was not associated with their sexual functioning. It appears to be the support provided by wives which mediates the impact of stress, rather than there being a relationship between male marital satisfaction, stress and sexual functioning.

Morokoff and Gillilland (1993) also found that there was a positive relationship between the experience of hassles and levels of sexual desire among both men and women. This surprising finding may be interpreted in one of two ways: the experience of minor hassles may lead both males and females to seek an escape from these events through seeking higher levels of sexual activity. Alternatively, the heightened arousal caused by the stress from the daily hassles may be interpreted as sexual desire, and so there are reported increased levels of sexual desire under conditions where arousal levels are somewhat elevated. This study demonstrates the complexity of the relationship between stress and sexual function. A major life event (unemployment) negatively influenced erectile capacity (but not desire) whereas elevated levels of daily hassles increased sexual desire but not sexual behaviour. It would appear that the respondents in this study were initially sexually functional, and so these same findings may not apply to sexually dysfunctional respondents in the same situation.

As discussed in the later section on the role of anxiety on sexual function, the association between heightened physiological arousal due to stress, levels of sexual desire and sexual arousal is not clear- cut. In addition to the nature of the stressful event, these relationships appear to be influenced by gender, level of sexual functioning and whether a subjective or physiological assessment is made of sexual response.

EFFECTS OF STRESS ON THE SEXUAL RESPONSE OF WOMEN

There has been a dearth of either empirical studies or theoretical formulations on the association between sexual function and stress among women. Herbert (1996) suggested that similar mechanisms operate among women as for men. However, among female monkeys dominance hierarchies are less easy to observe than for males, and the characteristics that define a dominant female are less easy to identify. It is, therefore, more difficult to pinpoint sources of social stress. Among primates it appears that reproduction is extremely sensitive to social stress, with females not ovulating until they leave the family group, although they are physically mature in other ways (Abbott & Hearn, 1978). Once having left the family group, the factors which lead to social stress are less clear. However, it is apparent that the less dominant females, who may be seen to be more stressed due to their social position, respond in different ways from their more dominant counterparts. Bowman, Dilley and Keverne (1978) found that these subordinate females remained insensitive to hormonal changes that would normally induce ovulation. This situation favoured the more dominant females in terms of both sexual activity and reproductive success. This led to an enhanced social position for these dominant females, with a corresponding reduction in social stress. These results show a clear negative relationship between social stress and sexual function among female monkeys, but the effect on sexual function of more general forms of stress has not been explored.

There have been few studies which have investigated the relationship between either physical stress or social stress and sexual function among human females, and the results are not as clear as they are for males. Morokoff and Gillilland (1993) found no relationship between unemployment and sexual dysfunction among women (although their only measure of sexual dysfunction was orgasmic frequency). However, this sample of women was largely comprised of women who were unemployed by choice, and so unemployment may not be accompanied by the high levels of stress that would be experienced by single-parent mothers who are financially dependent upon employment for the economic welfare of both themselves and their children. This study also did not evaluate the role of other life stressors in women's sexual functioning: unemployment is simply one of a myriad of stress factors which may impact on how women view their lives and on their sexual functioning. More importantly, neither this study nor any other studies have examined the role of social stress on the sexual functioning of women. Interpersonal relationships, and the quality of these relationships, play a central role in the lives of women, and problems in these relationships would be expected to have a significant effect on stress levels. This is an important aspect of factors influencing sexual functioning in women which requires further attention.

Clearly, more research needs to be conducted which explores the relationship between various aspects of stress and sexual function in men and women. In the absence of such studies, the literature on the association between anxiety and sexual functioning will be reviewed below. Since anxiety is frequently an aspect of the stress reaction, these data will provide some insight into the nature of the relationship between stress and sexual dysfunction, and the way in which males and females may differ in their response to stress.

Tentative conclusions about the association between stress and sexual function can be drawn from the literature regarding relationships between anxiety and sexual function. These findings reveal a very complex picture, which demonstrates that gender, level of sexual functioning, type of anxiety and measure of sexual responding all influence the conclusions that are drawn.

ROLE OF ANXIETY ON SEXUAL FUNCTION

The interrelationship between anxiety and sexual arousal involves a complex interplay among a range of variables. These variables include gender, whether or not the person currently experiences a sexual dysfunction (that is, difficulties with sexual desire, erection or ejaculation for males, and difficulties with sexual desire, arousal or orgasm for females), the nature of the anxiety experienced by the individual, and whether subjective or physiological indices of sexual arousal are assessed. The influence of each of these factors on sexual response within an anxiety provoking situation will be discussed below.

Historically, anxiety has been viewed as a major factor contributing to low sexual arousal and the development of sexual dysfunction in both men and women. Masters and Johnson (1970) cited anxiety as one of the strongest contributors to sexual dysfunction due to its effect on inhibiting sexual response and distracting the individual from attending to sexual stimuli. Likewise Kaplan (1974, 1988) has consistently claimed that anxiety impedes physiological response, which in turn lowers the subjective appraisal of sexual arousal. However, the data on which these conclusions are drawn are somewhat limited, and the subject populations are largely sexually dysfunctional respondents. It is therefore necessary to examine the literature more broadly to assess whether these claims stand the test of empirical validation, and whether anxiety impedes the sexual functioning of sexually functional as well as sexually dysfunctional respondents.

Role of Anxiety in Men

Anxiety may stem from a number of different sources within the sexual situation. An individual may experience anxiety simply as a result of being in a sexual situation, with the accompanying expectation that sexual interaction is likely to occur. The sexual anxiety which is generated in this situation is frequently accompanied by other negative emotions, for example, guilt, fear, anger and disgust. The source of the anxiety response comes from the difficulty the individual experiences with being involved in sexual activities. There have been few studies that have explored the influence of sexual anxiety on sexual arousal, although Bozman and Beck (1991) demonstrated that there were decreased levels of sexual desire and decreased levels of penile tumescence among sexually functional males when they were in a situation which evoked anger. Although these results demonstrated reduced physiological response when the respondents were angry, there was no measure of subjective levels of sexual arousal recorded. Kaplan (1979) has claimed that sexual anxiety lowers sexual arousal among both males and females, but no data were presented to support this claim. From the data that are available it is difficult to ascertain whether males respond differently from females to sexual anxiety, and whether there is a different response between functional and dysfunctional respondents. However, the limited data that are available suggest that sexual anxiety has a negative effect on sexual functioning.

The second type of anxiety which may influence sexual responding is performance anxiety. This type of anxiety occurs when an individual experiences a demand to perform in a sexual situation. Bozman and Beck (1991) demonstrated that performance anxiety resulted in decreased levels of desire among sexually functional males in relation to a control condition where there was no anxiety, but there were no differences between the control condition and the performance anxiety condition in the level of tumescence. On the other hand, Hale and Strassberg (1990) found that physiological responding of functional males to erotica was significantly impaired when they were pre-exposed (as opposed to the concurrent exposure condition adopted by Bozman and Beck) to a situation which elicited performance concerns. In contrast, Barlow, Sakheim and Beck (1983) found that pre-exposure to instructions elicited to increase performance concerns led to enhanced sexual arousal among sexually functional males using physiological measures.

These findings indicate substantially different findings in relation to the effect of performance anxiety on erectile response for functional males. These differences would seem to be due to the timing of the performance anxiety, the nature of the performance anxiety, and the age of the respondents. College students seem to have their sexual performance enhanced under performance demands, whereas older respondents seem to experience a less positive response to these demands.

The impact of performance anxiety on subjective levels of arousal is also not clear. Most of the data that have been gathered on performance anxiety and sexual functioning have focussed on physiological erectile response. Respondents have not been asked about their subjective levels of arousal, and so it is not possible to determine whether or not increased performance demands enhance or detract from subjective feelings of sexual arousal. It is interesting to note that within all of this discussion of sexual function among males, sexual response is defined in terms of erectile response: levels of interest in sex or ejaculatory response are not evaluated in terms of subjective or objective measurement.

Studies indicate that sexually dysfunctional males respond negatively to all performance demands in terms of their physiological erectile response (Beck, Barlow, & Sakheim, 1983; Heiman & Rowland, 1983), but subjective experiences of sexual response have not been assessed.

Similar results to the above have been found for general anxiety, which is the most common type of anxiety. This type of anxiety stems from difficulties in coping with stressors from general life events and daily hassles. When sexually functional men are in a situation of heightened arousal due to a general anxiety provoking situation, their sexual functioning at a physiological level is enhanced, whereas the sexual functioning of dysfunctional males is impeded (Barlow et al., 1983; Beck et al., 1983). As Barlow (1986) concluded, 'anxiety seems to affect functional and dysfunctional in very different ways' (p. 142).

In summary, it would appear that sexually functional and dysfunctional men respond differently to anxiety within a sexual context. Whereas sexually functional men seem to experience the heightened state of arousal that stems from anxiety as facilitating to their sexual response, dysfunctional men find that this experience of heightened arousal impedes their sexual response. Sexually functional men experience a positive emotional response in a sexual situation, whereas dysfunctional men experience negative emotions. Sexually functional men would seem to cognitively label their heightened state of arousal as a heightened sexual response when they are in a sexual situation. This labelling both facilitates their physiological sexual response and stems from their observation of their heightened physiological response. On the other hand, sexually dysfunctional men seem to experience negative emotions alongside their anxiety response, and so label their heightened levels of arousal in a negative manner when they occur in a sexual context. This cognitive reaction impedes subjective feelings of arousal, which in turn, impedes physiological arousal. At the same time, diminished physiological arousal also leads to lowered subjective feelings of sexual arousal.

Since there is a clear indicator of levels of physiological sexual arousal among men, the concordance between subjective and objective measures of arousal is very high. Among functional males, there is a feedback process whereby both subjective and physiological parameters enhance one another, the reverse process occurs among dysfunctional males.

Role of Anxiety in Women

There have been even fewer studies conducted on the effects of anxiety on the sexual functioning of women than there have been with men. The results also do not concord with the results that have been found for men. Wincze, Hoon and Hoon (1976) found that sexually functional women were more physiologically responsive than dysfunctional women when exposed to a situation which evoked high levels of general anxiety. However, there was no difference in the subjective response of the two groups of women, with all respondents indicating a decrement in their sexual response. These results will be interpreted below within a social learning model of sexual response.

In contrast to these findings, Morokoff and Heiman (1980) found that in an anxiety provoking situation functional and dysfunctional women experienced similar physiological responses but reported different subjective responses, with functional women reporting higher levels of sexual arousal. These results would suggest that anxiety leads to heightened levels of physiological arousal, including sexual arousal in all women. However, sexually functional women attend more closely to their physiological response and label their heightened state of arousal as sexual arousal and so report heightened subjective sexual arousal. In contrast, sexually dysfunctional women may fail to detect their heightened state of physiological sexual arousal and also label their arousal state as a negative emotional condition. As a result anxiety leads to a decrease in their subjective report of sexual arousal. Similar results to those of Morokoff and Heiman (1980) were also obtained by Hoon, Wincze and Hoon (1977) among sexually functional women.

In contrast to the above findings, Palace and Gorzalka (1990) found that general anxiety pre-exposure enhanced genital responding for both sexually functional and dysfunctional women, although the magnitude of this response was greater for sexually functional women. Surprisingly, both sexually functional and dysfunctional women reported lower levels of subjective sexual arousal following an anxiety provoking event. These results would seem to suggest that both sexually functional and dysfunctional women physiologically respond to anxiety in a similar manner (although dysfunctional women showed less response); a heightened state of general physiological arousal leads to increased vasocongestion, independent of whether or not the woman experiences a dysfunction. However, all women reported a subjective decrease in sexual arousal in the anxiety situation. These findings demonstrate less concordance between physiological sexual response and subjective response among women than among men; penile tumescence is more readily observed than vaginal vasocongestion, and so men have more apparent cues of their sexual arousal than women.

An interesting finding from this study was that both groups of women indicated that they experienced lowered levels of sexual arousal in the anxiety situation. These results contrast with those with men, where functional men experienced heightened sexual arousal in an anxiety provoking situation and dysfunctional men experienced diminished arousal. A social learning perspective can be used to explain these findings. Women, regardless of whether they are sexually functional or dysfunctional, are subject to social dictates that indicate the unacceptability of too strong a sexual response in women. In a situation which generates anxiety, the subjective response of lowered sexual arousal is likely to be evoked. In contrast, men experience societal endorsement of a strong and immediate sexual response, no matter what the situation. In situations which evoke anxiety, functional men are likely to label their increased arousal as sexual arousal, whereas dysfunctional males, who may be concerned about their sexual abilities, are likely to experience negative emotions which detract from their subjective experience of sexual arousal.

EVALUATION AND INTERVENTION

The literature reviewed in this chapter indicates that stress and anxiety influence the sexual function of men and women. The nature of this relationship varies for males and females, and is different for sexually functional and dysfunctional respondents.

Stress and anxiety enhance the physiological and subjective sexual response of functional males. Heightened general physiological arousal due to stress or anxiety leads to heightened sexual physiological arousal. This heightened general and sexual arousal is associated with a subjective sense of increased sexual arousal. These findings demonstrate that there is a strong positive interaction between stress/anxiety, physiological sexual response, and the cognitive labelling of the heightened sense of arousal.

This same process operates among sexually dysfunctional males. However, rather than the heightened state of general arousal being interpreted in a positive manner, it is associated with negative emotions (for example, anger, guilt, disgust) which diminish physiological sexual arousal and detract from the subjective experience of sexual arousal.

In order to enhance sexual functioning among dysfunctional males, it is important to lower stress/anxiety so that these associations do not occur. Once the male experiences confidence in his sexual performance, sexual response will also be improved by these males reinterpreting their response to stress/anxiety. The positive cognitive labelling that then occurs will facilitate a positive physiological response. In the treatment of sexually dysfunctional males, it is therefore important to alter the way in which stress/anxiety is perceived, as well as lowering the levels of stress/anxiety in the lives of these people.

Sexually functional and dysfunctional women appear to respond in a similar manner to stress/anxiety, although the results from studies are far from consistent and certainly not very convincing. Although women seem to respond positively at a physiological level to the heightened arousal stemming from stress/anxiety, their subjective sexual response to stress/anxiety is generally negative. An interpretation of these results is that women experience ambivalent feelings about their sexual responding. In a stressful or anxiety provoking situation, the negative aspects of these feelings are enhanced, which leads women to experience negative emotions in association with their heightened levels of arousal, and so lowered subjective sexual arousal.

It is important that women learn to feel comfortable with themselves as sexual beings, so that these feelings of ambivalence about their sexual response can be resolved. In this way, stress/anxiety is likely to facilitate rather than impede their sexual feelings and arousal.

This discussion demonstrates the complexity of the relationship between stress/anxiety and sexual function. It also highlights the number of areas in which there is a dearth of data and where further studies are necessary to understand more fully these interrelationships. The conclusions drawn in this chapter are often speculative, based on the data that are available. However, further research will allow these speculations to be tested and conclusions which are based on more substantive data to be drawn.

References

Abbott, D. H. & Hearn, J. P. (1978) Physical, hormonal and behavioural aspects of sexual development in the marmoset monkey. *Journal of Reproductive Fertility*, **53**, 155–164.

Barlow, D. H. (1986) Causes of sexual dysfunction: The role of anxiety and cognitive interference. *Journal of Consulting and Clinical Psychology*, **54**, 140–148.

Barlow, D. H., Sakheim, D. K. & Beck, J. G. (1983) Anxiety increases sexual arousal. *Journal of Abnormal Psychology*, **92**, 49–54.

Beck, J. G., Barlow, D. H. & Sakheim, D. K. (1983) The effect of attentional focus and partner arousal on sexual responding in functional and dysfunctional men. *Behaviour Research and Therapy*, **21**, 1–8.

Bowman, L. A., Dilley, S. R. & Keverne, E. B. (1978). Suppression of oestrogen-induced LH surges by social subordination in female talapoin monkeys. *Nature*, **275**, 56–58.

Bozman, A. W. & Beck, J. G. (1991) Covariation of sexual desire and sexual arousal: The effects of anger and anxiety. *Archives of Sexual Behavior*, **20**, 47–60.

Hale, V. E. & Strassberg, D. S. (1990) The role of anxiety on sexual arousal. *Archives of Sexual Behavior*, **19**, 569–581.

Heiman, J. R. & Rowland, D. L. (1983) Affective and physiological sexual response patterns: The effect of instructions on sexually functional and dysfunctional men. *Journal of Psychosomatic Research*, **27**, 105–116.

Herbert, J. (1996) Sexuality, stress and the chemical architecture of the brain. *Annual Review of Sex Research*, **7**, 1–43.

Hoon, P. W., Wincze, J. P. & Hoon, E. F. (1977) A test of reciprocal inhibition: Are anxiety and sexual arousal in women mutually inhibitory? *Journal of Abnormal Psychology*, **86**, 65–74.

Kaplan, H. S. (1974) *The New Sex Therapy*. New York: Bruner/Mazel.

Kaplan, H. S. (1979) *Disorders of Sexual Desire*. New York: Bruner/Mazel.

Kaplan, H. S. (1988) Anxiety and sexual dysfunction. *Journal of Clinical Psychiatry*, **49**(Suppl. 10), 21–25.

Lazarus, R. S. & Folkman, S. (1984) *Stress, Appraisal and Coping*. New York: Springer.

Masters, W. H. & Johnson, V. E. (1970) *Human Sexual Inadequacy*. Boston: Little, Brown.

Morokoff, P. J., Baum, A., McKinnon, W. R. & Gillilland, R. (1987) Effects of chronic unemployment and acute psychological stress on sexual arousal in men. *Health Psychology*, **6**, 545–560.

Morokoff, P. J. & Gillilland, R. (1993) Stress, sexual functioning, and marital satisfaction. *The Journal of Sex Research*, **30**, 43–53.

Morokoff, P. J. & Heiman, J. R. (1980) Effects of erotic stimuli on sexually functional and dysfunctional women: Multiple measures before and after sex therapy. *Behaviour Research and Therapy*, **18**, 127–137.

Palace, E. M. & Gorzalka, B. B (1990) The enhancing effects of anxiety on arousal in sexually dysfunctional and functional women. *Journal of Abnormal Psychology*, **99**, 403–411.

Schiari, R. L., White, D., Mandeli, J. & Levine, A. C. (1997) Effect of testosterone administration on sexual behavior and mood in men with erectile dysfunction. *Archives of Sexual Behavior*, **26**, 231–241.

Wincze, J. P., Hoon, E. F. & Hoon, P. W. (1976) Physiological responsivity of normal and sexually dysfunction women during erotic stimulus exposure. *Journal of Psychosomatic Research*, **20**, 445–451.

Yodyengyuad, U., Eberhart, J. A. & Keverne, E. B. (1982) Effects of rank and novel females on behavior and hormones in male talapoin monkeys. *Physiology and Behavior*, **28**, 995–1005.

Zumoff, B., Rosenfeld, R. S., Friedman, M., Byers, S. O., Rosenman, R. H. & Hillman, I. (1984) Elevated daytime urinary excretion of testosterone glucuronide in men with type A behavior pattern. *Psychological Medicine*, **46**, 223–225.

Chapter 8

WHY *MIGHT* STRESS MANAGEMENT METHODS BE EFFECTIVE?

F. Joseph McGuigan, PhD

OVERVIEW

I want to first survey a sample of stressful situations that we meet in life in order to assess the nature of some of the problems that professionals in stress management face. Then I will consider the variables professionals employ to instruct others as to how to face stressors. Those variables may be classified as either nonspecific, common to many methods, or specific to a given method. In either case, the question is, how do we institute such variables to attempt to achieve the self-control necessary for coping with stressors? Finally, whatever the method, we must consider how the voluntary muscles are effectively used, as it is with them that we behave as we attempt to cope with the stressful experiences of life.

INTRODUCTION

The word 'might' in the title is emphasized because often the validity of a particular method is assumed *a priori*. Before any stress management method, or any psychological method for that matter, is offered to the public, it should be presented with substantial validating data. Otherwise, a disclaimer to the public should state that 'the method has not been validated'.

However, if a particular method *has* been empirically established as effective, professionals should ask the next question, an analytical one: What are the relevant variables that control the behavior that effectively manages 'stress'? To be concrete about stress management methods, let us first set the problem by considering a sample of stressors that people face in everyday life.

Some Stressful Situations

Consider examples from the workplace. One is the common situation of an overloaded secretary in an office, answering telephones while trying to help executives, keeping computer and other demands on the desk organized and functioning. An executive, similarly overloaded, intermittently talking on the intercom and the telephone as the pile of work on his desk accumulates, and in the middle of all this someone enters and interrupts him, adding to his load. The effect of such work stressors can accumulate to the point of losing control and the victim may 'blow his or her stack'.

Not uncommon experiences are potentially painful such as having a vaccination or visiting a dentist wherein a person overtenses muscles with anticipatory pain, thereby exacerbating the discomfort of a mere needle prick, a tooth filling, etc.

A variety of other stressful situations that are frequently encountered include such as a crowded freeway when people become frustrated, reckless and dangerous in driving; the stress in living in an overcrowded environment; and a home-bound mother facing the day that includes problems with an irate husband, in-laws, being isolated, unruly children, etc.

In addition to such daytime stressors, there are stressors that we experience at night when the body is so active during dreams. The data show that the rate of heart attacks, for instance, is disproportionately high during sleep relative to waking life.

What can we learn from assessing such common stressful experiences?

Rational Versus Reflexive Responding

A preliminary answer is that in each case the individual should first be capable of maintaining tranquil behavior rather than immediate, reflexive responding. That provides the opportunity to rationally decide on an effective course of action. Then, one can behave in a manner that is sufficiently efficient to accomplish the purposes at hand. For instance, in the previous examples, one needs to be able to exert *control* over behavior so as to guide work smoothly, calmly and productively; accept the vaccinating needle or dentist's drill in a relaxed manner; drive safely in traffic with a relaxed, joyful attitude; ignore the pressures of a crowded environment and make the home environment a pleasant, constructive one.

Some Goals for Stress Management Methods

To enlarge on what stress management methods might seek to accomplish, I took a small sample of what graduate students thought should be the goals of stress management procedures. Some responses were: to improve the quality of life by relaxing, to eliminate unwanted racing thoughts, to keep from getting sick, to know your body when it is stressed out, to become less emotional and more relaxed when you are arguing, to reduce fatigue, to increase productivity and efficiency, to manage time efficiently, to set appropriate priorities, and to sleep well.

How do we program such behaviors?

CONTROLLING BEHAVIOR

To accomplish such goals as we have enumerated, two basic control strategies were long ago specified by John Watson: We can either re-engineer the environment to solve a behavioral problem or we can modify the behavior. His advice was to employ the first, if feasible, for it is usually the simplest.

Environmental Control

There are many ways that one can reduce or eliminate stressors and make the environment conducive to effective behavior. One example I recall from Watson was to remove the lamp from the coffee table rather than try to teach the infant to avoid it.

In the workplace, organizational stress management procedures have often focused on changing the environment to provide the worker an increased amount of control. For example, participation in decision making allows workers to improve environmental conditions such as in helping to allocate work assignments, to get some control over the pace of work, to provide rest breaks, and so forth. Other successful workplace efforts have been to reduce role stress through goal setting, increase job and work schedule autonomy, reduce conditions conducive to burn out, reduce factors causing work/family conflict, improve working conditions through job design, disseminate information, foster educational conditions, and so on. There are many reports that such organizational interventions into the work environment are indeed successful. There are successful interventions into other environments that can help us in stress management, such as when one reorganizes a personal schedule to prevent overloading.

While such environmental variables can be effective, behavioral issues constitute our primary problem—they are, as previously developed, how to consistently, effectively control ourselves when we meet stressors.

Behavioral Control

We are all aware of the numerous methods that are offered to the public for this purpose. Many are given in the outstanding book by Lehrer and Woolfolk (1993), covering about every stress management method of which I am aware. But *precisely* how do these methods help one to deal with such stressors as we have illustrated?

To elaborate, when confronting stressors, the immediate goal is to momentarily exert self-control to relax so as to act rationally, rather than reflexively (unless, of course, the stressor is an oncoming truck in your path). One can thus assess the situation thoughtfully, consider alternative modes of responding and select among them so as to effectively deal with the problem. A basic question is how do stress management methods teach one to so control oneself in the face of the stressors of life? Furthermore, what is the behavior that might transfer from the learning situation to when one copes with an actual stressor? A sample of the rationale that some methods have asserted accomplish such purposes is as follows. In one, the learner is instructed in arousal reduction techniques so as to build resistance to stressors: mentioned were relaxation, biofeedback, meditation, and breathing management. In another, one is instructed on how to modify ineffective 'coping techniques'. One method advocated 'cognitive restructuring' so that *perceptions* of work and personal stressors are changed—one learns how to more generally perceive life to be less stressful. Munz and Kohler (1997) have shown that past participators in stress management programs and volunteers in new ones are similarly aware of the work stressors that they face. However, the experienced workers perceive a lessor amount of stress. Thus, such stress management programs help lessen the psychological and physical strain of daily living, but their purpose is not to reduce the stressors that one encounters at work—past participants simply do not allow the stressors to bother them so much. Some studies have found that the nature of one's personality may affect how one reacts to stressors (e.g., Bolger and Zuckerman, 1995). Thus, stress management programs might be effective in part because constitution, ability, etc., influence the behavior of the learner.

Non-specific and Specific Variables for Control

In considering how various stress management approaches might be effective, we shall consider two general classes of variables for controlling behavior. Non-specific variables are those that are common to a number of methods, while specific variables are unique to a given method.

Non-specific Variables
One non-specific variable that some use to control behavior for stress management is *suggestion* that the given method really works as in the famous placebo effect. For instance, one is told that their hands are getting very warm, as in autogenic training; that we should use the power of positive thinking; or I am reminded of the famous French psychiatrist Coué who told us that the way to improve our condition was to repeatedly say that 'every day and in every way I get better and better'. We don't hear much about Coué these days and can question the effectiveness of his suggestion method.

While we are considering suggestion, psychologically we know that it does affect behavior. What is next of importance is how does it influence one? Physiologically and psychophysiologically, what is happening within us when suggestion causes changes in behavior? How stable are the behaviors and internal events generated by suggestion? These questions remain a major mystery that we should continue to investigate—a start has been made for the use of suggestion and hypnosis. The scientific strategy was to physiologically or to psychophysiologically explicate the phenomenon. Some model research has studied alpha and beta brain waves and p300 amplitudes of evoked potentials. Through electromyographic study, changes in the neuromuscular system often result from a specific state of suggestive hypnosis. Sustained psychophysiological research using sound experimental methodology could eventually lead to an understanding of what does happen within the body as a result of suggestive influences.

Suggestion is necessarily a non-specific variable, present to some extent in all methods (even if one tries to eliminate it), and most seek to capitalize on it. Just as when ones takes a pill that is inert, one's belief that a prescribed method of stress management will help does produce some positive consequences.

But *should* stress management methods, as well as psychotherapies in general, explicitly rely on suggestion? Or should methods be applied with a minimum of suggestion that a patient or other learner will improve their coping techniques? Edmund Jacobson (1938) pointed out 33 reasons that suggestion should be minimized. One reason was that by relying on suggestion, the body does not reeducate itself habitually for long-term versus only short-term improvement. Another reason is that suggestion may impair learning of muscle relaxation because one might think that the muscles are relaxed when they are not; consequently, the learner does not actually learn precise muscle control skill. Jacobson's goal was to test relaxation therapy, not suggestion therapy—he sought to find the causes of disorders. While suggestion might help a patient to improve, it will not allow the specification of the causes of complaints. Jacobson said that he recognized that he was operating at a distinct disadvantage by momentarily not helping patients with suggestions that they would improve. But he thereby validated his method and helped more patients in the long run. To appreciate this reasoning, as we shall shortly develop, to develop self control one needs to be able to systematically tense and relax the striated muscles to accomplish one's purpose. To be able to volitionally tense a muscle one needs to be able to observe its contracted state—tension is defined as the shortening of striated muscles. Relaxation is the absence of tension, which occurs when muscle fibers are elongated.

Another non-specific variable that may operate to help a stress management method be effective is the reduction of external environmental stimulation, resulting in a decrease in general bodily arousal. Merely going into a quiet room reduces external stimulation which can have positive effects by temporarily reducing agitation or calming the body. Many methods use this approach, seeking arousal reduction as the goal. In fact, some are actually called stress *reduction* techniques. Better, though, we should seek stress *control* techniques because sometimes we should increase a low level of 'stress', to optimize it for better performance in accordance with a modified version of the famous Yerkes-Dodson law. However, if methods for reducing excessive arousal are effective, that must only be a general, quieting effect on the body—it cannot lead to specialized behavioral control to carry out a particular response strategy; furthermore, any favorable effects are probably only temporary and not generalizable to everyday life.

Specific Variables for Control
Many specific variables have been advocated, such as the stress expert who referred to 'caffeine intoxication', stating that caffeine makes one 'more stressed out'. A reverse suggestion that he made was that eating fruits and vegetables can have a calming effect. Ingesting other substances such as medications like muscle relaxants can have beneficial effects on one's internal environment and decrease general bodily arousal, if only temporarily.

One category of specific variables is wherein efforts are made to calm the body by instructing the learner to engage in a unique behavioral act. One recommendation was to engage in deep breathing at least five times a day. A related method has the learner think of the words 'gold' and 'blue' successively while respectively inhaling with only one nostril and then exhaling with the other.

A different strategy is for one to talk to oneself by repeating a meaningless term. Such verbal behavior, which engages the speech and other muscles, however, must have something of a muscle arousing effect; if carried out in a quiet environment, the arousal may be somewhat counteracted.

Sometimes one can instruct oneself by subvocalizing a self-instruction to calm down and behave reasonably. No doubt telling oneself to behave in a certain way can sometimes be effective, but one must know how to carry out the self-instruction and actually be able to exert such self-control. This may happen when one learns certain coping skills and instructs oneself to use them. For example, for time management one sets out a schedule prioritizing tasks to be accomplished that day; the question is, can the person exert sufficient self control to actually carry out the schedule. In psychotherapy or in stress management training programs, one might obtain 'insights' as to how to more effectively behave. To the extent to which one can actually carry out such self-instructions, behavior might be modified; if one can then successfully implement the 'insight' then one can more effectively cope with stressors or adjust so that the behavioral problem is alleviated.

While we may have many insights or learn all of the coping skills in the world, that does us no good unless we can actually use them. It is one thing to tell a person what to do, but another for that person to learn and implement the behavior.

IMPLEMENTING BEHAVIOR

Behavior (both overt and covert) is the systematic tensing (contracting) and relaxing (lengthening) of striated muscles—we act with our muscles. Hence, to control behavior, as well as many internal functions (Jacobson, 1938; McGuigan, 1994), one needs to learn how to judiciously use those muscles. Fortunately, Sir Charles Bell (1842) discovered that one can become aware of subtle striated muscle contractions, the well-known muscle sense of Bell. Since then we have learned how to use that sense to help guide behavior. But unlike the senses of vision and audition, the muscle sense must be cultivated, which requires diligent practice in observing it and then using it to program behavior. For this, Jacobson's (1938) method of Progressive Relaxation is an excellent model: One first learns to control a given set of muscles by overtly contracting them, observing the resulting muscle signal, the muscle sense of Bell, and then relaxing those muscles. Through continued practice, control is gained over that set of muscles, i.e., one can contract (tense) and lengthen (relax) it at will. This physiologically simple method is then extended so that control over the entire striated musculature (all 1,030 or so muscles) is achieved.

Studying Covert Behavior

Gradually in successive practice periods of Progressive Relaxation, one diminishes the amplitude of the highly localized muscle contraction (a specific response) until it becomes covert, whereupon an external observer cannot see the response with the naked eye (it is electromyographically observable though). Once the individual learns to internally observe the covert behavior as a small scale muscle tension, it too is relaxed away. The decrease in amplitude of a response is accomplished with the Method of Diminishing Tensions as developed by Jacobson (1929, p. 53).

To repeat, with this method, one decreases the amplitude of a muscular contraction in successive sessions until it is extremely slight. For instance, in the first practice position in Progressive Relaxation while supine, one raises the hand vertically (at a 90° angle) at the wrist. If one is successful in observing the muscular tension (it is in the dorsal surface of the forearm), on the next practice one raises the hand half as high, at a 45° angle. In the next practice session the hand is only raised half that much at about a 23° angle, and so on until the hand is not visibly raised at all, producing minimal muscular contraction. Such covert behaviors typically have amplitudes in the low microvolt region, as electromyographically measured.

Long ago the famous psychophysiologist R. C. Davis (1957), as well as many others, pointed out the importance of such covert behaviors; for one, covert behaviors, he said, are far more numerous than overt behaviors, those on which psychologists have traditionally concentrated. Becoming aware of covert responses is of extreme importance for gaining control over behavior. One reason is that they serve critical functions in the generation of cognitive activities (Jacobson, 1938; McGuigan, 1978, 1991).

Controlling Behavior

Once the learner acquires control over covert behavior generated by the striated musculature, the learner next programs behavior for controlling responses that are desired. What is required for this is a methodologically sound strategy for exercising volition, for providing an individual with specific causal variables by which other specific behaviors can be controlled.

For this, the great Russian physiologist Ivan Michailovich Sechenov (1863) provided the general paradigm that a muscle response (R_1) that produces sensory stimulation (afferent neural feedback, can control a later response (R_2): R_1 —— s —— R_2. It is through Progressive Relaxation that we learn how to institute R_1, though that response may be covert (r_1), viz, Jacobson emphasized the relatively great importance of covert speech and eye muscle controls (Jacobson, 1938; Also see McGuigan, 1992, 1994). That is, through verbal self instruction (overt or covert) and through visual imagery, the speech and eye muscles respectively can volitionally contract so as to direct other muscles to respond—the speech and eye muscles are the primary causal variables. The pioneering research of Jacobson (e.g., 1932) well documents the electrographic recording of such covert behaviors, for instance, numerous parts of the body covertly respond to instructions to imagine that they are engaged in appropriate activites. The instruction to imagine hitting a nail with a hammer a specific number of times evokes that number of covert responses in the preferred arm. Confirmation of such recordings of covert behavior are numerous (McGuigan, 1978). In addition, those covert behaviors are highly differentiated such as in the eye responses (McGuigan & Pavek, 1972) or the covert speech behavior (e.g., McGuigan & Winstead, 1974). Covert speech and eye responses are also important causal variables in pathological conditions, participating in a variety of psychiatric and psychosomatic disorders (e.g., McGuigan, 1994). A relevant anecdotal demonstration has occurred a number of times in my classes in which an instruction to slightly tense the eye muscles has evoked headaches in some of my students—the lesson is obvious to them that if they can so produce a headache they can allieviate or prevent it by relaxing the eye muscles.

Eventually, through continual practice, automaticity may be developed so that one need not volitionally, consciously institute R_1 or r_1 to evoke the desired response R_2 or r_2.

Behaving in Stressful Situations

The successful learner can apply these principles in stressful situations so that they can behave in accordance with self-instructions issued either overtly or covertly (McGuigan, 1992, 1994). In achieving this, one has first learned through relaxation to reduce or eliminate heightened bodily arousal typical of stressful situations so that one can better detect and study the stimulus signals (s) generated by the musculature contractions. By thus reducing excessive arousal, achieving momentary tranquility, one can program oneself to behave in a strategic, well thought out manner. It is important to emphasize that while the controlling response can be overtly issued as in speaking aloud, so telling oneself to behave in such and such a way, it is more frequently issued silently (covertly), neither of which changes the general principle. Either way the muscle sense of Bell is generated by contracting muscles (r_1), so that the desired response is evoked by the relevant stimulus signal (s) and brought under control.

Problems of Self Control and Generalization

I should highlight two of the major difficulties in stress management and indeed in psychotherapy in general, viz, how to develop self-control and how to generalize that behavioral change outside of the learning environment—the goal is to be able to execute specific behaviors in every day life on verbal and non verbal (e.g., visual imagery) command. That is, a successful stress management method is one that leads to generalized ability to control behavior in any situation—rather than reflexively responding to threats, the 'stress is managed'. The essence of stress management is thus embodied in the concept of self-control, as denoted in the journal *Biofeedback and Self-Regulation*, in Self-Operations Control, Jacobson's (1964) synonym for Progressive Relaxation, and elsewhere. Control should generalize to everyday living twenty-four hours a day, which includes restful sleep.

Specific Variables Again

We have seen that to achieve control of specific muscles in a stress management situation, one must be able to institute the appropriate, specific R_1 or r_1 and thereby evoke the appropriate, specific R_2 or r_2. If a stress management method has only non-specific effects on the body, it cannot lead to such specialized control of R_2 or r_2. Progressive Relaxation is a method that can institute Sechenov's paradigm effectively, especially where covert behaviors are concerned.

Achieving Generalization

Jacobson's method of Differential Relaxation is designed for generalizing self control from the learning situation to everyday life, which consists of driving, reading, writing, talking, etc. In learning Differential Relaxation, one comes to be able to *optimally* contract only those muscles necessary to achieve a given purpose, relaxing all irrelevant muscles. Thus, one is able to sit comfortably, for instance, without fidgeting, dangling a foot at the crossed knee, with hands and arms comfortably relaxed in the lap.

By following these methods a great deal of energy can be saved and redirected efficiently for the accomplishment of a person's goals. All of the usual components of stress management programs follow naturally from these principles. For example, one naturally sets priorities, not wasting energy on low priority or unessential tasks, one manages time well so as to explicitly direct energies on worthwhile work, and so on.

No doubt approaches other than Progressive Relaxation can result in some degree of generalized self-control and the use of any method that has positive results is certainly encouraged. But at least it has been well established that Jacobson's Methods of Diminishing Tension and Differential Relaxation are effective for those purposes. So far, though, if one wishes to develop effective control over one's body, including one's cognitive processes (e.g., McGuigan, 1991), no short cuts have been found in the over seven decades in which Jacobson searched for them.

Common sense uses of the term 'stress' vary widely, but a common one is that 'I am stressed out'. In the immediate context that often means a state of general hyperarousal of the body produced by excessive muscular tension, often only covert. Those who are able to exercise sufficient, highly-generalized bodily control would consistently generate optimal striated muscle tensions; they thus would not be victimized by a condition of being 'stressed out'—they would generalize behavioral control to all phases of life with optimal tension of only those muscles required to perform given acts.

The topics of Jacobson's numerous books also indicate the widespread applicability (generalization) of Progressive Relaxation, e.g., Teaching and Learning, Modern Treatment of Tense Patients, You Must Relax, The Human Mind, Anxiety, How to Sleep Well, Biology of Emotions, Relax and Have your Baby, and Tension Control for Businessmen.

CONCLUSION

Everything we do, we do with our striated muscles, which is why they have long been called 'voluntary muscles', the instrument of the will (e.g., see Bain, 1855, 1859). To the extent that any stress management method is effective, it must rely on muscle control, whether or not it explicitly recognizes that—as I have emphasized behavior is a muscular (effector) phenomenon, intimately generated by interacting systems of the body. As has been documented in research since the early part of this century, only one method thoroughly reeducates those muscles, the original stress management method, Progressive Relaxation—so for maximum effectiveness that is the method of preference.

References

Bain, A. (19855) *The Senses and the Intellect*. London: Parker.

bain, A. (1859) *The Emotions and the Will*. London: Parker.

Bell, Sir C. (1842) On the necessity of the sense of muscular action to the full exercise of the organs of the senses. Proceedings of the Society of Edinburgh, 361–63.

Bolger, N. & Zuckerman, A. A. (1995) Framework for studying personality in the stress process. *Journal of Personality and Social Psychology*, **69**, 890–902.

Davis, R. C. (1957) Response patterns. *Transactions of the New York Academy of Sciences*, **19**, 731–39.

Jacobson, E. (1929) (rev. edn., 1938). *Progressive Relaxation*. Chicago, IL: University of Chicago Press.

Jacobson, E. (1932) Electrophysiology of mental activities. *American Journal of Psychology*, **44**, 677–694.

Jacobson, E. (1964) *Self-operations Control*. Philadelphia: Lippincott.

Lehrer, P. M. & Woolfolk, R. L. (eds.) (1993) *Principles and Practice of Stress Management*. New York, NY: Guilford.

McGuigan, F. J. (1978) *Cognitive Psychophysiology: Principles of Covert Behavior*. Englewood Cliffs, NJ: Prentice-Hall.

McGuigan, F. J. (1991) Control of normal and pathological cognitive functions through neuromuscular circuits. In *International Perspectives on Self-Regulation and Health*, edited by J. Carlson and R. Seifert. New York, NY: Plenum.

McGuigan, F. J. (1992) *Calm Down: A Guide for Stress and Tension Control*. Dubuque, IA: Kendall-Hunt.

McGuigan, F. J. (1994) *Biological Psychology: A Cybernetic Science*. Englewood Cliffs, NJ: Prentice-Hall.

McGuigan, F. J. (1997) A neiromuscular model of mind with clinical and educational applications. *The Journal of Mind and Behavior*, **18**(4), 351–370.

McGuigan, F. J. & Pavek, G. V. (1972) On the psychophysiological identification of covert nonoral language processes. *Journal of Experimental Psychology*, **92**, 237–45.

McGuigan, F. J. & Winstead, C. L., Jr. (1974) Discriminative relationship between covert oral behavior and the phonemic system in internal information processing. *Journal of Experimental Psychology*, **103**, 885–90.

Munz, D. C. & Kohler, J. M. (1997) Do worksite stress management programs attract the employees who need them and are they effective? *International Journal of Stress Management*, **4**, 1–11.

Sechenov, I. M. Reflexes of the Brain. In *Selected Works*, edited by I. M. Sechenov. Moscow and Leningrad: State Publishing House for Biological and Medical Literature, 1935. Originally published in St. Petersburg, 1863. In *A Source Book in the History of Psychology*, edited by R. J. Herrnstein & E. G. Boring. Cambridge, MA: Harvard University Press, 1965.

Chapter 9

BIOFEEDBACK AND STRESS

Michael G. McKee, PhD and Jerome Kiffer, MA

Biofeedback uses instruments, primarily electronic ones, to help people learn to control bodily processes. The electronic instruments sense and display (feedback) information about the ongoing activity of various body (biological) processes, usually outside of one's awareness, that are either naturally involuntary or have become involuntary because of disease or accident. The goals of biofeedback therapy are to help one acquire voluntary control of such processes. Stress responses are ideal targets for biofeedback treatment. Instruments can feed back a wide variety of data about systems in the body that are in varying degrees of hyper-arousal or relaxation. Biofeedback is used in helping to diagnose and treat a wide range of psychophysiologic, performance, and habit disorders that are stress related.

Precisely because the stress response is a psychophysiologic response, biofeedback therapy for stress-related disorders usually overlaps with clinical and health psychology processes such as psychological assessment, cognitive-behavioral and coping strategies, stress management and psychotherapy. The American Psychological Association has identified 'Biofeedback: Applied Psychophysiology' as one of its first two proficiencies. Proficiencies are subspecialties requiring special training and measurable knowledge and skills that deserve to be recognized through certification. Designating biofeedback as a proficiency reflects the fact that there are knowledge and skills specific to biofeedback and applied psychophysiology which include: instrumentation and electronics; psychophysiological recording; autonomic nervous system interventions; and neuromuscular interventions.

Biofeedback, as it is used today in clinical settings, stems from laboratory studies in the 1960s that yielded a sizeable body of literature (Barber, DiCara & Kamiya, 1971; Birk, 1973) showing that human subjects could develop and exert voluntary control over many physiological parameters, including aspects of vasomotor, electromyographic, electroencephalo-graphic, electrodermal and cardiac activity. The outcomes literature on biofeedback since that time has been summarized in a number of works; see especially Hatch, Fisher, and Rugh (1987), Basmajian (1989), Gatchel and Blanchard (1993), Lehrer and Woolfolk (1993), and Schwartz and Associates (1995). The studies reviewed are mixed in rigour and goals. They include case reports, clinical series, and controlled outcomes studies, some with comparisons to alternative treatments.

INSTRUMENTATION

By definition, biofeedback training requires biofeedback instrumentation. These are typically electronic devices that monitor bodily information and provide feedback in a variety of ways, mainly visual and auditory. Self-regulation approaches that do not use instrumentation are not biofeedback, such as meditation, autogenic training, progressive muscle relaxation, and yoga. These training programs are often used in combination with biofeedback.

The most widely used biofeedback modality is surface electromyo-graphic (EMG) recording. EMG recordings are taken by applying sensors to the skin over the surface of muscles. Continuous recording of EMG fluctuations is displayed to the patient in the form of audio and/or visual feedback. EMG biofeedback training goals can be to reduce EMG amplitudes to low microvolt levels, as in generalized muscle relaxation training, or to increase EMG wave form activity, as in neuromuscular re-education.

EMG biofeedback is a powerful tool in treating stress-related problems. Excessive muscle tension ranks as one of the most frequent stress symptoms reported by the general population. EMG feedback has immediate and intuitive meaning that can enlist the patient to attend to and change muscle activity. For this reason, EMG procedures have been effectively used with individuals of all ages, including very young children.

Because of the importance of muscular functioning in overall health, EMG biofeedback is a procedure used in a wide variety of professional health-care disciplines, especially by psychologists, physical therapists and medical doctors. The most frequent direct use of EMG biofeedback training is in muscle tension headache syndromes. EMG training has also been fully integrated into the treatment team approach for rehabilitation, chronic pain syndromes and muscle re-education.

The second most frequently used biofeedback modality is skin temperature biofeedback (TBF), measured by sensors taped to the skin. Peripheral skin temperature is thought to be correlated with general sympathetic activity. Peripheral vasoconstriction, manifest in cool extremities and low peripheral temperature, is thought to be part of a high

stress reaction. By contrast, warm extremities and high peripheral temperature reflecting peripheral vasodilation are indicative of a high degree of
relaxation and of low sympathetic nervous system activity. TBF is used in
isolation for specific learning (as in Raynaud's Disease and Raynaud's
Phenomenon). Most often, however, TBF is used as part of general
relaxation training to cultivate states of low arousal, within a context of
broader stress management training and psychophysiologic psychotherapy.

Another frequently used form of biofeedback is monitoring the galvanic
skin response (GSR) and its counterpart, the skin conductance level (SCL).
Like TBF, GSR and SCL are thought to be associated with autonomic
nervous system activation. The most direct use of GSR/ SCL feedback is in
hyperhidrosis, excessive sweating and activation of sweat gland activity.
More generally, however, GSR/SCL biofeedback, like TBF, is used as part of
a program for reducing autonomic activation as part of a stress-reduction
program. Sensors for TBF and GSR/SCL are attached to the skin, usually
the fingertips.

Cardiovascular monitoring can also be done by biofeedback equipment.
The most frequently monitored variables are heart rate, blood pressure, and
pulse volume using a photoplethysmograph. Heart rate and photoplethys-
mographic readings are dynamic and continuous recordings. Systolic and
diastolic blood pressure can only be measured every two to three minutes.
Technological improvements are needed to enable recording continuous
systolic and diastolic blood pressure activity in a non-invasive modality.
Cardiovascular variables are directly used in training for blood pressure
reduction and sometimes for electrocardiographic abnormalities, especially
arrhythmias. However, as with TBF and GSR/SCL biofeedback,
cardiovascular variables are most often used as measures of autonomic
activity and employed in training for lowered arousal.

Respiratory activity can also be monitored using biofeedback equipment.
The two most frequently used methods are CO_2 capnometry and measurement of thoracic and diaphragmatic breathing using strain gauges. Capnometry is used most directly in disorders involving pulmonary variables,
such as asthma and hyperventilation. Again, however, breathing retraining
is most often used to train for lowered arousal, to reduce stress reactions.

The latest, burgeoning subfield of biofeedback training is neurofeedback.
Electroencephalographic (EEG) biofeedback equipment allows on-line,
immediate monitoring of several channels of EEG activity. The most
frequently used EEG biofeedback applications have been in Attention
Deficit-Hyperactivity Disorder (ADHD) (Lubar, 1995). Through EEG
biofeedback, several aspects of brain activity can be selected for
modification. EEG monitoring allows direct recording of beta, alpha,
sensorimotor, theta, and delta wave-form activity. Both frequency and
amplitude can be monitored and training schedules can be developed so
that one frequency can be enhanced or diminished while simultaneously
reducing or augmenting the amplitude of another frequency.

THEORETICAL AND TREATMENT MODELS

Biofeedback training follows one of two models:

1. A feedback learning model in which the goal is to learn control of one specific bodily function.
2. Learning to control the level of low arousal.

The first model makes straightforward use of feedback as a necessary condition of learning. The four conditions that must be met for effective learning to occur are:

1. the learner must have the capacity to appropriately respond;
2. the learner must be sufficiently motivated to learn;
3. the learner must be reinforced (rewarded for learning); and
4. the learner must be given accurate information about the results of each learning effort.

Straightforward biofeedback learning is typically employed to treat disorders that are not generally considered stress related. Examples are Raynaud's Disease and Raynaud's Phenomenon, severe peripheral vasoconstriction precipitated by exposure to a cold environment or emotional stress. These vasospastic attacks produce a painful blanching and cyanosis, followed by a reactive hyperemia accompanied by throbbing and paresthesias. Freedman (1993) reported that Raynaud's Disease patients who received TBF alone had a decrease of 67% to 92% in the number of vasospastic symptoms, improvements which were maintained at follow-ups two and three years later.

Additional disorders that appear to respond to biofeedback training in the feedback learning model are fecal incontinence (Whitehead, 1992), rehabilitation of neuromuscular disorders (Basmajian, 1989), and musculoskeletal and myofascial pain syndromes (Cram & Associates, 1990; Donaldson, Pow & Gossen, 1995).

Training for lowered arousal is usually indicated for anxiety disorders, performance disorders, and many stress-related psychophysiologic disorders. At the simplest level, the modality of feedback is selected that appears to correlate most with the symptom, which varies with degree of autonomic arousal. Feedback training to achieve lowered arousal usually consists of some combination of TBF, surface EMG and GSR/SCL biofeedback. In the simplest model, the goal is to master the ability to bring about lowered arousal, and treatment is considered successful when the individual reaches specific training goals (such as fingertip skin temperature above 95 degrees Fahrenheit). Much more frequently, because anxiety, impaired performance, and psychophysiologic symptoms are related to stress, people have to learn how to change patterns of thinking and feeling and acting in order to create less stress for themselves and in order to react to stressors in different ways physiologically. For this reason, stress management and psychotherapy interventions have been conjoined with biofeedback training in modifying the cognitive and emotional factors perpetuating stress-related disorders.

Often it is difficult to isolate the specific contribution of biofeedback in such a treatment program. For example, a typical clinical biofeedback session with a man recently discharged from the hospital following recovery from an uncomplicated myocardial infarction, a Type A personality with high blood pressure, could be summarized as follows: Harry was monitored during therapy with temperature biofeedback equipment, his initial finger temperature being approximately 78°F. The following dialogue is a brief summary of an hour's interaction (McKee, 1978). (Reprinted with permission from Slack, Inc. [*Psychiatric Annals*, October 1978].)

Harry: I can't relax.
Therapist: Why?
Harry: I've got to get back to work. I've got things to do, and I'm angry that they won't let me go back yet. I get very angry, and I can't do anything about it, and I can't express it.
Therapist: What do you mean you can't do anything? You can, too. In fact, you could tell people that you're angry; you could relax; you have many choices.
Harry: Well, I know we've been talking about that a lot, but I'm not sure that I can exercise those choices.
Therapist: Well, let's try simply letting go now. Let's realize that hurting your body further is not helping you get back to work. Just picture yourself in a very calm setting, at the beach. Recognize that you can be calm if you want to. You have control over your life. You have choices, but you also have responsibilities. One of those responsibilities may be to keep yourself calm, to assert your rights, and to take control over your own life rather than just reacting, rather than being bound up in anger or anxiety. Let yourself be very deeply calm and know that your mind is open when you're deeply calm. (A 15-minute relaxation period follows.)

As Harry relaxes deeply, his finger temperature goes up into the 90s [°F.].

Harry: That felt good, but now I've got to go back into the real   world.
Therapist: It sounds as if you're not sure whether you want to use these relaxation skills or not.
Harry: You're right. I'm not sure I do just want to relax. I want to get things done.
Therapist: You know that you're going to get things done only if you live, so relax. Being angry and being uptight is not going to get you back to work any earlier. Don't you think you could produce more in this relaxed state than you could the way you came in?
Harry: Yeah, I guess you're probably right.

Therapist: Take this book to read. It will help you learn how to identify your angry feelings, how to anticipate situations that lead to your getting angry. Learn how to respond to them differently. And I want you to practice this relaxation exercise twice a day.

If we study the dynamics of that session, we can ask what process was operating. Was it:

1. Operant conditioning of smooth muscles surrounding arterioles in the fingers, with success in increasing skin temperature (as fed back visually and auditorially) representing immediate positive reinforcement?
2. Feedback learning, with the biofeedback equipment representing imposition of an external psychophysiologic feedback loop upon already existing internal feedback loops, directly affecting blood flow to the fingers?
3. Feedback learning, with the biofeedback equipment affecting general arousal through impact on already existing feedback loops of the homeostatic adaptive control systems?
4. Learning relaxation via imagery and cognitive exercises?
5. Modifying assumptions, attitudes, and expectations that lead to psychophysiologic stress reactions?
6. Enhancing self-awareness in general, including awareness of bodily functioning, by getting specific information about bodily functioning and experimenting with the relationship of physiologic functioning to thought patterns?
7. Resolving conflicts by discussing them with a therapist, thus reducing self-generated stressors leading to psychophysiologic reactions?
8. Responding to hypnotic suggestion of greater well-being while in an altered state of consciousness induced by narrowing of attention?
9. Faith healing, with belief in the process being a curative agent leading to placebo healing?
10. Changing behavior to reduce stressors, in response to specific counseling of the therapist?
11. Experiencing an increase in self-esteem secondary to warmth, genuineness, and empathy of the therapist, thereby reducing stress?
12. Emulating a relaxed therapist who is not upset thinking about and discussing emotionally-laden topics?
13. Articulating values and shifting them to enable attitudinal, behavioral, and emotional changes?
14. A cathartic re-experiencing and emotional release that reduces stress?
15. Changing the locus of control so that Harry takes responsibility for his own well being, with Harry starting to realize he is in charge of his life?

All of the above processes possibly are operative over many

psychophysiologic therapy sessions. In clinical biofeedback therapy, the client develops greater awareness of psychological and physiologic functioning and an early warning system of his or her own unique stress response, then learns an idiosyncratic stress-management technique under tutelage of an experienced therapist. With the aid of the therapist, one modifies patterns of thinking, feeling, and acting in order to reduce stressors and to enable application of new stress-control techniques.

The complexity of the process of psychophysiological psychotherapy, in which biofeedback monitoring is added to a traditional psychotherapeutic process, confounds research. Most of the reportable research controls but a small number of factors. When efforts are made to do clinical research studies across multiple sites to measure outcomes of biofeedback therapy, the efforts break down because biofeedback is embedded within a complex multimodal diagnostic and therapeutic process. Another example of the complexity is reflected in the clinical case of a middle-aged woman presenting with chronic headaches (McKee, 1991). Psychological diagnosis and treatment of her headaches were enhanced by adding physiologic monitoring to biofeedback. The physiologic data displayed to the patient fostered insight by identifying patterns of emotional arousal pointing to stressors and conflicts not previously labeled as causes of emotional upset. Awareness of physiologic reactivity enabled greater understanding of emotional triggers for her headaches and also guided, reinforced, and confirmed learning of self-regulation skills enabling headache control. The biofeedback monitoring helped refine the diagnostic impression of what cause and effect chains contributed to physiologic arousal. The case highlights use of biofeedback equipment in clinical practice for problem identification and patient education as well as diagnosis and treatment. It perhaps also highlights why there are strong commonalities between the practice of biofeedback and the general field of clinical health psychology, as suggested by a survey of members of the American Psychological Association, Division of Health Psychology. Of 270 respondents, 151—or 56 percent—used biofeedback at least for assessment. The 151 respondents using biofeedback instruments were more than those mentioning use of any of 20 paper and pencil measures except the Minnesota Multiphasic Personality Inventory (MMPI) (Piotrowski & Lubin, 1990).

Clinical biofeedback therapy is typically a learning process rather than a treatment in which something is done to the patient. Learning to control physiologic arousal is like learning a foreign language, with the biofeedback equipment functioning roughly analogously to a language lab. Thus, much of the research that evaluates simple biofeedback training and its impact on syndromes is of limited usefulness in evaluating the effectiveness of complex psychophysiologic psychotherapy, which in turn is difficult to evaluate because it is very hard to construct reasonable control or even comparison groups.

Trying to measure the specific effects of biofeedback as part of multimodal treatment is difficult. Measuring patient satisfaction is not. In our department, there are multiple specialties and subspecialties providing inpatient and outpatient psychological and psychiatric services. Consistently, in surveys of patient satisfaction, the biofeedback program is rated number one in terms of helpfulness, understanding of patient's problem, and providing useful strategies for change. In two inpatient programs, those for chronic pain and substance abuse, biofeedback is one of many treatments provided in a multimodal inpatient or day patient treatment program. There too, biofeedback has consistently ranked number one in customer satisfaction. We believe that the wide use of biofeedback among health psychologists, and the high degree of acceptance by clients and patients, reflects the obvious value of adding timely, accurate, and relevant feedback to the self-regulation process, to stress management.

A review of the literature on biofeedback in treatment of selected stress-related syndromes and disorders follows.

HYPERTENSION

Hypertension is a very common problem in the United States. The Joint National Committee on Detection, Evaluation, and Treatment of High Blood Pressure (1993) defines the disorder as a systolic blood pressure of 140 mmHg or higher, or a diastolic blood pressure of 90 mmHg or higher. Hypertension is of great concern because it is a significant risk factor for disorders which cause more than half of the deaths in the United States: myocardial infarction, congestive heart failure, and stroke.

Essential hypertension is the most common form of high blood pressure, meaning that there is sustained blood pressure with no specific cause identified. While some cases of hypertension represent specific diseases, including adrenal tumors and kidney disease, most high blood pressure represents genetic, physiologic and psychologic factors in complex interactions.

Pharmacotherapy is the standard medical treatment for hypertension, but the 1993 report of the Joint National Committee gives special attention to the role of 'lifestyle modification', including psychophysiologic and biofeedback approaches. The report is more definitive about the role of stress in raising blood pressure than of stress management techniques in lowering blood pressure.

Published reports on efficacy of applied psychophysiologic and biofeedback are ambiguous. Early studies (Fahrion, Norris, Green, Green & Snarr, 1986; Patel, Marmot & Terry, 1981) were quite positive. Blanchard et al. (1986) reported successful use of TBF as an effective substitute for sympatholytic medication in moderate hypertension in patients on two drugs, yet Blanchard et al. (1993) failed to confirm those earlier findings. Combining biofeedback-assisted relaxation and pharmacotherapy may lead to an increase in treatment effects. Jurek, Higgins and McGrady (1992) reported that biofeedback-assisted relaxation combined with a diuretic produced blood pressure decreases greater than that from just the diuretic. Goebel, Voil and Orabaugh (1993) used a research design constituting an incremental model to isolate specific effects of behavioral treatments in essential hypertension, and found that outpatient veterans with borderline or moderate essential hypertension had significant decreases in blood pressure secondary to behavioral techniques, including biofeedback, in contrast to comparison groups that showed non-significant and small changes. McGrady (1994) reported significant blood pressure reductions in 49% of a treatment group of essential hypertension patients receiving group relaxation training and TBF. Thirty-seven percent maintained the ability to meet blood pressure criterion at 10-month follow-up. In the Joint USSR-USA Behavioral Hypertension Project (Wittrock, Blanchard, McCoy, McCaffrey & Khramelashvil, 1995), there were no differences pre- or post-treatment between TBF and autogenic training as treatments for mild essential hypertension, but both outcome and efficacy expectations were related to relapse over the three months following completion of treatment. Blanchard et al. (1996) also found no differences at any point between groups receiving TBF training and those doing home monitoring of blood pressure, the subjects being unmedicated mild hypertensives. Hunyor et al. (1997) found that in a sample of untreated, mildly hypertensive individuals, almost half could lower systolic pressure at will for short intervals, and that this capability was independent of the real or placebo nature of the feedback signal, the conclusion being that there was no specific short-term biofeedback pressure-lowering capability in hypertensive individuals.

It may be that selection of individuals is critical. With biofeedback alone or with biofeedback-assisted relaxation, Jurek et al. (1992) found that blood pressure decreases mediated by the combined approach of biofeedback-assisted relaxation and a diuretic were associated with high pre-treatment blood pressure, low finger temperature, and high/normal plasma renin activity. McGrady and Higgins (1989, 1990) found that individuals characterized by a high chronic level of response to stress, as indicated by high/normal cortisol levels and high anxiety scores, and those characterized by high autonomic overactivity responded better to self-regulation than those without the high chronic level of response to stress. Weaver and McGrady (1995) conclude that response to biofeedback-assisted relaxation is not uniform among hypertensive individuals, finding that a regression model derived from five variables (heart rate, finger temperature, forehead muscle tension, plasma renin response to furosemide, and mean arterial pressure response to furosemide) provided significant predictive power for blood pressure response. This model needs validation.

Reviewers of studies vary in their conclusions about the efficacy of biobehavioral treatments of hypertension. Eisenberg et al. (1993)

identified only 26 of 800 published works on biobehavioral treatment of hypertension as worthy of review, and reported, 'Cognitive interventions for essential hypertension are superior to no therapy but not superior to credible sham techniques or to self-monitoring alone'. The Joint National Committee (1993) concluded, 'The available literature does not support the use of relaxation therapies for definitive therapy or prevention of hypertension'. Linden and Chambers (1994), in a meta-analysis comparing psychological with pharmacological treatments of blood pressure, reported the two kinds of treatment led to similar reductions in blood pressure when adjustments were made for baseline differences. Lehrer, Carr, Sargunaraj, and Woolfolk (1993), reviewing the literature on stress management in the treatment of hypertension, conclude, 'The balance of the evidence indicates that some form of stress management training should play a role in the treatment of hypertension'. Rosen, Brondolo, and Kostis (1993) conclude that, 'Relaxation and stress management approaches have produced inconsistent results in the studies to date'. This conclusion most clearly summarizes the research.

INSOMNIA

Insomnia is a very prevalent symptom experienced by as many as one-third of adults. Insomnia is a symptom of a wide range of medical and psychological conditions. Once an underlying medical illness or psychiatric/psychological illness is ruled out, the most common type of insomnia that presents to a clinician is psychophysiological insomnia. It is this form of insomnia for which biofeedback approaches have been used.

Psychophysiological insomnia is caused by increased cognitive activation and excessive physiological activation. Behavioral factors are important in contributing to this type of insomnia. Poor sleep hygiene, consisting of irregular sleep-wake cycles, afternoon napping, and stimulant intake are typically involved in perpetuating chronic psychophysiologic insomnia.

Biofeedback approaches have been tried both separately and in conjunction with other behavior therapy approaches. Behavioral treatments include relaxation training, stimulus-control training, strict scheduling of sleep time, and sleep restriction. Biofeedback is one form of behavioral treatment that has been used to augment relaxation training. A study comparing three types of biofeedback approaches for psychophysiologic insomnia found no differential improvement in the biofeedback approaches (Hauri, 1981). EMG feedback was no better than combined EMG and theta EEG feedback, or sensorimotor rhythm EEG feedback in improving sleep. A study comparing EMG biofeedback training to a cognitively-focused program found no difference between the two groups; both showed improvement in sleep quality (Sanavio, 1988). A study that compared progressive relaxation, EMG biofeedback, and biofeedback placebo in the treatment of sleep-onset insomnia found no significant differences among the three treatments, although each produced improvement (Nicassio, Boylan & McCabe, 1982). There have been several studies that have shown significant, positive effects of biofeedback and behavioral therapy approaches for insomnia. (See Turner, 1986, for review.)

The recommended non-pharmacologic treatment for insomnia is a behavioral approach (Bootzin & Perlis, 1992). Clinical presentation of chronic insomnia finds a high number of people reporting difficulty relaxing. When relaxation training is indicated as part of a behavioral approach, biofeedback training can facilitate the acquisition of relaxation skills. Muscular relaxation training along with autonomic relaxation continue to be the preferred biofeedback approaches.

TEMPOROMANDIBULAR DISORDERS

Temporomandibular disorders (TMD) are a collection of disorders characterized by facial and jaw pain. The majority of TMD cases involve problems in the facial and head muscles, the temporomandibular joint (TMJ), or difficulties involving the bony structures of the jaw. TMD is sometimes called TMJ disorder.

Dental professionals recognize psychological factors as playing key roles in the etiology, perpetuation and treatment of TMD (Dworkin et al., 1992). There are several reviews of the literature on the psychophysiological and psychological aspects of TMD (Flor & Turk, 1989; Gevirtz, Glaros, Hopper & Schwartz, 1995; Glaros & Glass, 1993). Of the psychological and behavioral factors associated with TMD, excessive muscle tension responses (such as clenching and grinding of the teeth) play a significant part in ongoing pain and symptomatology. Muscle tension affects the TMD patient in three ways. First, a TMD patient may have higher levels of facial/jaw muscle activity than non-TMD patients. Second, TMD patients may react to stress with increased facial/jaw muscle tension which contributes to ongoing pain. Third, TMD patients may be less aware and less able to control their facial muscles than non-TMD patients.

The masseter muscles are most commonly used for EMG biofeedback in treatment of TMD (Mealiea & McGlynn, 1987). The lateral pterygoids are also sites for EMG biofeedback and an intra- oral EMG device for recording this muscle has been reported in the literature (Gevirtz, 1990). These muscles are typically painful to palpation on clinical exam, and it is unknown whether this is a primary or secondary mechanism for TMD pain. EMG biofeedback has been found to be effective along with traditional dental interventions such as intraoral splints and bite-guards (Gevirtz, Glaros, Hopper, & Schwartz, 1995). Often, EMG biofeedback procedures are part of a broader behavior approach that involves learning muscle relaxation skills, interrupting habits of bruxism, and acquiring stress management techniques. When a multimodal approach is used along with EMG biofeedback in TMD, significant reductions in physical, psychosocial, and behavioral symptoms can be accomplished (Turk, Rudy, Kubinski, Zaki & Greco, 1996).

HEADACHES

Migraine Headache: Migraine headache is typically experienced as unilateral, pulsating pain, often accompanied by nausea, vomiting, sensitivity to sound and light, and inability to perform normal activities. Epidemiological studies estimate a lifetime prevalence of migraine headache of about 8 percent for males and 25 percent for females (Solomon, 1993). The standard biofeedback approach to migraine combines TBF aimed at volitional warming with relaxation training. There are many pharmacological approaches to treating migraine, with beta blockers such as propranolol commonly used for prophylaxis. Holroyd and Penzien (1990) reported a meta-analysis of the comparative efficacy of propranolol and thermal biofeedback/ relaxation based on 25 studies of propranolol treatment and 35 studies of thermal biofeedback/relaxation training. Over all types of outcome measures, the two interventions yielded similar average improvements in headache activity of approximately 55 percent. The improvement for the two active interventions was substantially greater than placebo medication (14 percent improvement) or no treatment (3 percent improvement). In sum, both pharmacological and biofeedback prophylaxis result in substantial and equivalent improvement in migraine headache activity, which implies that the choice of intervention can be determined by such factors as patient preference, relative cost and long-term benefits of the two treatments.

Tension-Type Headache: Tension-type headache (TTH) is experienced as a bilateral pressing or tightening pain of mild to moderate severity that may interfere with but usually does not prevent daily activities. TTH is ubiquitous. Over 90 percent of the population report at least one such headache yearly. Approximately 36 percent of the population suffer from recurrent TTH, and 3 percent meet criteria for chronic TTH (Solomon, 1993).

The pathophysiology of TTH is not well characterized. Although abnormal activity in facial, paracranial, and posterior neck muscles cannot be ruled out, both central mechanisms and peripheral vascular activity may also be contributory (Schwartz & Associates, 1995). There have been conflicting results as to whether excessive EMG activity can differentiate headache patients from non-headache controls (Schwartz & Associates, 1995). Additionally, people who suffer with tension-type headaches often have EMG levels that are not differentiated in the headache and no-headache phase (Lichstein et al., 1991). These conflicting results on EMG levels are a major reason the nomenclature now calls such headaches Tension-Type Headaches rather than Tension Headaches.

Pharmacological treatment for TTH includes analgesics or analgesic/sedative combinations to abort recurrent TTH, and antidepressants for prophylaxis of chronic TTH (Solomon, 1993). The standard biofeedback intervention for TTH is EMG biofeedback from frontal and other paracranial sites. In early biofeedback treatment of headache, the frontal EMG site was the most frequently-used placement. As biofeedback instrumentation developed into multi-channel capabilities, and as research studies became more advanced, multiple areas in the face, neck and shoulders were studied. Hudzinski and Lawrence (1988, 1990) studied the frontal-posterior neck placement for EMG monitoring and reported that this site was the most discriminating between headache and non-headache activity. Schwartz and Associates (1995) also report that this is a more useful site than traditional frontalis placement. Limited understanding of underlying mechanisms has undoubtedly impeded the development of optimal treatments for tension-type headache. Nevertheless, a variety of behavioral interventions, including biofeedback, relaxation training, and cognitive-behavioral therapy are known to be effective (Blanchard, 1992; Martin, 1993).

SUMMARY

Biofeedback is a behavioral technology that can be used in treating stress-related disorders. Biofeedback training is often embedded in a variety of other therapy approaches. It is most widely used to augment relaxation training and psychotherapy where there is a stress component.

Despite mixed results and equivocal findings in biofeedback outcomes research, biofeedback is increasingly used in medical and psychological treatment settings and is well received by patients. Biofeedback training techniques will continue to be part of 'clinical packages' for certain stress-related conditions. Biofeedback is a useful technology and process that has survived infancy and adolescence and is now gaining greater maturity in a wide variety of applications, with research support lagging significantly behind provider and patient acceptance.

References

Barber, T. X., DiCara, L. V. & Kamiya, J. (1971) *Biofeedback and Self-control*. Chicago: Aldine-Atherton.

Basmajian, J. V. (ed.) (1989) *Biofeedback: Principles and Practice for Clinicians* (3rd edn). Baltimore: Williams & Wilkins.

Birk, L. (ed.) (1973) *Biofeedback: Behavioral Medicine*. New York: Grune and Stratton.

Blanchard, E. B. (1992) Psychological treatment of benign headache disorders. *Journal of Consulting and Clinical Psychology*, **60**(4), 537–551.

Blanchard, E. B., Eisele, G., Gordon, M. A., Cornish, P. J., Wittrock, D. A., Gilmore, L., Vollmar, A. J. & Wan, C. (1993) Thermal biofeedback as an effective substitute for sympatholytic medication in moderate hypertension: A failure to replicate. *Biofeedback and Self-Regulation*, **18**, 237–253.

Blanchard, E. B., Eisele, G., Vollmer, A., Payne, A., Gordon, M., Cornish, P. & Gilmore, L. (1996) Controlled evaluation of thermal biofeedback in treatment of elevated blood pressure in unmedicated mild hypertension. *Biofeedback and Self-Regulation*, **21**(2), 167–190.

Blanchard, E. B., McCoy, G. C., Musso, A., Gerardi, M. A., Pallmeyer, T., Gerardi, R. J., Cotch, P. A., Siracusa, K. & Andrasik, F. (1986) A controlled comparison of thermal biofeedback and relaxation training in the treatment of essential hypertension: Short-term and long-term outcome. *Behavior Therapy*, **17**, 563–579.

Bootzin, R. R. & Perlis, M. L. (1992) Nonpharmacologic treatments of insomnia. *Journal of Clinical Psychiatry*, **53**(6, Suppl.), 37–41.

Cram, J. R. & Associates (1990) *Clinical EMG for Surface Recordings, vol 2*. California: Clinical Resources.

Donaldson, S., Pow, R. & Gossen, L. (1995) Myofascial pain syndromes. In *Clinical Applications of Biofeedback and Applied Psychophysiology*, pp. 39–40. Wheat Ridge, CO: Association for Applied Psychophysiology and Biofeedback.

Dworkin, S. F. & LeResche, L. (eds.) (1992) Research diagnostic criteria for tempomandibular disorders: Review, criteria, examinations and specifications, critique. *Journal of Craniomandibular Disorders: Facial and Oral Pain*, **6**, 301–355.

Eisenberg, D. M., Delbanco, T. L., Berkey, C. S., Kaptchuk, T. J., Kupelnick, B., Kuhl, J. & Chalmers, T. C. (1993) Cognitive behavioral techniques for hypertension: Are they effective? *Annals of Internal Medicine*, **118**, 964–972.

Fahrion, S., Norris, P., Green, A., Green, E. & Snarr, C. (1986) Biobehavioral treatment of essential hypertension: A group outcome study. *Biofeedback and Self-Regulation*, **11**, 257–278.

Flor, H. & Turk, D. (1989) Psychophysiology of chronic pain: Do chronic pain patients exhibit symptom-specific psychophysiological responses? *Psychological Bulletin*, **105**, 215–259.

Freedman, R. R. (1993) Raynaud's disease and phenomenon. In *Psychophysiological Disorders: Research and Clinical Applications*, edited by R. J. Gatchel & E. B. Blanchard, pp. 245–267. Washington, DC: American Psychological Association.

Gatchel, R. J. & Blanchard, E. B. (1993) *Psychophysiological Disorders: Research and Clinical Applications*. Washington, D.C.: American Psychological Association.

Gevirtz, R. N. (1990) Recording the lateral pterygoid in MPD patients. *Biofeedback*, **18**(1), 45–47.

Gevirtz, R. N., Glaros, A. G., Hopper, D. & Schwartz, M. S. (1995) Temporomandibular disorders. In *Biofeedback: A Practitioner's Guide*, edited by M. S. Schwartz & Associates, pp. 411–428. New York: Guilford Press.

Glaros, A. G. & Glass, E. G. (1993) Temporomandibular disorders. In *Psychophysiological Disorders*, edited by R. Gatchel & E. Blanchard, pp. 293–355. Washington, DC: American Psychological Association.

Goebel, M., Voil, G. & Orabaugh, C. (1993) An incremental model to isolate specific effects of behavioral treatments in essential hypertension. *Biofeedback and Self-Regulation*, **18**, 255–280.

Hatch, J. P., Fisher, J. G. & Rugh, J. D. (eds) (1987) *Biofeedback: Studies in Clinical Efficacy*. New York: Plenum Press.

Hauri, P. (July 1981) Treating psychophysiologic insomnia with biofeedback. *Archives of General Psychiatry*, **38**(7), 752–758.

Holroyd, K. A. & Penzien, D. B. (1990) Pharmacological versus nonpharmacological prophylaxis of current migraine headache: A meta-analytic review of clinical trials. *Pain*, **42**, 1–13.

Hudzinski, L. G. & Lawrence, G. S. (1988) Significance of EMG surface electrode placement models and headache findings. *Headache*, **28**, 30–35.

Hudzinski, L. G. & Lawrence, G. S. (1990) EMG surface electrode normative data for muscle contraction headache and biofeedback therapy. *Headache Quarterly, Current Treatment and Research*, **1**(3), 23–28.

Hunyor, S. N., Henderson, R. J., Lal, S. K., Carter, N. L., Kobler, H., Jones, M., Bartrop, R. W., Craig, A. & Mihailidou, A. S. (1997) Placebo-controlled biofeedback blood pressure effect in hypertensive humans. *Hypertension*, **29**(6), 1225–1231.

Joint National Committee on Detection, Evaluation, and Treatment of High Blood Pressure (JNC-V). (1993). Fifth report. *Archives of Internal Medicine*, **153**, 154–183.

Jurek, I. E., Higgins, J. T., Jr. & McGrady, A. (1992) Interaction of biofeedback-assisted relaxation and diuretic in treatment of essential hypertension. *Biofeedback and Self-Regulation*, **17**, 125–141.

Lehrer, P. M., Carr, R., Sargunaraj, D. & Woolfolk, R. L. (1993) Differential effects of stress management therapies in behavioral medicine. In *Principles and Practice of Stress Management*, edited by P. M. Lehrer & R. L. Woolfolk, (2nd edn.) (pp. 571–605). New York: Guilford Press.

Lehrer, P. M. & Woolfolk, R. L. (eds.) (1993) *Principles and Practice of Stress Management* (2nd edn). New York: Guilford Press.

Lichstein, K. L., Fischer, S. M., Eakin, T. L., Amberson, J. I., Bertorini, T. & Hoon, P. W. (1991) Psychophysiological parameters of migraine and muscle-contraction headaches. *Headache*, **31**, 27–34.

Linden, W. & Chambers, L. (1994) Clinical effectiveness of non-drug treatment for hypertension: A meta-analysis. *Annals of Behavioral Medicine*, **16**, 35–45.

Lubar, J. L. (1995) Neurofeedback for the management of Attention Deficit/ Hyperactivity Disorder. In *Biofeedback: A Practitioner's Guide*, edited by M. S. Schwartz & Associates. New York: Guilford Press.

Martin, P. R. (1993) *Psychological Management of Chronic Headaches*. New York: Guilford Press.

McGrady, A. (1994) The effects of group relaxation training and thermal biofeedback on blood pressure and related psychophysiological variables in essential hypertension. *Biofeedback and Self-Regulation*, **19**, 51–66.

McGrady, A. (1995) Biofeedback in essential hypertension. In *Clinical Applications of Biofeedback and Applied Psychophysiology*, pp. 21–25. Wheat Ridge, CO: Association for Applied Psychophysiology and Biofeedback.

McGrady, A. & Higgins, J. T., Jr. (1990) Effect of repeated measurements of blood pressure on blood pressure in essential hypertension: Role of anxiety. *Journal of Behavioral Medicine*, **13**, 93–101.

McGrady, A. & Higgins, J. T., Jr. (1989) Prediction of response to biofeedback-assisted relaxation in hypertensives: Development of a hypertensive predictor profile (HYPP). *Psychosomatic Medicine*, **51**, 277–284.

McKee, M. G. (1978) Using biofeedback and self-control techniques to prevent heart attacks. *Psychiatric Annals*, **8**(10), 92–99.

McKee, M. G. (1991) Contributions of psychophysiologic monitoring to diagnosis and treatment of chronic head pain. *Headache Quarterly*, **11**(4), 327–330.

Mealiea, W. L. & McGlynn, F. D. (1987) Temporomandibular disorders and bruxism. In *Biofeedback: Studies in Clinical Efficacy*, edited by J. P. Hatch, J. G. Fisher & J. D. Rugh, pp. 123–151. New York: Plenum Press.

Nicassio, P. M., Boylan, M. R. & McCabe, T. G. (1982) Progressive relaxation, EMG biofeedback and biofeedback placebo in the treatment of sleep onset insomnia. *British Journal of Medical Psychology*, **55**, 159–166.

Patel, C., Marmot, M. G. & Terry, D. G. (1981) Controlled trial of biofeedback-aided behavioral methods in reducing mild hypertension. *British Medical Journal*, **282**, 2005–2008.

Piotrowski, C. & Lubin, B. (1990) Assessment practices of health psychologists: Survey of APA Division clinicians. *Professional Psychology, Research and Practice*, **21**(2), 99–106.

Rosen, R. C., Brondolo, E. & Kostis, J. B. (1993) Nonpharmacologic treatment of essential hypertension: Research and clinical applications. In *Psychophysiologic Disorders: Research and Clinical Applications*, edited by R. J. Gatchel & E. B. Blanchard, pp. 63–110. Washington, DC: American Psychological Association.

Sanavio, E. (1988) Pre-sleep cognitive intrusions and treatment of onset-insomnia. *Behavior Research and Therapy*, **26**(6), 451–459.

Schwartz, M. S. & Associates (eds.) (1995) *Biofeedback: A Practitioner's Guide*. New York: Guilford Press.

Solomon, G. D. (1993) Headache. In *Clinical Preventive Medicine*, edited by R. N. Matzen & R. N. Lang, pp. 988–1002. St. Louis: Mosby-Year Book.

Turk, D. C., Rudy, T. E., Kubinski, J. A., Zaki, H. S. & Greco, C. M. (1996) Dysfunctional patients with temporomandibular disorders: Evaluating the efficacy of a tailored treatment protocol. *Journal of Consulting & Clinical Psychology*, **64**(1), 139–146.

Turner, R. M. (1986) Behavioral self-control procedures for Disorders of Initiating and Maintaining Sleep (DIMS). *Clinical Psychology Review*, **6**(1), 27–38.

Weaver, M. T. & McGrady, A. (1995) A provisional model to predict blood pressure response to biofeedback-assisted relaxation. *Biofeedback & Self-Regulation*, **20**(3), 229–240.

Whitehead, W. E. (1992) Biofeedback treatment of gastrointestinal disorders. *Biofeedback and Self-Regulation*, **17**(1), 59–76.

Wittrock, D. A., Blanchard, E. B., McCoy, G. C., McCaffrey, R. J. & Khramelashvil, W. (1995) The relationship of expectancies to outcome in stress management treatment of essential hypertension: Results from the Joint USSR-USA Behavioral Hypertension Project. *Biofeedback and Self-Regulation*, **20**(1), 51–63.

Chapter 10

STRESS MANAGEMENT: What Can We Learn from the Meditative Disciplines?

Johann Martin Stoyva

The term 'meditative disciplines' covers a rich variety of techniques and traditions. Accordingly in the interests of both coherence and brevity, our focus will be confined simply to three related procedures or practices drawn from two of the major meditative traditions within Buddhism. These traditions are, respectively, the Vipassana (or Mindfulness) tradition and the Zen approach to meditative experience.

In this paper we propose certain techniques drawn from these two traditions can be utilized to cope with some of the adverse psychological reactions associated with an excessive response to stress. These techniques have evolved in more or less pragmatic fashion over many centuries and thus already enjoy a measure of empirical support. It is also significant to note, especially in view of Western stereotypes regarding 'oriental mysticism', that many meditative practices are surprisingly operational in character. There are specific skills to be learned, and specific training steps to be followed in their acquisition.

The three techniques, or practices, to be discussed are as follows:

1. The use of a relaxed, abdominal breathing response. This procedure, which derives from the Vipassana tradition of meditation, can be used to moderate situational and performance anxiety.
2. A basic Zen exercise: learning to pay quiet attention to respiratory sensations. Skill in this technique enables the individual to reduce or eliminate extraneous mental activity, an ability that is helpful in overcoming certain common types of insomnia.
3. An exercise derived from Mindfulness (task-absorption) meditation. This method may have considerable potential for countering performance anxiety, as well as for reducing the tendency to excessive rumination.

Recent empirical studies show that the latter tends to exacerbate anxiety and depressive reactions, as well as compromise performance under stress (Nolen-Hoeksema, 1996).

THEORY

Our theoretical orientation concerning stress is to view the stress response as a co-ordinated reaction pattern made up of physiological, behavioural, and cognitive components—psychological hyperarousal being part of the cognitive component ('Stress Defined as a Three-Systems Phenomenon'; Stoyva & Carlson, 1993, pp. 727–729).

In this paper we propose that the techniques, or **practices** mentioned above can be used to moderate two major components of the stress reaction. These components are (1) the heightened **physiological arousal** characteristic of this reaction; and (2) **psychological hyperarousal**, a condition in which thinking is often fragmented, scattered, and unfocused.

Research and practice over many decades have shown that various relaxation methods are efficacious in reducing the physiological hyperarousal associated with excessive stress reactions (see Lehrer & Woolfolk, 1993 for detailed discussion of the various techniques). The reduction of **psychological** hyperarousal, however, has been a less successful endeavour. In particular, the phenomenon of 'mental chatter', 'an inability to stop thinking', is a persistent and elusive difficulty that frequently manifests itself in the acquisition of a thorough relaxation response. The same problem occurs in the meditative disciplines, which have long recognized it as a major impediment to progress. References to such things as 'the chattering monkey mind' or to a 'grasshopper consciousness' appear frequently in the meditation literature. It would be no exaggeration to say that, for centuries, a major preoccupation within the various meditative traditions has been the question of how to cope with intruding thoughts.

RESEARCH REVIEWS

Valuable reviews of empirical research findings regarding meditation and its clinical usefulness can be found in Benson (1975), Carrington (1993), Patel (1993), and Sheppard (1989). Kabat-Zinn (1990) focuses on the therapeutic usefulness of mindfulness meditation, as well as on its application to daily living.

Carrington's (1993) review is especially useful for its sophisticated description of the experiential aspect of meditation, an aspect often ignored by Western investigators. Sheppard (1989) summarizes empirical data from research studies regarding various types of meditation, and also offers a number of interesting observations based on personal visits to meditators in various parts of the world.

In a series of clinically-oriented experiments conducted over more than twenty years, Patel (1993) has examined the effect of Yoga-based relaxation and meditation techniques on various measures of cardiovascular system activity. These studies, mainly carried out with hypertensives, have repeatedly shown that the previously-mentioned Yoga-based techniques exhibit a favourable impact on essential hypertension. In a carefully-designed study by Patel and Marmot (1988), hypertensives were randomly assigned to various relaxation and control groups. General practitioners and their nurses were trained to administer the (Yoga-based) relaxation and stress management techniques. At the 1-year follow up, blood pressure changes in the relaxation groups were significantly more favourable than in the control groups. A related observation of great interest was that the subgroup that stopped taking antihypertensive drugs, and then commenced relaxation training, successfully maintained lowered blood pressure levels. In contrast, the subgroup that stopped taking medications, but did not engage in relaxation training, showed significant increases in both systolic and diastolic pressure.

A study by Kabat-Zinn, Lipworth, and Burney (1985) examined mindfulness meditation techniques in the treatment of chronic pain patients. Over a 10-week program, 90 chronic pain patients received training in mindfulness meditation, relaxation, and stress reduction methods. Significant decreases in pain and pain-related affect were observed in the treatment group. A control group of 21 patients given only customary medical treatment failed to show significant reductions in their pain measures.

In this paper, rather than summarizing research studies, our main purpose is to describe three meditative techniques we have found useful in clinical practice, especially with patients suffering from anxiety problems or classical insomnia. The three procedures described below can be useful in reducing 'mental chatter' and in 'quieting the mind'. As already mentioned, each of these exercises derives from a major type of meditative practice utilized within the Buddhist tradition.

PRACTICE I: ABDOMINAL BREATHING EXERCISE

A specific technique drown from the Vipassana tradition of meditation emphasizes relaxed, abdominal breathing in combination with paying quiet attention to the tiny muscular sensations in the abdominal muscles that accompany this respiratory pattern.

The Vipassana tradition, like several other meditative disciplines, makes explicit use of a relaxed, abdominal breathing technique. The three components of this technique which are readily identified and readily taught to patients consist of the following:

1. An erect but relaxed sitting posture.
2. A relaxed abdominal breathing procedure in which the abdomen rises gently on the in-breath and falls on the out-breath.
3. The use of a 'mental-quieting device'. Specifically, during the exercise, the patient quietly attends to the faint muscular sensations accompanying expansion and contraction of the abdomen. As an additional reminder to help in steadily focusing one's attention, the patient repeats quietly and subvocally, the words 'rise' on the in-breath and 'fall' on the out-breath.

WHAT ABOUT DIFFICULTIES IN LEARNING?

These generally are minimal. Probably the most frequently-encountered problem is that patients forget to employ the manoeuvre in the very situation where it is most needed. Under the pressure of extreme situational anxiety, he or she remains locked into the old reaction pattern. In such cases, it is useful to recommend not only practising the exercise several times during the day, but also to use it in various everyday situations that are only moderately stressful. In this way, the exercise becomes a more robust response, and is less likely to be derailed or forgotten under conditions of extreme emotion. (For a review of research on the physiology and psychophysiology of respiration, see Fried, 1993.)

EMPIRICAL WORK: APPLICATION TO PERFORMANCE ANXIETY

In our clinic, the abdominal breathing exercise has been used as an adjunct to systematic desensitization with 16 medical student patients suffering from performance anxiety associated with examinations or with public speaking situations. Six of the sixteen patients with performance anxiety reported the abdominal breathing exercise as being the most useful single procedure available to them during their encounter with the anxiety-evoking situation. An additional three said the abdominal breathing exercise was one of several skills that helped them during the stress episode. (In other words, at least 50 percent of our patient group reported the abdominal breathing exercise as being useful during their encounter with the anxiety-arousing situation.)

Three additional patients reported the abdominal breathing exercise to be helpful in 'decreasing background levels of tension', thus reducing anticipatory anxiety. One patient did not find the exercise useful in any way. Another three patients made good progress with their initial relaxation training, but then discontinued treatment prior to the introduction of either the abdominal breathing exercise or systematic desensitization.

ADVANTAGES OF THE EXERCISE

Several advantages of the abdominal breathing exercise are worth noting:

1. Its three components, posture, breathing pattern, and focus of attention, can be described to the patient in clear, operational terms.
2. The exercise does not take long to explain, and is quickly learned. Patients usually get 'the feel of it' within a few minutes (or over two or three episodes of practice).
3. The procedure is a tool that can be deliberately employed during the anxiety situation itself. Moreover, it is highly flexible and can be utilized in various situations the patient finds stressful.

PRACTICE II: MENTAL QUIETING EXERCISE

The abdominal breathing manoeuvre just-described constitutes a key part of another very useful exercise. This second exercise is a fundamental practice of both Zen Buddhism and in the Vipassana Mindfulness tradition of South-East Asia. Essentially, it involves paying close and continuing attention to certain sensations accompanying respiration. As this skill becomes stronger, the meditator uses it to bring about a cessation of mental activity, i.e. the paying of 'quiet attention' to respiratory sensations serves to interrupt the ordinary flow of images, thoughts, and feelings that comprise our normal (and unceasing) 'stream of consciousness'. (For comments on research pertaining to mental quieting, see Carrington, 1993, p. 143.)

This foregoing manoeuvre, which we refer to as the Mental Quieting Exercise, can be useful both in moderating anxiety-provoking thought processes, and especially in providing patients suffering from psychophysiological-type insomnia with a means of dealing with 'mental chatter'. Such chatter is usually the primary complaint in this kind of insomnia.

It is important to note that, although this exercise sounds disarmingly simple, attaining a high degree of skill takes a good deal of practice. Paying attention to a neutral stimulus for 100 percent of the time, and not being episodically derailed by intruding thoughts, can be an elusive and exasperating task. Accordingly, in keeping with behaviour therapy precepts, we make the task easier, at least initially. So instead of being instructed to pay attention to one's respiratory sensations 100 percent of the time, the guidelines are simply to "pay attention to the breathing sensations in your nose on **every in-breath**. Simply note the cool-air sensation in your nostrils as the air flows in. On the out-breath, just let your attention 'float'. Then on the next in-breath return to the cool-air sensation. As you become better at noticing the cool-air sensation, the thoughts begin to evaporate".

The instructions for this exercise overlap considerably with those for the abdominal beginning exercise. Indeed, the first two-parts, the posture and the breathing pattern, are identical. For the third and mental part, however, instead of attending to the tiny abdominal muscle sensations which accompany breathing, the patient focuses on sensations in the respiratory tract. These sensations, which are easily noticeable in the nose, for example, constitute a neutral stimulus that begins to service as a gentle 'anchor' for one's attention. Instructions for this third part of the exercise proceed approximately as follows:

> First, note the coolness in your nose as you breathe in. Next, on the out-breath, just let your attention 'float'. Then, on the next in-breath, again note the cool-air sensation on the in-breath, that's okay. Just make sure to make at least a brief return to the coolness sensation on every in-breath. With practice, your attentional focus gets steadier. The 'mental chatter' becomes softer, and you begin to quiet down mentally, kind of a nice condition.

For some fairly agitated patients, sustaining this kind of attentional focus can be a taxing business; it may be something they've never tried before. With such patients it is useful to apply the shaping concept. We recommend that they at 'first do the sequential-focusing on the in-breath for only three breath cycles in a row. Rest for a few seconds, then do a sequence of three once more. Then, as your attentional ability strengthens, increase the number to six breaths in a row, then later to twelve. After reaching twelve, simply repeat the cycle'.

Patients also generally find it more effective to practice this exercise with their **eyes closed**. The same holds for the Mental Quieting and the Mindfulness exercises to be described in the second half of this paper. (Parenthetically, however, it should be noted that in Zen meditation the eyes are kept half open, although this is something that exposes the beginner to more distractions).

EMPIRICAL WORK: APPLICATION TO INSOMNIA

Becoming skilled at this exercise is often helpful for patients suffering from classical, or psychophysiological, insomnia. Hauri, a leading authority on sleep disorders, indicates that both relaxation and meditation techniques are often useful in treating this type of insomnia (Hauri, 1991; Hauri & Linde, 1990).

In psychophysiological insomnia, probably the commonest presenting complaint pertains to an inability to bring about a cessation of racing thoughts. ('The harder I try to stop the thoughts, the more persistent they become'). Often, the patient's failure in the attempt to bring about sleep can lead to irritation, anger, or anxiety, none of which is conducive to sleep onset! Overall, the situation may be viewed as one in which the patient is locked into a psychophysiological feedback loop of continuing high arousal. First, a trickle of thoughts begins to trigger physiological arousal (e.g. skeletal muscle tension). Then, proprioceptive impulses from the muscles feed back into the CNS, thereby leading to increased cortical arousal and an accelerated surge of thoughts. The latter, in turn, trigger further physiological arousal.

A specific insomnia treatment program based upon the concept of a self-perpetuating vicious circle has been described by Steinberg (1991). In his view:

> The vicious circle of insomnia typically begins with incidents of emotional upset and acute stress. These experiences, in turn, create physiological tension and arousal and, consequently, insomnia. At this point, the person often feels tension and anxiety when preparing for bed and spends time in bed engaging in nonsleep activities and worry, behaviours that are contradictory to sleep (Steinberg, 1991, p. 157).

Over time, these nonsleep activities become associated with the bedroom and preparation for sleep. The outcome is a learned insomnia pattern.

Steinberg's therapy focuses on interrupting the vicious circle. Interventions can be made at each of several points in the sequence, and each patient usually receives interventions at more than one point in the cycle. Psychotherapy or systematic desensitization can be used to moderate the emotional reaction; relaxation and mental quieting techniques are used to reduce physiological as well as subjective arousal. Behaviour management techniques are used to reassociate bedtime and the bed with the state of sleep.

In our own work with insomniacs (referred by the Sleep Disorders Center at the University of Colorado Health Sciences Center), we have found the mental quieting technique to be a key intervention in interrupting the insomniac's psychophysiological feedback loop.

For some patients, a good muscle relaxation technique is sufficient to break into this loop. But there are many who complain that the 'racing thoughts' persist even when they are deeply relaxed. Such patients frequently benefit from the mental quieting procedure. For many patients, simply knowing they have mastered a technique for eliminating intruding thoughts and promoting sleep-onset serves to defuse anxiety about their problem.

A useful set of techniques for the insomniac is the following three-step sequence. This sequence can be employed either at sleep-onset, before a daytime nap, or when one wishes to make it easier to return to sleep after a nocturnal awakening. The instructions can be summarized as follows:

1. Do a brief progressive relaxation exercise, going from your toes and feet and arms up to your shoulders and neck.
2. Continue the relaxation, (as in the Jacobson sequence) up through your facial muscles. Be careful to relax all of your face muscles, including the muscles around your eyes, mouth, tongue and throat. (An important property of the facial muscles is that relaxation of these muscles is closely associated with a reduction in ideation and in emotional experience.) (Stoyva & Budzynski, 1993).
3. After doing the body and face muscle relaxation, shift to the mental quieting exercise, i.e. paying attention to the cool-air sensations on every in-breath. Repeat the three-step sequence several times if necessary. This technique can also be used to return to sleep after night-time awakenings.

Note that after the mental-quieting exercise has been well-learned, the patient may prefer to proceed directly to attending to respiratory sensations, thereby omitting the two muscle relaxation steps.

Many patients with psychophysiological insomnia report that this exercise clearly helps them in returning to sleep. It gives them a specific tool to use in the problem situation, and one which is directly relevant to their main presenting symptom. But, this said, two qualifying remarks are in order.

1. The technique is helpful for patients with insomnia of the psychophysiological type (usually characterized by sleep-onset difficulties in resuming sleep after frequent nocturnal awakenings). However, for insomnia of the early morning awakening type, typically associated with either clinical depression, or the ageing process, it may not be particularly efficacious. In this kind of insomnia, biochemical determinants are probably a key part of the phenomenon.
2. The exercise is usually offered in the context of providing other behavioural self-management interventions that are known to exert a demonstrable impact on sleep. These techniques include such things as (a) getting up at a fixed time in the morning, (b) avoiding the practice of daytime naps, (c) keeping busy during the day, (d) not going to bed too early in the evening, and (e) not remaining in bed for excessive amounts of time. These last two items are methods for consolidating (and deepening) the patient's sleep pattern (see Hauri and Linde, 1990).

PRACTICE III: THE PRACTICE OF MINDFULNESS

The practice of mental quieting just described leads to a consideration of mindfulness meditation. Indeed, the mental quieting exercise, in which one cultivates a steady and unforced attention to the regularly-recurring sensations that accompany breathing, constitutes a fundamental practice utilized in teaching this third kind of meditation.

A principal goal of mindfulness meditation, which is said to be a tradition going back to the original teachings of Gautama Buddha, is to foster a mental state characterized by a non-verbal present-mindedness. This state is very much a Here-and-Now condition. While cultivating it, the practitioner remains fully aware of what is going on, including his or her sensory and social surroundings, as well as the stimuli from within, such as thoughts, feelings, and perceptions. The critical skill is to note any thoughts that occur, and then to let go of them. A major point of emphasis is not to let oneself become fixated or absorbed in any particular thought, fantasy, emotion, or association. Instead, one gently lets go of each thought that occurs, then notes what comes up next to the 'mental screen'. One quietly notes the next thought, then lets go of it, and so on.

In mindfulness meditation, the individual remains wholly absorbed in the present task or situation, and at the same time, is aware of being thus absorbed. The practitioner is not wool-gathering, engaged in fantasies, whether pleasant or unpleasant, ruminating over the past, or worrying about the future. Thich Nhat Hanh, the Vietnamese poet and Zen master, uses the homely example of washing dishes:

> While washing the dishes one should only be washing the dishes, which means that while washing the dishes one should be completely aware of the fact that one is washing the dishes … If while washing the dishes, we think only of the cup of tea that awaits us, thus hurrying to get the dishes out of the way as if they were a nuisance, then we are not washing the dishes to wash the dishes. What's more, we are not alive during the time we are washing the dishes … If we can't wash the dishes, the chances are we won't be able to drink our tea either.

As Thich Nhat Hanh puts it, this mental habit of not-being-where-you-are means that 'we are sucked away into the future, and we are incapable of actually living one minute of life' (Thich Nhat Hanh, 1987, p. 5).

Similarly, Gunaratana (1993), a Buddhist priest trained in the Vipassana tradition, and also the holder of a Western doctorate in theology, offers the following descriptions:

> Mindfulness is the observance of the basic nature of each passing phenomenon. It is watching the thing arising and passing away (Gunaratana, 1993, p. 153).

You just notice exactly what arises in the mind, then you notice the next thing. 'Ah, this … and this … and now this' (Gunaratana, 1993, p. 156).

He also notes that mindfulness is a mental condition already present in consciousness at least part of the time. One place it manifests itself is in the initial stages of perception:

> When you first become aware of something, there is a fleeting instant of pure awareness just before you conceptualize the thing, before you identify it. That is a stage of mindfulness. It is the purpose of Vipassana meditation to train us to prolong that moment of awareness (Gunaratana, 1993, p. 150).

Practitioners in this tradition often speak of cultivating 'bare attention', i.e. conscious experience as it exists before it becomes encrusted with words and dismembered into concepts.

In order to cultivate mindfulness one engages in two related meditative practices. First, one learns to pay attention to breathing sensations (a procedure we have already described). This kind of practice helps develop ability at the requisite kind of concentration. Second, one engages in mindfulness meditation itself, and in the manner described in the above passages. Finally, one begins carrying the practice of mindfulness into everyday life.

A particular activity designed to bring mindfulness into the tasks of everyday life is the practice of walking meditation. Thich Nhat (1987) describes several variants of this exercise. One example would be hiking in the mountains. The hiker attends closely to the natural setting surrounding him. But if he notices that his thoughts have wandered away to what is not present, he then switches for a time to paying attention to breathing sensations. As the wandering thoughts begin to settle and then vanish, he again turns his attention to the natural setting, and to his direct impressions of it. This walking meditation exercise provides a means of fostering a calm and collected state of consciousness even during activity.[1]

For more details about the exercises described in this section, see Thich Nhat Hanh (1987, pp. 79–89, and pp. 11–14) and Gunaratana (1993, pp. 51–58, pp. 65–68, pp. 75–85, and pp. 149–183).

Another excellent source concerning this tradition of meditation is the volume by Kornfield (1993). Prior to becoming a clinical psychologist, Kornfield spent many years in southeast Asian monasteries studying the Theravada mindfulness tradition. In his clinical work, he combines mindfulness training with psychotherapy.

EMPIRICAL WORK AND SOME POTENTIAL APPLICATIONS OF MINDFULNESS MEDITATION

Observations from several independent sources, both eastern and western,

---

[1] It is possible that biofeedback technology could assist in some aspects of learning mindfulness meditation. For example, in biofeedback relaxation training, most subjects report that low frontal EMG (electromyogram) levels are associated with non-effort and with an absence of thinking of the directed, problem-solving type.

suggest the potential utility of the mindfulness techniques, or of closely-related procedures, as means of moderating the reaction to stress. In particular, it seems likely that techniques drawn from mindfulness meditation could be used both to minimize extraneous mental activity, and to help the individual keep his or her attention on-task during stressful situations. Several pertinent sources of evidence are the following:

1. **Sport and Fitness Research**
   An experimental investigation by Brown et al. (1995) examined the impact on psychological well-being of regular walking combined with mindfulness meditation. Their total of 135 subjects was divided into four different comparison groups and one control group. Training went on for 16 weeks. In the main comparison of interest, Brown et al. found that women who combined regular **low-intensity walking** with mindfulness techniques experienced significant reductions in feelings of tension, depression, anger, and total mood disturbance, as opposed to the pattern shown by the other groups without the mindfulness component.

2. **The Martial Arts**
   The martials arts can be described as focusing on one particular type of stressful interpersonal encounter, namely, hand-to-hand combat. For many centuries, in both China and Japan, meditative disciplines have been employed as an integral part of martial arts training. One beneficial result of meditation is deemed to be an enhancement of physical and mental tranquillity. Another benefit is thought to be an improvement in one's ability to pay close attention to events transpiring in the Here-and-Now, a skill of direct relevance, for instance, to the martial art of swordsmanship. In the Samurai art of swordsmanship, for example, a significant part of the discipline is learning to focus well during the martial encounter. The desired kind of concentration, moreover, is to be of an effortless kind.[2]

3. **The Stanislavki System of Acting**
   In the writings of Stanislavski, probably the most influential theatre director of the twentieth century, one sees clear-cut statements indicating that absorption in the present task constitutes an effective way of reducing performance anxiety, or stage fright. On the basis of observations on himself, and on fellow members of the Moscow Art Theatre, Stanislavski concluded that anxiety was closely associated both with increased muscular tension, and also with poor concentration.

---

[2] Something akin to mindfulness probably occurs in certain sports. In downhill skiing, for example, one must pay close attention to the present situation, including the next several hundred feet of slope. Or, again, in racquet sports, it is necessary to attend closely to the behaviour of the ball if one wishes to remain in the game. It may be that the deeply engaged quality of attention fostered by certain sports is an important part of the satisfaction they offer.

Anxiety and concentration were inversely related. The poorer one's concentration, the greater the anxiety, and the worse the performance.

In Stanislavski's view, the actor possesses two main weapons to draw upon in countering performance anxiety, 'relaxation and concentration'. Accordingly, Stanislavski first taught his actors to relax well muscularly, a skill that was to become near-automatic. Secondly, the actors were taught ways to improve their concentration. For instance, the actor was instructed to 'think of your action, not of your feelings. You will feel at ease and relaxed if you concentrate on action' (Moore, 1976, 26).

4. **Stress Research Literature**

At least two observations in the Western scientific literature attest to the idea of mindfulness skills as being relevant to the goal of moderating the stress reaction. One observation concerns the trait of job-involvement, a characteristic long regarded as a prominent part of the Type A coronary-prone behaviour pattern, and something that presumably implies a high degree of task absorption. But curiously, even though Type A and 'workaholic' are colloquially often used as synonymous terms, it appears that a high level of job involvement may actually diminish the likelihood of a coronary event (Dembroski, Weiss, Shields, Haynes & Fenleib, 1978).

Similarly, Flanagan (1987) in a survey aimed at determining the major and best empirically-documented coping strategies of stress-resistant individuals, identified the capacity for task involvement as one leading characteristic of such persons. (Three other important categories were: a sense of personal control; the presence of positive health practices, such as regular exercise and relaxation, along with low use of stimulants such as caffeine and nicotine, and utilization of social supports.)

5. **Rumination as an Impediment to Successful Coping Responses**

Another potential application of mindfulness meditation may be decreasing the tendency of some individuals to excessive rumination. Recent empirical work by Nolen-Hoeksema and her associates shows that the tendency to engage in rumination works both to impair performance under stress, as well as to impede psychological recovery after experiencing an episode of great stress. It seems probable that certain procedures drawn from the meditative disciplines could be used both to reduce extraneous mental activity and to help keep the individual's attention on-task.

As Nolen-Hoeksema (1996, p. 498) defines the term, rumination 'involves isolating ourselves to think about how badly we feel, worrying about the consequences of the stressful event of our emotional state, or repetitive talking about how bad things are without taking any action to change them'. Several studies conducted by Nolen-Hoeksema, and her coworkers over the past decade, support the idea that ruminative activity is a variable adversely contributing to the ability to cope with stress.

One of their investigations can fairly be described as 'an experiment of nature'. In this study, the researchers looked at emotional coping responses both before and after the San Francisco Bay Area earthquake of 1989. Just by chance, the investigators happened to have already taken measurements of depression, anxiety, and emotion-focused coping tendencies in a large group of college students two weeks prior to the day of the earthquake. The same students were then reassessed on these three measures at both ten days and seven weeks subsequent to the earthquake (Nolen-Hoeksema & Morrow, 1991).

Individuals who had exhibited a ruminative emotional coping style before the disaster were more likely to be depressed and anxious at both the ten day interval and at seven weeks after the earthquake. Those using alcohol or other drugs also did more poorly at follow-up. The shortest and least intense periods of depression were seen in the students who had engaged in various pleasant activities as a means of regaining a sense of personal control and emotional equilibrium after the earthquake.

An additional experimental study by this group suggests that rumination may interfere with effective problem-solving. In a laboratory study of depressed persons, it was found that depressed individuals who first engaged in ten minutes of rumination before turning to a task of problem-solving did worse than a comparably-depressed group who spent ten minutes occupied with a 'distraction task' before turning to the problem-solving task (Lynbomirsky & Nolen-Hoeksema, 1991). In a related study, it was noted that persons who engage in ruminative coping are less likely to utilize active problem-solving following a stress episode. Contrariwise, people who use pleasant activities (such as some form of distraction) to gain respite from their moods, and from emotional turmoil, were also more likely to employ some form of active problem-solving in coping with stressors.

In summary, it seems highly probable that methods drawn from the meditative disciplines could be used to reduce the tendency to ruminate. Such a goal seems eminently feasible when we consider that a principal emphasis within various forms of meditation has been to bring about a state of consciousness which is clear and tranquil, but in which verbal, analytical, and conceptual thinking are absent.

CONCLUDING REMARKS

Important issues for further investigation in this area are:

(a) learning more about the physiological substrate of particular meditative procedures;

(b) determining the therapeutic impact of a particular meditative procedure taken singly (i.e. used by itself);
(c) assessing combined effects, i.e. finding out which other stress management techniques can be fruitfully combined with the meditative procedure in question. For example, certain EEG biofeedback techniques may be useful in training aspects of attention—such as in teaching a patient to shift voluntarily from an analytical, problem-directed mode of consciousness to a mentally-quiet state;
(d) determining what kind of patient, and which disorders, are most amenable to treatment techniques based on meditation procedures.

In conclusion: the meditative disciplines, as we have attempted to show in this paper, have much to offer in expediting the task of stress management. To be sure, we should not expect miracles from these procedures. They are not the psychological counterpart of penicillin. Nonetheless, for those willing to learn and practice the requisite skills, the benefits can be substantial.

References

Benson, H. (1975) *The Relaxation Response*. New York: Moscow.

Brown, D. R., Wang, Y., Ward, A., Ebbeling, C. B., Fortlage, L., Puleo, E., Benson, H. & Rippe, J. M. (1995) Chronic psychological effects of exercise and exercise plus cognitive strategies. *Medicine & Science in Sports & Exercise*, **27**, 765–775.

Carrington, P. (1993) Modern forms of meditation. In *Principles and Practice of Stress Management*, (2nd edn) edited by P. M. Lehrer & R. L. Woolfolk, pp. 139–168. New York: Guilford.

Dembroski, T. M., Weiss, S., Shields, J. L., Haynes, S. & Feinleib, M. (eds) (1978) *Coronary-Prone Behavior*. New York: Springer Verlag.

Fried, R. (1993) The role of respiration in stress and stress control: Toward a theory of stress as a hypoxic phenomenon. In *Principles and Practice of Stress Management*, (2nd edn) edited by P. M. Lehrer & R. L. Woolfolk, pp. 301–331. New York: Guilford.

Gunaratana, H. (1993) *Mindfulness in Plain English*. Boston: Wisdom Publications.

Hauri, P. J. (ed.) (1991) *Case Studies in Insomnia*. New York: Plenum.

Hauri, P. & Linde, S. (1990) *No More Sleepless Nights*. New York: Wiley.

Kabat-Zinn, J. (1990) *Full Catastrophe Living*. New York: Delacorte Press.

Kabat-Zinn, J., Lipworth, L. & Burney, R. (1985) The clinical use of mindfulness meditation for the self-regulation of chronic pain. *Journal of Behavioral Medicine*, **8**, 163–190.

Kornfield, J. (1993) *A Path with Heart: A Guide through the Promises and the Perils of Spiritual Life*. New York: Bantam Books.

Lehrer, P. M. & Woolfolk, R. L. (eds.) (1993) *Principles and Practice of Stress Management* (2nd edn). New York: Guilford.

Lynbomirsky, S. & Nolen-Hoeksema, S. (1991) Effects of self-focused rumination on negative thinking and interpersonal problem-solving. *Journal of Personal and Social Psychology*, **69**, 176–190.

Moore, S. (1976) *The Stanislavski System: The Professional Training of an Actor*. New York: Penguin.

Nolen-Hoeksema, S. (1996) Coping skills. In *Hilgard's Introduction to Psychology* (12th edn), edited by R. L. Atkinson, R. C. Atkinson, E. E. Smith, D. J. Bem & S. Nolen-Hoeksema, pp. 497–499. Fort Worth, Texas: Harcourt Brace. (Pages 497–499 of this text provide a useful summary of Nolen-Hoeksema's research.)

Nolen-Hoeksema, S. & Morrow, J. (1991) A prospective study of depression and distress following a natural disaster: The 1989 Loma Prieta earthquake. *Journal of Personality and Social Psychology*, **61**, 105–121.

Patel, C. (1993) Yoga-based therapy. In *Principles and Practice of Stress Management* (2nd edn), edited by P. M. Lehrer & R. L. Woolfolk, pp. 89–137. New York: Guilford.

Patel, C. & Marmot, M. G. (1988) Can general practitioners use training in relaxation and management stress to reduce mild hypertension? *British Medical Journal*, **296**, 21–24.

Sheppard, J. L. (1989) Relaxation and meditation as techniques for stress reduction. In *Advances in Behavioural Medicine*, edited by J. L. Sheppard, Vol. 6, pp. 137–157.

Steinberg, N. (1991) Breaking the vicious circle of insomnia. In *Case Studies in Insomnia*, edited by P. Hauri, pp. 155–174. New York: Plenum.

Stoyva, J. M. & Budzynski, T. H. (1993) Biofeedback in the treatment of anxiety and stress disorders. In *Principles and Practice of Stress Management* (2nd edn), edited by P. M. Lehrer & R. L. Woolfolk, pp. 263–300. New York: Guilford. (See pages. 276–277 concerning relationship between frontal EMG and sleep onset).

Stoyva, J. M. & Carlson, J.G. (1993) A coping/rest model of relaxation and stress management. In *Handbook of Stress: Theoretical and Clinical Aspects* (2nd edn), edited by L. Goldberger & S. Breznitz, pp. 724–756. New York: Free Press/Macmillan.

Thich Nhat Hanh (1987) *The Miracle of Mindfulness: A Manual on Meditation*. Boston: Beacon Press.

Chapter 11

BEHAVIOR CHANGE FOLLOWING AFFECT SHIFT: A
Model for the Treatment of Stress Disorders

John L. Sheppard, PhD

A wide range of psychotherapies has emerged to deal with stress disorders that have a high anxiety component (Frank & Frank, 1991). Such disorders have become quite prevalent in our society, and have led to considerable reduction in human effectiveness, both in the workplace and in the home. Much research has now focused in this area, such as on traumatic stress syndromes (Wilson & Raphael, 1993). Studies have been conducted to test the value of particular therapies for particular aspects of disorder. While these therapies distinguish themselves by their unique characteristics, they hold nonetheless some common conceptual features. For example, a central experience by clients in many therapies is claimed to be an emotional catharsis and a movement from negative to positive emotion. This experience can be found in techniques that have very different orientations, theoretical background, purpose, credibility, scientific grounding, and cultural origin. An examination of the different sources of change can yield commonalities that point to core features. In this context I will consider eight different approaches.

(1) EYE MOVEMENT DESENSITIZATION AND REPROCESSING

Since 1989 a new technique has been reported by Francine Shapiro (Shapiro, 1989a, 1989b, 1990, 1991a, 1991b, 1992a, 1993, 1995, 1996a, 1996b, 1997; Shapiro & Forrest, 1997; Shapiro, Solomon & Kaufman, 1991; Shapiro, Vogelmann-Sine & Sine, 1994; Solomon & Shapiro, 1997) for treating victims of trauma and stress who had developed severe symptoms of anxiety. It is called Eye Movement Desensitization and Reprocessing (EMDR), and although controversial (Hammond, 1991, 1992; Metter & Michelson, 1993; Penzel, Ricciardi & Baer, 1992; Shapiro, 1993), is now widely practised in the

USA. In her training courses, Shapiro acknowledges how EMDR draws on the work of others, such as Joseph Wolpe's (1969) systematic desensitization, yet has its unique characteristics.

A substantial body of literature on EMDR is rapidly developing, thereby fulfilling an aim set by Shapiro (1992b). Initial studies investigated post traumatic stress disorder. Some of the research has become controversial, and there have been critiques of research designs used (Acieno, Hersen, Van Hasselt, Tremont et al., 1994; deBell & Jones, 1997; Herbert & Mueser, 1992; Lohr, Kleinknecht, Tolin & Barrett, 1995; Shapiro, 1996a, 1996b; Tolin, Montgomery, Kleinknecht & Lohr, 1995; Van Omeren, 1996). Lipke and Botkin (1992) reported mixed results with case studies on five PTSD veterans, but pointed out that their subjects presented with severe symptoms. Working with 30 PTSD veterans divided into a treatment EMDR group and two control groups, Boudewyns, Stwertka, Hyer, Albrecht, and Sperr (1993) reported reduced distress resulting for the EMDR group when dealing with traumatic memory material, but without significant change on physiological measures. Wilson, Becker and Tinker (1995; 1997) successfully used 4–5 hours of EMDR to treat traumatized subjects, achieving gains on several indices at posttreatment and at   18-montth follow-up. Carlson, Chemtob, Rusnak and Hedland (1996) found marked clinical improvements from EMDR in three out of four case study combat veterans with moderate to severe symptoms but not improvements on physiological measures. Jensen (1994), however, obtained negative results with veterans. A methodological difference between the Carlson et al. (1996) study and the Jensen (1994) is that in the former there was close attention to procedures, with Shapiro being used as a research advisor, and applying 12 treatment sessions with experienced therapists, while the latter used two sessions only, with therapists who were much less experienced. In a later study, Carlson, Chemtob, Rusnak, Hedland and Muraoka (1998) compared EMDR to biofeedback assisted progressive relaxation, with a control of routine clinical care, working with 35 combat veterans who had posttraumatic stress disorder. Relaxation and clinical care did not lead to improvements on indices used, but EMDR produced gains on a number of measures taken at posttreatment, as well as at 3-month and 9-month follow-up. Similar gains were found at posttreatment and 3-month follow-up by Rothbaum (1997) working with 21 PTSD female sexual assault victims. Experimental subjects improved significantly more than wait-list control subjects.

While EMDR has been used in the management of posttraumatic stress disorder (Shapiro, 1996a, 1997), it has also by now been applied successfully to depression (Shapiro, 1995; Shapiro & Forrest, 1997), sexual abuse (Shapiro, 1995; Shapiro & Forrest, 1997), dissociative disorders (Paulsen, 1995), Complex Personality Disorders (Fensterheim, 1996), grief (Solomon & Shapiro, 1997), substance abuse (Shapiro, Vogelmann-Sine & Sine, 1994), pain (Hekmat, Groth & Rogers, 1994), pathological gambling (Henry, 1996), phobia (Shapiro, 1995; Shapiro & Forrest, 1997), and panic attack (Goldstein & Feske, 1994).

EMDR is a psychotherapy in which typically a client with severe anxiety is asked to imagine an original trauma scene while tracking the eyes from left to right and right to left as the therapist moves a hand laterally across the client's visual field. This is done repeatedly during a session, and the client reports on thoughts, feelings, and body awareness, rating level of distress at the beginning and end on a scale 0–10 called a Subjective Units of Disturbance Scale (SUDS), and similarly rating how far one is towards one's self-image goal on a 7-point scale called a Validity of Cognition Scale (VoC). At some point during the sessions it is claimed there is a sudden change in feelings about the trauma. There is an acceptance, the anxiety disappears, and is replaced by considerations of a positive coping program developed by the client. If there has been a perpetrator of harm, forgiveness may appear. Clients can develop a sense of responsibility for their own actions, realise that they are now stress-free, safe, and not under threat, and are in a position to make quite capable choices about their future. There is an internal spontaneity to these changes, sometimes with a sense of surprise being experienced, but the therapist does guide the process, and may move from one area of pain to another when one area has been desensitized. The Reprocessing in the name Eye Movement Desensitization and Reprocessing applies to the spontaneous cognitive reconstruction that goes on in the client as the trauma is being worked on, that then leads on to the Desensitization of affect. All of this produces a new sense of identity in the person.

Shapiro has developed a theoretical explanation of EMDR in terms of neural networks, which she calls the Accelerated Information Processing model (Shapiro, 1995). When the client brings up memories or current stimuli each of these is a node or target in the neural network for the therapist to apply eye movements. EMDR links the cognitive with the affective, by opening up painful memories that have been blocked or frozen because of trauma, linking up neural networks that have been kept separated (adult information linking with child information). The eye movements are seen as having the capability of unfreezing an excitatory/inhibitory imbalance in the brain so that the memories may now undergo adaptive information processing (Shapiro, 1995).

Other explanations have also been suggested. Waters (1997) proposes that the eye movements lead to a process of resolute perception, a deliberate sustained focus of attention, designed to achieve clarity, and suggests a research design to test the theory (see Carlson & Chemtob, 1997 for a reply). On the other hand, Dyck (1993) suggests a distraction hypothesis, whereby deconditioning occurs as the client cannot concentrate on the image because of the distracting eye movements. Shapiro (1995) examines this claim and finds insufficient support for it in clinical and experimental findings. Andrade, Kavanagh, and Baddeley (1997) propose that the eye movements reduce the vividness and emotiveness of traumatic images via the visuospatial sketchpad of working memory, based on a research study. Nicosia (1995) contradicts a proposal that the eye movements may have a hypnotic effect, and considers on the basis of EEG monitoring that the EMDR state is qualitativeley different from the hypnosis state, showing EEGs within normal range and not differing from the waking state. This supports the views of Shapiro (1995). Greenwald (1995) proposes that the rapid integration of a traumatic memory occurring with the eye movements shows strong similarity to the process of dreaming and therapeutic dreamwork. Shapiro (1995) examined the idea that eye movements may be like REM sleep patterns, but found insufficient existing support for it. Yet another conceptualization sees EMDR as a form of exposure therapy, akin to techniques used with phobias (Carlson, Chemtob, Rusnak & Hedlund, 1996; Fulcher, 1994; Puk, 1991; ten Broeke & de Jongh, 1995). Patients are kept exposed to their trauma while the eye movements are occurring, and they come to find that they can be relaxed and not suffer. This leads them to a more rational approach to their circumstances rather than an emotional one. Shapiro (1995) draws attention to the fact that exposure studies require much more time than EMDR to be effective, and prefers an accelerated processing explanation. Just what is really going on in EMDR is not yet clear, and we can expect to see further explanations developed.

(2) AUTOGENIC NEUTRALIZATION

Anxiety reduction has been produced as a result of a special form of abreaction in a technique termed Autogenic Neutralization, an approach not widely known or utilized, although Autogenic Training is widely known, utilized, and researched (Linden, 1990, 1994; Linden & Lenz, 1997). The theoretical and practical details of this method were developed by Luthe (1969) and have been advocated by his student Adler (1992) who uses it in his psychiatric private practice for treatment of some stress disorders. During the 1970s in Montreal and San Francisco, Adler was a student of Wolfgang Luthe, who in turn was a student and colleague of Johannes Schultz (Schultz, 1953; Schultz & Luthe, 1959). Luthe has described Autogenic Neutralization in Volumes V and VI of his six volume work (Luthe, 1969). Using visualization and imagery, coupled with verbalization, brain-directed phenomena, and sensori-motor or visceral discharges under therapist guidance over an extended period of time with many sessions, patients finally develop a shift into a sense of well-being that replaces a previous state of tension, and have a sense of acceptance of the circumstances that have led to the development of their anxieties. There is a strong cognitive component to the therapy, but there is also a strong emotional effect, that becomes a clear motivator to the development of new positive adaptive behavior. The abreactions are believed to be triggered by primarily unconscious (e.g. post-traumatic) features of the patient's personal history. The method evolved from work in traditional Autogenic Training (Luthe, 1969) when certain patient-specific recurring discharges were found to be followed by symptom relief. It is, however, not the same as Autogenic Training.

Although the technique is difficult to master, Adler (1994) considers it is one of the most powerful available for quieting stressful traumatic memories and percepts, whether psychosomatic, physiologic, or psychological. In Adler's terms, the word 'neutralization' refers to its capacity to reduce the pathogenetic force of these influences via repeated discharge of the memories and their patient-specific symbols in a technique where the process is believed to be directed, even one might say choreographed, by subcortical mechanisms in the patient's brain. It is seen as being brain-directed, rather than therapist-directed. As such it not only operates with sophistication (as seen in dreams) but has built-in safety valves that protect the patient from overload, much like circuit breakers.

To be more specific, Adler (1994) has said, the technique includes the following procedures. After conducting Autogenic Training, an explanation of it is given to the patient in general terms, emphasizing that there is a building up of arousal in various areas of the brain that leads to the brain providing its own release when the person reaches the autogenic state and verbalizes his or her experiences. Standard instructions are then given as: "Would you now please develop the attitude of a spectator observing everything what flows through your stream of consciousness with an attitude of passive acceptance towards it, and in a continuous fashion would you please describe all that you see or feel or think." Eyes are closed, and the person does not move. The therapist does not make intellectual connections for the patients, but mainly offers help to keep the flow going, when it is seen that there is a blockage; e.g. "Do you think you can describe X a little more?"

Adler (1994) has said that he describes neutralization as occuring after the discharge of memories, and the brain has finished what was unfinished, so the pressure causing anxiety and associated behaviors is quieted down. There may be some crying and physical movements. When something very powerful has been discharged the patients may experience a phenomenon of extreme brilliant bright light with euphoria for several minutes. At the end, patients are often in a deep state of well being, with tension gone, and there is a reintegration, with acceptance.

What are the similarities to EMDR? Both techniques use visualization and imagery of memories, have a meditative repetitive aspect, cognitive working of the material, emotional catharsis, and a major moving from negative to positive emotion, ending with positive coping.

(3) TIBETAN PROSTRATIONS

There is a particular Tibetan Buddhist practice of grand prostrations (Blofeld, 1987; David-Neel, 1984, p. 188), a procedure only to be adopted when approved by one's teacher (Lama Chime Rinpoche, 1992). It consists of prostrating oneself on the ground 100,000 times, usually in a special room, on the floor of which have been placed some thin mattresses or cushions. In EMDR one moves the eyes back and forth from left to right, while here one is moving the body back and forth from up to down, in a repetitive pattern. While prostrating the devotee meditates and visualizes. One might do this for an hour at a time, or for longer periods. If practised every day the minimum completion time to get to 100,000 is a little under two years, and usually takes longer. You take it at your own pace. As time goes on, and one does more and more prostrations, one's thoughts narrow down, become more focused, and old ideas and images come forward from within one's depths, to the point where one becomes aware of strong emotions that can last sometimes for long periods, days or even weeks, to be followed ultimately by their reversal.

These emotions are particularly sexual desire (lust), anger (hatred), questioning of one's faith and feeling upset with its tenets or its proponents (ignorance), feeling very superior to others, to the point of possibly being offensive in one's behavior towards others (pride), feeling very acquisitive and wanting to have possessions (envy), to the point of possibly stealing small things belonging to someone else.

After a period, these negative emotions undergo a shift, a swing into the opposite, associated with a sense of calm and peace. The emotions and their shifts may be experienced one by one, not all at once.

In Buddhist teaching, there is to be a cleansing of 'the five main desire-passions of man, namely lust, hatred, ignorance, pride and envy' (Chang, 1963, p. 78). One can see that these are precisely the emotions I have just outlined. Table 11.1 lists the emotions before and after the shift from negative emotion to positive. In Buddhism, emotions of this kind are classified and referred to in different ways (sometimes varying which

Table 11.1 List of emotions in the cleansing of the five desires, with a shift from the negative to the positive

Emotions	
Before the shift	After a shift into the opposite
Lust; sexual desire	Detachment, absence of desire
Hatred; anger	Compassion, loving-kindness
Ignorance, doubt; questioning	Wisdom, faith
Pride; feeling superior	Renunciation, self-denial
Envy, jealousy; acquisitive of others' things	Giving, altruism

emotions or states are listed) by different authors, such as the Five Hindrances (Hanh, 1987, pp. 120–122, Yupho, 1984, p. 60), Styles of Imprisonment (Trungpa, 1976), the five internal evils that are contrasted to the five ways of righteousness (Yupho, 1984, p. 9), the five Kilesa (Mahaniranonda, undated, pp. 33–34; Nanasanvara, 1984, pp. 7–9, 16–19; Yupho, 1984), and the Ten Fetters or Samyojana (Humphreys, 1976, p. 166).

So this Tibetan practice has a basis in dogma. The shift in emotions, which may be of lasting effect, appears to be the same kind of emotional shift that Luthe and Adler speak about, and that is found in Eye Movement Desensitization and Reprocessing.

We have here a technique, developed many hundreds of years ago, that has similar psychotherapeutic effects to EMDR. Naturally, the efficacy of these effects can really only be checked by controlled research studies, and these have not been conducted. I would hope, however, that practices from the East will be investigated by Western researchers, and this is an example.

(4) KUNDALINI

Another concept that comes from the East is called the Kundalini rising or awakening, a notion emanating from Indian religions in the Hindu tradition, with an age-old history (Greenwell, 1991; Krishna, 1976; Swami Muktananda, 1978, 1979; Swami Vishnu Tirtha, 1962; Woodroffe, 1973). Experienced under the guidance of a guru, it is a progressive set of powerful sensations that begin in the lower part of the person's abdomen, work their way upward, and finally rise to the cranium, with a feeling that a force has shot out through the top of the head. It can be 'bestowed' on a person by a guru through a process called 'Shaktipat', or it may come more gradually. It is likened to a serpent (Swami Satyananda Saraswati, 1982; Woodroffe, 1973) uncoiling its way up from the base of the spine to the crown of the head.

Prior to Kundalini awakening, there has been a period of preparation, that normally includes meditation practices of a wide range of forms, but usually involving a concentration on doing good works or living a good life, thinking good or pure thoughts. Meditative visualization is often used. Images include deities or symbols (e.g. Shiva), the elements (e.g. a fire, a candle alight), objects in nature, the chakras (particular points aligned generally vertically in the body), and sounds (e.g. om; the chakra sound symbols).

Meditations may produce spontaneous visualization and imagery involving life experiences. Coming from a culture that believes in reincarnation these memories are often seen as being from past lives, even as far back as a thousand years or more. Many are about stressful events, of unpleasant things happening.

Kundalini awakening is viewed as a process of purification that brings many emotions to the fore, often in exaggerated intensity. 'Blockages ... give rise to such feelings as aversion, hatred, lethargy, dullness and greed, and these qualities also disappear when ... washed by the Kundalini' (Swami Muktananda, 1979, p. 34). This process is reminiscent of the subjective experience reported during the Tibetan practice of prostrations.

Together with the cleansing of emotions, there is believed to be a cleansing of the body through a range of Kundalini-induced body movements called kriyas. 'One may experience involuntary movements of the body, such as shaking and movements of the arms and legs. The head may even begin to rotate violently' (Swami Muktananda, 1979, p. 26). This is similar to the experiences that can occur in autogenic neutralization (Luthe, 1969), and in powerful abreactions in psychotherapy. The kriyas are believed to lead to a dissolution of the destructive and impure emotions, and a dissolution of the connection between unconscious memories and these emotions, leading to a state of bliss. This state of bliss may be accompanied by awareness of a blinding light (Krishna, 1976; Swami Muktananda, 1978, 1979), a feature which again is reminiscent of autogenic neutralization (Luthe, 1969).

The many emotions and imagery experiences, the movements, lights and visualizations that appear in meditation, usually prove to be matters for reflection. Some of the experiences are very stressful, and people begin to wonder what is happening, why it is happening, and ask questions about themselves generally. In other words, a person experiencing Kundalini has much cognitive working of material.

Proponents of Kundalini warn that there are distinct dangers when the practice is adopted without a guide. Indeed, even with a guru the individual may experience severe difficulties. These dangers have been described by Indians (Krishna, 1976; Swami Muktananda, 1978), but also by scholars in the West, where people have taken up the Eastern practices but without appropriate help, or where health workers have decided that misdiagnosed psychosis or neurosis is really a problematic manifestation of Kundalini awakening requiring therapeutic support (Fox, 1993; Greenwell, 1991; Greyson, 1993; Grof & Grof, 1986, 1990; Ossoff, 1993; Sanella, 1978; Thalbourne & Fox, 1993).

When problems are resolved, a wide range of positive experiences is described as resulting from the final stages of the working of the Kundalini. These include positive emotions (especially happiness and a love for others), friendliness, a strong belief in one's own inner self, knowledge and wisdom, and successful coping behavior (such as being creative) (Krishna, 1976; Swami Muktananda, 1979).

The Kundalini experience can therefore be seen to share all the six commonalities that we have highlighted: visualization and imagery of memories, meditation, emotional catharsis, cognitive working of material, moving negative emotions to positive, and final positive coping.

(5) EEG BIOFEEDBACK

Recently electroencephalographic biofeedback has been used to treat addictions, alcoholism, and Post Traumatic Stress Disorder. This research, like EMDR, is controversial (Cowan, 1993; Ochs, 1992; Rosenfeld, 1992; Wickramasekera, 1993; Wuttke, 1992), but there has been a great upsurge of interest in it (Peniston, 1994b) especially by clinicians since it was first reported (in 1989 like EMDR) by Peniston & Kulkosky (1989).

Peniston (1992, 1994a, 1996; Peniston & Kulkosky, 1989, 1990, 1991b; Saxby & Peniston, 1995) has been one of the major proponents in this area, and others have followed his procedure successfully (Byers, 1992; Fahrion, Walters, Coyne & Allen, 1992). He trained his subjects to produce a relaxed alpha state, then to go into theta, accessing stressful past memories and repressed material. Then they would go back to alpha to relax. He has found that if alcoholics were first given some temperature autogenic feedback training sessions, producing a relaxed state, followed by 15 sessions of rewarding feedback when they were producing more alpha frequency (8–12 hertz) and then later more theta wave (4–7 hertz) EEG feedback, they eventually developed a major change in drinking behavior, and did not want to drink.

During the feedback training they visualized themselves in an alcohol rejection scene. After training, most developed successful self-control of their drinking behavior. The initial research study had small samples and needed replicating, but the changes were striking: only 2 out of the 10 in the experimental biofeedback training group relapsed after 3 years, while 8 out of the 10 in a traditional medical therapy group relapsed. In a later study, Saxby and Peniston (1995) used the same training protocol for 20 sessions with 14 adults suffering chronic alcohol abuse. The Beck Depression Inventory showed marked reductions in depression, and a 21 month follow-up showed those who completed the training did not relapse.

The technique has also been used successfully with Vietnam veterans suffering Post Traumatic Stress Disorder (Peniston, 1990, 1992, 1994a, 1996; Peniston & Kulkosky, 1991a, 1991b). Patients have reported a marked reduction in nightmares and flashbacks.

We again have here a sudden emotional shift to the positive arising from switching between calm alpha and emotional theta. I suggest that this shift is the same kind that Luthe and Adler speak about, that happens with the Tibetan prostrations, as with Kundalini, and that is found in EMDR.

The salient elements in the procedure include visualization and imagery, a meditative, repetitive aspect in the many trials of the alpha/theta training, emotional catharsis, cognitive working of the material, and a shift from negative emotion to positive coping.

Peniston and Kulkosky (1991b, p. 7) state that their EEG biofeedback training 'optimized the surfacing of abreactive imageries' in Post Traumatic Stress Disorder patients. This highlights a feature in yet another therapy: traditional psychotherapy.

(6) ABREACTIONS IN TRADITIONAL PSYCHOTHERAPY OR PSYCHOANALYSIS

In psychoanalysis (Freud, 1922, 1933), the process of therapeutic change is typically dependent on the development of transference, that may be either positive and idealised, or negative. Freud has described transference in the following way. 'Every time that we treat a neurotic psycho-analytically, there occurs in him the so-called phenomenon of *transference*, that is, he applies to the person of the physician a great amount of tender emotion, often mixed with enmity, which has no foundation in any real relation, and must be derived from the old wish-fantasies of the patient which have become unconscious. Every fragment of his emotive life ... is accordingly lived over by the patient in his relations to the physician .... The symptoms ... can only be dissolved in the higher temperature of the experience of transference' (Rickman, 1953, p. 38).

Healing in this form of therapy occurs when, through a process of uncovering, the unconscious becomes conscious, the conflict between wishes and fears is understood and resolved, and the transference is worked through to a point of experienceing a more balanced emotional tone. Says Freud (1949, p. 138), 'When, in the course of an analysis, we have given the ego assistance and have put it in a position to abolish its repressions, it recovers its power over the repressed id and can allow the instinctual impulses to run their course as though the old situations of danger no longer existed'.

During therapy, patients transfer onto the analyst their childhood conflicts and feelings that arose in relation to their parent, in whose place the analyst now stands. Childhood images and visualizations are explored, examined cognitively, re-shaped cognitively, and some old emotions are re-experienced. Sometimes these emotions become intense, and abreaction occurs, in which there is emotional release. Says Freud (1949, pp. 161–162), "a danger-situation is a recognized, remembered and expected situation of helplessness. Anxiety is the original reaction to helplessness in the trauma and is reproduced later on in the danger-situation as a signal for help .... The ego ... now repeats it actively in a weakened version, hoping to have the direction of it in its own hands .... If this is meant by 'abreacting a trauma' we can have nothing to urge against the phrase".

It is not hard to see that once again we have a similar set of features here to what we have been describing in the earlier approaches. We have visualization and imagery of memories, a washing out of emotions that produces a numbing effect so that those emotions are no longer troublesome, a cognitive working of material, a shift of emotion to the opposite emotion, and an element of surprise in patients. It is not apparent how it has a repetitive, meditative aspect, other than perhaps in the fact that in classical psychoanalysis one is lying down in a relaxed pose, with eyes closed, thereby providing ample opportunity to go over and over aspects of one's conflicts.

(7) NEUROLINGUISTIC PROGRAMMING

NLP has been used for a wide range of stress disorders, including anxiety conditions, Post Traumatic Stress Disorder, results of abuse, and phobia (Angell, 1996; Barnett, 1990; de Luynes, 1995; Hoenderdos & van Romunde, 1995; House, 1994; Macdonald, 1997; Sterman, 1991). As with EMDR, the theoretical basis to the technique has yet to be fully examined, and is controversial (Baddeley, 1989; Baddeley & Predebon, 1991; Beyerstein, 1990; Coe & Scharcoff, 1985; Elich, Thompson & Miller, 1985; Jupp, 1989a, 1989b; Monguio-Vecino & Lippman, 1987; Starker & Pankratz, 1996; Wertheim, Habib & Cumming, 1986; Wilbur & Roberts-Wilbur, 1987). Use of the technique is widespread, with many reports of positive effectiveness (Beaver, 1989; Curreen, 1995; Duncan, Konefal & Spechler, 1990; Einspruch & Forman, 1988; Field, 1990; Holdevici, 1990, 1991; Hossack & Standidge, 1993; Konefal, Duncan & Reese, 1992; Masters, Rawlins, Rawlins & Weidner, 1991; Mayers, 1993; Shelden & Shelden, 1989; Stanton, 1989).

As described by the Bandlers, the Andreas and Grinder in a number of publications (Andreas & Andreas, 1989; Andreas & Andreas, 1987, 1992; Bandler, 1985; Bandler & Grinder, 1975, 1979, 1982; Cameron-Bandler, 1985; Dilts, Grinder, Bandler, Bandler, & DeLosier, 1980; Grinder & Bandler, 1976, 1981), there is a strong use of visualization and imagery of memories, childhood, old hurts and problem or feared stressful situations. The client may be asked to 'make a picture in your mind's eye', looking for childhood memories, then building onto them new memories by visualizing a positive version of the old hurt, changing negative images to a positive self-image. Clients report on their experience to the therapist, who guides the imagery into a positive direction, offering new perspectives, interacting many times with the client, who keeps reporting sensations from the imagery experiences. The therapist may take the client back to the initial problem situation and go over it again, this time without the problem emerging. When that happens therapy has been successful.

In addition to the client reports, the therapist watches body cues to inner experiences, particularly noting evidence of tension, relaxation, fear and anxiety, anger, happiness and joy. Sessions leading to change in emotion are reported as being as short as 10, 15 or 30 minutes, within which time the person's emotional state has moved to the reverse of what it was at the beginning, going from tension to calm, fear to acceptance, anger to peace. A technique of anchoring uses a physical 'mantra' which is very repetitive, and many NLP exercises use a repetitive switching.

Andreas and Andreas (1989) outline a procedure which 'neutralizes intense bad feelings' (p. 68) that have arisen from abuse and trauma, and describe how to 'reprocess' (p. 70) these experiences. We see here terminology reminiscent of Luthe's autogenic neutralization, and the reprocessing feature in the R of EMDR.

So once again we have a method that concentrates on visualization and imagery, causes a numbing effect on intense emotions which make a sudden shift from negative to positive, the numbing is like an emotional catharsis so their intensity is gone, and there is a very active cognitive working of the material, with a repetitive, meditative aspect.

(8) SUINN'S ANXIETY MANAGEMENT TRAINING

In 1971 Richard Suinn, at the University of Colorado in Fort Collins, developed a technique of self-control and self-regulation using applied relaxation and competence imagery (Suinn & Richardson, 1971; Suinn, 1990). Among many other conditions, he has found it useful in the treatment of hypertension, ulcers, stomach distress, nausea, diabetes, headaches, shoulder tension, insomnia, performance anxiety, Post Traumatic Stress Disorder (dealing with anxiety, panic attacks, nightmares, flashbacks, anger control), and other stress disorders (Suinn, 1992). By now there are over 50 research studies in the literature attesting to its effectiveness.

After an intake interview assessment session, the client in Anxiety Management Training (AMT) identifies an anxiety experience, preferably a recent one. Therapy consists of sequences of imagery about the anxiety scene (rated by the client on a scale of 0–100 for severity) coupled with relaxation produced through a revision of the technique of Wolpe and Lazarus (1966) used in systematic desensitization. The client engages in home practice and keeps a relaxation log and a stress log. In succeeding sessions the therapist guides a sequence of anxiety scene followed by relaxation repeatedly. In later sessions the client is instructed to remain in the anxiety scenes while producing the relaxation, rather than doing them sequentially. The technique clearly owes a debt to the systematic desensitization approach of Wolpe (1969, 1973), in turn derived from the progressive muscle relaxation technique of Jacobson (1938, 1970).

How does AMT fit within the constellation of techniques I have been describing? It uses visualization and imagery of memories, it has a repetitive meditative aspect (both through the use of a relaxation technique and by the repeated returning to an anxiety scene coupled with relaxation), there is cognitive working of the material, there is emotional catharsis, a numbing, a neutralization, a desensitization, and there is a shift from negative to positive emotion, leading to coping behaviour.

A THEORETICAL MODEL FOR THE TREATMENT OF STRESS DISORDERS: A VISUO-COGNITIVE AFFECT SHIFT (VCAS) MODEL

The same six essential features are to be found in eight separate therapies. These features have been represented in Figure 11.1 as a model for treatment. The model draws on Hegel's theory of the dialectic on the left, describes the steps of growth in the middle and categorizes their essential actions on the right.

The proliferation of therapies has prompted a number of authors to search for common elements. Patterson (1966) considered the three conditions proposed by Rogers (1957), empathic understanding, unconditional positive regard or respect, and congruence or therapeutic genuineness, to have generality across the therapies, but was later concerned (Patterson, 1977) at the divergence of approaches emerging. Karasu (1986) proposed three common features: affective experiencing, cognitive mastery, and behavioural regulation. The model in Figure 11.1 has an affinity with this approach. Phares (1988) proposed the list should contain the inner world, release of emotion, reciprocal communication between therapist and client, a special relationship between therapist and client, anxiety reduction, building competence, self-efficacy and professional competence and skill in the therapist role. Release of emotion and anxiety reduction both find an important place in the Figure 11.1 model, but indeed the features listed are all relevant to it.

Other proposals for commonalities have been made by Bohart and Todd (1988), Brady et al. (1980), Frank (1982), Goldfried (1980), Grencavage and Norcross (1990), Hobbs (1962), Kleinke (1994), Korchin and Sands (1983), Marmor (1985), Stiles, Shapiro and Elliott (1986), and Strupp (1986).

Frank and Frank (1991) proposed that all psychotherapies share four effective features: an emotionally charged, confiding relationship with a helping person; a healing setting; a rationale, conceptual scheme, or myth that provides a plausible explanation for the patient's symptoms and prescribes a ritual or procedure for resolving them; and that ritual or procedure requires active participation of both patient and therapist and is believed by both to be the means of restoring the patient's health. One of the functions of myth and ritual is arousing emotions, which makes an important contribution to attitude change. These two features are represented significantly in the Figure 11.1. model. While these commonalities of Frank and Frank were applied to Western therapies, they are relevant to all the eight techniques considered in the present chapter, including those from the Eastern traditions.

At the heart of the model of visuo-cognitive affect shift (VCAS) is a cognitive-affective dimension: the cognitive-working and the emotional divesting/shift. These processes are stimulated by triggers used in the preparation phase, and they result in behavioural mastery. The six features found common in the eight therapies can be reduced to four components: initial triggers, cognitive-working, emotional divesting/ shift, final behavioural mastery. These elements are the same as those proposed by Karasu (1986) except for the addition of the triggers.

Figure 11.1 shows that there is a preparation phase in all eight approaches, where the scene is set for the subsequent cognitive-working phase. Preparation is facilitated by providing a relaxed environment where

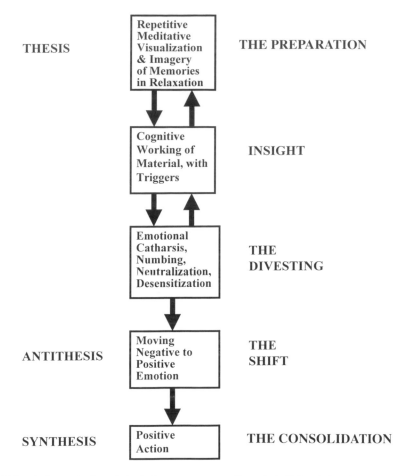

Figure 11.1 A theoretical model of visuo-cognitive affect shift (VCAS) for the treatment of stress disorders

the individual can feel safe, to re-experience past and current disturbing events. The preparation phase involves the 'healing setting' of Frank and Frank (1991) and the 'supportive atmosphere' of Marmor (1985). This starting point represents a thesis in the Hegelian dialectic sense, a statement of self-identity.

Preparation techniques include the practice of repetitive meditative visualization and imagery of traumatic memories in a state of induced relaxation. Many research studies show the effectiveness of these basic procedures for establishing psychological and physical health through stress reduction (Lehrer & Woolfolk, 1993; McGuigan, 1975, 1991; Pinkerton, Hughes & Weinrich, 1982; Sheppard, 1989). Five of the eight approaches to therapy appear to draw on the essential concepts involved in the systematic desensitization technique of Wolpe (1958, 1969), who reduced anxiety level by visualization of a feared object or event while practising relaxation, working through a progressive sequence of stimuli of increasing threat level. The impact of Wolpe's technique on therapeutic practice has been widespread. The three approaches which cannot draw on Wolpe are those developed before his time: psychoanalytic abreaction, Tibetan prostrations, and the Eastern kundalini phenomenon. Nonetheless, it has been shown that these all contain the esential elements of the preparation phase of the VCAS model, acting as triggers to the processes which follow.

In all eight techniques we have a facilitator helping set the healing process in motion and indeed continuing as a guide through that process. In none of the eight procedures does the person work alone; it is always with a helper, an external agent with whom there is a therapeutic relationship. These agents take many forms: for example, monk, guru, guide, psychotherapist, psychologist, psychiatrist. The person views the agent as a knowledgeable expert in their field, offering a safe environment for self expression and self-development. It was mentioned earlier that Phares (1988) regarded professional competence and skill in the therapist role, and a special relationship between therapist and client, as two of the commonalities across therapies.

All eight techniques involve the external agent as an expert, but in different ways. In eye movement desensitization and reprocessing the agent is primarily seen as a psychologically-skilled facilitator, in autogenic neutralization a psychologically-skilled or medically trained facilitator, in Tibetan prostrations a spiritual master, in Kundalini an awesome bestower of grace, in EEG biofeedback a highly trained behavioural technician, in psychoanalytic/psychotherapeutic abreaction usually a medically trained interpreter of the unconscious, in neurolinguistic programming a directive guide, in anxiety management training a psychologically-skilled facilitating guide. Despite the subtlety of the differences, all are seen by the person as holding a professional role of competence and special skill that they respect. Considering the fact that different therapeutic approaches can be effective, with somewhat different professional roles, the differences are not what are important, but the common features.

The therapeutic relationship between person and external agent described by Phares (1988) involves accepting, nonjudgemental revelations of one's inner life with warmth between both parties. The greatest differences among the eight approaches are between the Western and the Eastern therapies. Western therapies emphasize the therapist's genuineness, empathy, and unconditional positive regard of Rogers (1957), and the collaboration between therapist and client of Sullivan (1953) in a working alliance (Horvath & Symonds, 1991). Eastern and Western approaches both feature these characteristics, but in the Eastern there is a greater distance between the external agent and the person, with considerable veneration bestowed on the agent. Strupp (1986) speaks of the Western therapist as a mentor, model, or teacher in a collaboration. The Tibetan monk and the Indian guru are treated with higher respect than the Western therapist and are seen as teachers of great authority and wisdom who are the spiritual masters of the person, a follower of their way. However, despite these differences between East and West, the therapeutic relationship is a common feature, and as Yalom (1980) says, it is the relationship that heals. This is just as true of the Western position as it is of the Eastern.

While the external agent is important in the establishment and maintenance of a healing process, the nature of the preparation procedures is such that they set in motion a cognitive working that has an internal spontaneity to it, that is not totally dependent on an external agent like a therapist. The real work is going on 'inside' the person, that is, the 'inner world' of Phares (1988). The preparation procedures lead to insights and cognitive restructuring. The therapist is able to guide and facilitate this process, but does not directly 'cause' it to happen, as it is an internal change. This lack of an external agent is most dramatic in the case of the Tibetan prostrations.

Insights reached in the cognitive phase (compare with the 'cognitive mastery' of Karasu, 1986) may change the impact of the preparation activities so that they in turn lead to new insights in a loop effect that can cycle multiple times. The reverse arrows in Figure 11.1 are intended to represent this feature.

With the development of cognitive restructuring a further spontaneous internal event occurs, which the person does not 'create' or 'make happen', but which seems to the client to have a determinism of its own, namely, an emotional discharge. Describing commonalities, this is discussed by Karasu (1986) as 'affective experiencing', Phares (1988) as 'release of emotions', Frank and Frank (1991) as 'emotional arousal', and Bohart and Todd (1988) as 'arousal of emotion'. The cognitive and the emotive, thought and emotion, here come together in a unique whole. There is a divesting of the emotional attachments that have been dominant, whether they be fear, anxiety, jealousy, guilt, pain, hatred, anger, or aggression. There is a sense of them flowing out and away, leaving an emptiness where they have been, as they are no longer there. This emotional discharge or catharsis may be an intense experience, welling up within the person, bringing on tears or other abreactive expression of feelings, thereby releasing the emotions through a process of heightening them. Such discharge may in its turn lead to further cognitive restructuring, and is represented in Figure 11.1 by a reverse arrow. Indeed the cognitive working of the second phase in the model may not produce insight for the client, i.e. a conscious appreciation of new perspectives, but may directly trigger emotional catharsis, and cognitive change may occur after the emotional discharge. As with the first and second phases, there can be a feedback loop between the second and third phase.

Frank and Frank (1991) point out that strong emotional arousal is involved in traditional healing rituals of non-Western countries and in religious conversion in the West. They propose that one can group some techniques as abreactive therapies, and consider the commonalities they hold. Such treatments, now particularly used for the management of posttraumatic stress disorder, typically require the client to experience past traumatic events with intense emotional discharge. 'All require a highly supportive setting, a therapist who takes full charge, and various methods of encouraging the patient to remember or re-create the events in fantasy' (Frank & Frank, 1991, p. 234). These features all apply to the eight techniques from which the VCAS model is derived. The techniques are therefore not representative of psychotherapies in general, but are a subset relevant to the treatment of stress disorders.

After the divesting of emotion, the model indicates a shift into the antithesis of the original emotion attached to the visualized stressful memories, moving from a negative to a positive orientation. This is shown in Figure 11.1 as an antithesis according to the sequence of the Hegelian dialectic. This shift is also spontaneous. From the client's point of view, it is not that the person says: 'I now want to change my emotion'. Instead, it suddenly 'happens' to the person, who indeed may be quite surprised by it, wonder why or how it is happening, and question the whole event. Despite such questioning, there may develop a sense of 'What does it matter?' when contemplating the original visualized memory of stress, and an accepting, forgiving feeling towards those who had produced the original pain, replacing negative affect. This subjective pattern of change has not been particularly highlighted by writers seeking commonalities.

The changes in emotion follow such a fixed sequence that it suggests there is a natural process involved, with its own inherent momentum that has a self-healing quality. (Note that Friedman (1991) speaks of the existence of a 'self-healing personality'.) It can be compared to what happens when there is a healing process at the physical level, such as when one's skin is cut. We have a hard-wired natural process that deals with the lesion, by the coagulation of the blood to seal up the wound and by a knitting together of the folds of the skin, so that within some days the wound has healed. The auto-immune system is spontaneously triggered to defend the lesion, and a whole series of complicated natural processes follow. A similar sequence may be hypothesized for a psychological lesion, for which an autonomous, neurologically hard-wired system may be spontaneously triggered to repair, so that eventually the psychological stress wound has healed. The trauma is like the knife making the cut; the early negative affect is like the cut itself, the lesion that has been created by the trauma; the emotional discharge is like the flowing out of the blood; the numbing or desensitization effect is like the coagulation of the blood so there is no longer any flow; the reversal of affect from the negative to the positive is like the knitting of the skinfolds thereby obliterating the cut; final positive action is like making effective use of the affected limb or body part.

A neurologically hard-wired system in the treatment of stress response syndromes is proposed by Everly (1984, 1985, 1989) with a neurocognitive therapy, designed to produce neurologic desensitization (Everly, 1993), on the basis that the syndromes involve pathognomonic arousal and cognitive-affective processes which facilitate that arousal. Everly (1993) presents a neurophysiological model of posttraumatic stress disorder involving neurologic hypersensitivity and hyperexcitation, whereby a precipitating event leads to an interpretation that produces pathognomonic arousal and recollective ideation, both of which contribute to a numbing, withdrawal, and depression. Procedures which reduce arousal are advocated (Everly & Benson, 1989), as they lock into the neurologically hard-wired system of the disorder, where 'hypersensitivity is proposed to exist as a lowered functional threshold for depolarization of neurons within the limbic system and its immediate neurologic and neuroendocrine effector mechanisms (e.g. the sympathetic nervous system, the adrenal medullary catecholamine system, and even the adrenal cortical axis). The net result of this functional hypersensitivity is thought to be unusually high levels of excitation within the effector systems' (Everly, 1993, p. 799).

The Everly (1993) model's attention to arousal therefore lends support to the possibility of a neurologically hard-wired system involved in the emotion phases of the VCAS model, but one should also note that his model contains cognitive-affective processes that facilitate arousal. The respective importance of cognitive and affective aspects of therapy have been a matter of dispute (Lang, 1984; Rachman, 1981). Lazarus (1984) argued for the primacy of cognition, Zajonc (1984) for primacy of affect.

Kleinke (1994) lists nine common therapeutic processes, among which are establishing the corrective emotional experience, and allowing the experience of emotions. Phares (1988, p. 321) says 'some have stated that psychotherapy without anger, anxiety, or tears is no psychotherapy at all', while Frank and Frank (1991, p. 46) say 'emotional arousal is essential to therapeutic change'. Alexander and French (1946, p. 66) say a central goal in therapy is 'to reexpose the patient, under more favourable circumstances, to emotional situations which he/she could not handle in the past'.

Frank and Frank (1991, p. 239) consider 'abreactive therapies excel in their ability to change the patient's self-image from that of a person who is at the mercy of emotions to one who can withstand and eventually control them'. This implies that it is the emotional experience that comes before the cognitive one, the attitude change. The VCAS model acknowledges this sequence by the feedback loop.

Proponents of cognitive behaviour therapy consider emotional change is most effectively produced after cognitive-working (e.g. Lazarus, 1984). The rational-emotive therapy of Ellis (1962, 1973) establishes the cognition/emotion nexus in a technique which emphasizes confronting one's illogical thinking, and Beck's (1976) cognitive therapy targets on modifying dysfunctional thoughts. In the VCAS model cognitive-working is seen as a trigger to emotional discharge, and this may or may not be with insight at the beginning of the process. The mere act of cognitive-working can become a trigger to the emotional experience.

Kleinke (1994) proposes six goals relevant to almost all psychotherapies, and includes helping clients achieve insight, but says insight is neither necessary nor sufficient for therapeutic change, and Marmor (1990) points out one can achieve an intellectual insight into one's past and still not change. In the VCAS model the term insight has been used broadly, to include the cognitions resulting from emotional discharge as well those which produce it, the kinds of processes used by the cognitive behaviour therapists, and the traditional sense.

After the emotional shift phase, the person has an opportunity for positive change in behaviour, to move forward from the restricted lifestyle that the original conflicts and their attendant affects had produced. This is the 'behavioural regulation' of Karasu (1986), where behavioural change takes place, with a commitment to new patterns of practice. Such positive change is a consolidation of the whole process, synthesizing what has been learned, and is represented in Figure 11.1 as the synthesis stage in the Hegelian dialectic of the VCAS model.

To move in the direction of positive change, the person treads a path in search of self-efficacy (Bandura, 1977, 1982), a part of their identity (Kleinke, 1994). At the end of the trail the person has a reformulated identity, enhanced by behavioural mastery. The sense of self and self-worth (Linville, 1985, 1987) has been re-cast. The therapies touch on significant aspects of the person's being, and if they are to be effective then they must touch the person deeply. Major questions underlying the cognitive processing that is occurring include who, what, and where am I in this world?

Much has been written about the need for identity. Erickson (1968), for example, has described how it emerges during adolescence as a major developmental stage. But it is not something that is completed in adolescence, and is a struggle that a person may have all through life. It may recur during what has been termed the mid-life crisis period (O'Connor, 1981), for example. Maslow (1970) sees self actualization, preceded by self-esteem, as being at the top of his hierarchy of human developmental needs. The most fulfilled person is the one who has attained a clear sense of identity, and has a lifestyle that expresses that identity.

SUMMARY

Stress disorders with a high anxiety component have been treated by some therapies that have features in common. This chapter has addressed the question of why such therapies have led to purported successful treatment. Inspection of a number of different approaches reveals six common features: visualization and imagery of memories in relaxation, a repetitive meditative aspect, cognitive working of material with triggers, emotional catharsis with a numbing/neutralization/desensitization, and moving from negative emotions to positive, culminating in positive coping. The different approaches come from a diversity of perspectives, including the psychodynamic, learning theory, Eastern religious traditions, and theories of brain functioning. They have been applied in cases of shell shock, war neurosis, and combat produced post traumatic stress disorder, as well as rape, child abuse, torture, man-made disasters, and natural disasters. The commonalities isolated have been used to construct a theoretical model of visuo-cognitive affect shift for the treatment of stress disorders, creating a sequential pattern of behaviours.

References

Acieno, R., Hersen, M., Van Hasselt, V. B., Tremont et al. (1994) Review of the validation and dissemination of eye movement desensitization and reprocessing: A scientific and ethical dilemma. *Clinical Psychology Review*, **14**, 287–299.

Adler, C. S. (1992) *Fluctuating Awareness of Physiology During Different Types of Psychotherapy*. Paper presented at the 23rd Annual Conference of the Association for Applied Psychophysiology and Biofeedback, Colorado Springs, USA.

Adler, C. S. (1994) Personal communication.

Alexander, L. B. & French, T. M. (1946) *Psychoanalytic Therapy: Principles and Application*. New York: Ronald.

Andrade, J., Kavanagh, D. & Baddeley, A. (1997) Eye movements and visual imagery: A working memory approach to the treatment of post-traumatic stress disorder. *British Journal of Clinical Psychology*, **36**, 209–223.

Andreas, C. & Andreas, S. (1989) *Heart of the Mind*. Moab, Utah: Real People Press.

Andreas, S. & Andreas, C. (1987) *Change Your Mind—and Keep the Change*. Moab, Utah: Real People Press.

Andreas, S. & Andreas, C. (1992) Neuro linguistic programming. In *The First Session in Brief Therapy*, edited by S. H. Budman, M. F. Hoyt & S. Friedman, pp. 14–35. New York: Guilford.

Angell, G. B. (1996) Neurolinguistic programming theory and social work treatment. In *Social Work Treatment: Interlocking Theoretical Approaches*. (4th edn), edited by F. J. Turner, pp. 480–502. New York: Free Press.

Baddeley, M. (1989) Neurolinguistic programming: The academic verdict so far. *Australian Journal of Clinical Hypnotherapy and Hypnosis*, **10**, 73–81.

Baddeley, M. & Predebon, J. (1991) 'Do the eyes have it?': a test of neurolinguistic programming's eye-movement hypothesis. *Australian Journal of Clinical Hypnotherapy and Hypnosis*, **12**, 1–23.

Bandler, R. (1985) *Using Your Brain—for a Change*. Moab, Utah: Real People Press.

Bandler, R. & Grinder, J. (1975) *The Structure of Magic*, vol. 1. Palo Alto: Science and Behavior Books.

Bandler, R. & Grinder, J. (1979) *Frogs into Princes*. Moab, Utah: Real People Press.

Bandler, R. & Grinder, J. (1982) *Reframing: Neuro-Linguistic Programming and the Transformation of Meaning*. Moab, Utah: Real People Press.

Bandura, A. (1977) Social-efficacy: Toward a unifying theory of behavioral change. *Psychological Review*, **84**, 191–215.

Bandura. A. (1982) Self-efficacy mechanism in human agency. *American Psychologist*, **37**, 122–147.

Barnett, E. A. (1990) The contribution and influence of neurolinguistic programming on analytical hypnotherapy. *Australian Journal of Clinical Hypnotherapy and Hypnosis*, **11**, 1–14.

Beaver, R. (1989) Neirolinguistic programme as practised by an educational psychologist. *Educational Psychology in Practice*, **5**, 87–90.

Beck, A. T. (1976) *Cognitive Therapy and the Emotional Disorders*. New York: International Universities Press.

Beyerstein, B. L. (1990) Brainscams: Neuromythologies of the New Age. Special Issue: Unvalidated, fringe and fraudulent treatment of mental disorders. *International Journal of Mental Health*, **19**, 27–36.

Blofeld, J. (1987) *The Tantric Mysticism of Tibet*. Boston: Shambhala.

Bohart, A. C. & Todd, J. (1988) *Foundations of Clinical and Counselling Psychology*. New York: Harper & Row.

Boudewyns, P. A, Stwertka, S. A., Hyer, L. A., Albrecht, J. W. & Sperr, E. V. (1993) Eye movement desensitization for PTSD of combat: A treatment outcome pilot-study. *Behavior Therapist*, **16**, 29–33.

Brady, J. P., Davison, J. C., Dewald, P. A., Egan, G., Fadiman, J., Frank, J. D., Gil, M. M., Hoffman, I., Kempler, W., Lazarus, A. A., Raimy, V., Rotter, J. B. & Strupp, H. H. (1980) Some views on effective principles of psychotherapy. *Cognitive Therapy and Research*, **4**, 271–306.

Byers, A. P. (1992) The normalization of a personality through neurofeedback therapy. *Subtle Energies*, **3**, 1–17.

Cameron-Bandler, L. (1985) *Solutions*. Moab, Utah: Real People Press.

Carlson, J. G. & Chemtob, C. M. (1997) The role of 'resolute perception' in EMDR: Reply to Linda Waters. *Psychotherapy*, **34**, 100.

Carlson, J.G., Chemtob, C. M., Rusnak, K. & Hedland, N. L. (1996) Eye movement desensitization and reprocessing treatment for combat-relared PTSD. *Psychotherapy*, **33**, 104–113.

Carlson, J. G., Chemtob, C. M., Rusnak, K., Hedland, N. L. & Muraoka, M. (1998) Eye movement desensitization/reprocessing (EMDR) for combat-related posttraumatic stress disorder. *Journal of Traumatic Stress*, **11**, 3–24.

Chang, G. C. C. (1963) *Teachings of Tibetan Yoga*. Secaucus, N. J.: Citadel.

Coe, W. C. & Scharcoff, J. A. (1985) An empirical evaluation of the neurolinguistic programming model. *International Journal of Clinical and experimental Hypnosis*, **33**, 310–318.

Cowan, J. D. (1993) Alpha-theta brainwave biofeedback: The many possible theoretical reasons for its success. *Biofeedback*, **21**, 11–16.

Curreen, M. P. (1995) A simple hypnotically based NLP technique used with two clients in criminal justice settings. *Australian Journal of Clinical and Experimental Hypnosis*, **243**, 51–57.

David-Neel, A. (1984) *Magic and Mystery in Tibet*. London: George Allen & Unwin.

DeBell, C. & Jones, R. D. (1997) As good as it seems? A review of EMDR experimental research. *Professional Psychology—Research and Practice*, **28**, 153–163.

de Luynes, M. (1995) Neuro linguistic programming. *Educational and Child Psychology*, **12**, 34–47.

Dilts, R., Grinder, J., Bandler, R., Bandler, L. & DeLosier, J. (1980) *The Study of the Structure of Subjective Experience. Neuro-Linguistic Programming*, vol. 1. Cupertino, CA: Meta Publications.

Dooley, K. O. & Farmer, A. (1988) Comparison for aphasic ande control subjects of eye movements hypothesized in neurolinguistic programming. *Perceptual and Motor Skills*, **67**, 233–234.

Duncan, R. C., Konefal, J. & Spechler, M. M. (1990) Effects of neurolinguistic programming training on self-actualization as measured by the Personal Orientation Inventory. *Psychological Reports*, **66**, 1323–1330.

Dyck, M. J. (1993) A proposal for a conditioning model of eye movement desensitization treatment for posttraumatic stress disorder. *Journal of Behavior Therapy and Experimental Psychiatry*, **24**, 201–210.

Einspruch, E. L. & Forman, B. D. (1988) Neiro-linguistic programming in the treatment of phobias. *Psychology in Private Practice*, **6**, 91–100.

Elich, M., Thompson, R. W. & Miller, l. (1985) Mental imagery as revealed by eye movements and spoken predicates: A test of neurolinguistic programming. *Journal of Counseling Psychology*, **32**, 622–625.

Ellis, A. (1962) *Reason and Emotion in Psychotherapy*. New York: Lyle Stuart.

Ellis, A. (1973) *Humanistic Psychotherapy: The Rational-emotive Approach*. New York: McGraw-Hill.

Erickson, E. H. (1968) *Identity: Youth and Crisis*. New York: Norton.

Everly, G. S. (1984, December) *A Neurocognitive Analysis of Stress Response Syndromes Associated with Trauma*. Paper presented to the FEMA/NIMH Conference on Role Conflict and Support for Emergency Workers, Washington, DC.

Everly, G. S. (1985, April) *Neurocognitive Therapy and Rehabilitation of Psychiatric Syndromes in Response to Stress*. Paper presented to the International Conference on Stress and Behavioral Emergencies, Balto.

Everly, G. S. (1989) *A Clinical Guide to the Treatment of the Human Stress Response*. New York: Plenum.

Everly, G. S. (1993) Neurophysiological considerations in the treatment of posttraumatic stress disorder. A neurological perspective. In *International Handbook of Traumatic Stress Syndromes*, edited by J. P. Wilson & B. Raphael, pp. 795–801. New York: Plenum.

Everly, G. S. & Benson, H. (1989) Disorders of arousal. *International Journal of Psychosomatics*, **36**, 15–22.

Fahrion, S. L., Walters, D. E., Coyne, L. & Allen, T. (1992) Alterations in EEG amplitude, personality factors and brain electrical mapping after alpha theta brain wave training: A controlled case study of an alcoholic in recovery. *Alcoholism: Clinical and Experimental Research*, **16**, 547–552.

Fensterheim, H. (1996) Eye movement desensitization and reprocessing with complex personality pathology: An integrative therapy. *Journal of Psychotherapy Integration*, **6**, 27–38.

Field, E. S. (1990) Neirolingvistic programming as an adjunct to other psychotherapeutic/hypnotherapeutic interventions. *American Journal of Clinical Hypnosis*, **32**, 174–182.

Fox, B. (1993) Kundalini—Alive—but is it well in Australia? *Consciousness*, Aug/Sept, 7 & 14.

Frank, J. D. (1982) Therapeutic components shared by all psychotherapies. In *The Master Lecture Series: Vol. 1. Psychotherapy Research and Behavior Change*, edited by J. H. Harvey & M. M. Parks. Washington, DC.: American Psychological Association.

Frank, J. D. & Frank, J. B. (1991) *Persuasion and Healing: A Comparative Study of Psychotherapy*, (3rd edn). Baltimore: Johns Hopkins University Press.

Freud, S. (1922) *Introductory Lectures on Psycho-Analysis*. London: George Allen & Unwin/International Psycho-Analytical Institute.

Freud, S. (1933) *New Introductory Lectures on Psycho-Analysis*. London: Hogarth/Institute of Psycho-Analysis.

Freud, S. (1949) *Inhibitions, Symptoms and Anxiety*. London: Hogarth/Institute of Psycho-Analysis.

Friedman, H. S. (1991) *The Self-healing Personality*. New York: Henry Holt.

Fulcher, G. (1994, February) *The Impact of Trauma and the Development of Post-traumatic Stress Disorder*. Paper presented at the Cross District Counselling and Mental Health Services Forum, Bateman's Bay, Australia.

Goldfried, M. R. (1980) Psychotherapy as coping skills training. In *Psychotherapy Process: Current Issues and Future Directions*, edited by M. J. Mahoney. New York: Plenum.

Goldstein, A. J. & Feske, U. (1994) Eye movement desensitization and reprocessing for panic disorder: A case series. *Journal of Anxiety Disorders*, **8**, 351–362.

Greenwald, R. (1995) Eye movement desensitization and reprocessing (EMDR): A new kind of dreamwork? *Dreaming: Journal of the Association for the Study of Dreams*, **5**, 51–55.

Greenwell, B. (1991) *Energies of Transformation: A Guide to the Kundalini Process*. Cupertino, CA: Shakti River.

Grencavage, L. M. & Norcross, J. C. (1990) Where are the commonalties among the therapeutic common factors? *Professional Psychology: Research and Practice*, **21**, 372–378.

Greyson, B. (1993) The physio-kundalini syndrome and mental illness. *The Journal of Transpersonal Psychology*, **25**, 43–58.

Grinder, J. & Bandler, R. (1976) *The Structure of Magic*, vol. 2. Palo Alto: Science and Behavior Books.

Grinder, J. & Bandler, R. (1981) *Trance-formations: Neuro-Linguistic Programming and the Structure of Hypnosis*. Moab, Utah: Real People Press.

Grof, C. & Grof, S. (1986) Spiritual emergency: The understanding and treatment of transpersonal crisis. *ReVision*, **8**, 7–20.

Grof, C. & Grof, S. (1990) *The Stormy Search for the Self*. Los Angeles: Tarcher.

Hammond, D. C. (1991) EMDR: Critique and cautionary notes. *American Society of Clinical Hypnosis Newsletter*, **32**.

Hammond, D. C. (1992) Letter to the Editor—EMDR. *American Society of Clinical Hypnosis Newsletter*, **32**.

Hanh, T. N. (1987) *The Miracle of Mindlessness. A Manual on Meditation*. Boston: Beacon.

Hekmat, H., Groth, S. & Roger, D. (1994) Pain ameliorating effect of eye movement desensitization. *Journal of Behavior Therapy and Experimental Psychiatry*, **25**, 121–129.

Henry, S. L. (1996) Pathological gambling:Etiological considerations and treatment efficacy of eye movement desensitization/reprocessing. *Journal of Gambling Studies*, **12**, 395–405.

Herbert, J. D. & Mueser, K. T. (1992) Eye movement desensitization: A critique of the evidence. *Journal of Behavior Therapy and Experimental Psychiatry*, **23**, 169–174.

Hobbs, N. (1962) Sources of gain in psychotherapy. *American Psychologist*, **17**, 741–747.

Hoenderdos, H. T. W. & van Romunde, L. K. J. (1995) Information exchange between client and the out-side world from the NLP perspective. *Communication and Cognition*, **28**, 343–350.

Holdevici, I. (1990) Neurolinguistic programming: A form of mental training in high-performance shooting. *Revue Roumaine des Sciences Sociales—Serie de Psychologie*, **34**, 169–173.

Holdevici, I. (1991) Neurolinguistic programming: A form of mental training in high-performance shooting. *Revista de Psihologie*, **37**, 75–79.

Horvath, A. O. & Symonds, B. D. (1991) Relation between working alliance and outcome in psychotherapy: A meta-analysis. *Journal of Counseling Psychology*, **38**, 139–149.

Hossack, A. & Standidge, K. (1993) Using an imaginal scrapbook for neurolinguistic programming in the aftermath of a clinical depression: A case history. *Gerontologist*, **33**, 265–268.

House, S. (1994) Blending NLP representational systems with the RT counseling environment. *Journal of Reality Therapy*, **14**, 61–65.

Humphreys, C. (1976) *A Popular Dictionary of Buddhism*, (2nd Edn). London: Curzon.

Jacobson, E. (1938) *Progressive Relaxation*. Chicago: University of Chicago Press.

Jacobson, E. (1970) *You must Relax*. New York: McGraw Hill.

Jensen, J. A. (1994) An investigation of eye movement desensitization and reprocesing (EMD/R) as a treatment for posttraumatic stress disorder (PTSD) symptoms of Vietnam combat veterans. *Behavior Therapy*, **25**, 311–325.

Jojart, J. & Revenstorf, D. (1986) Theoretical foundations of Bandler and Grinder's linguistic metamodel. *Hypnose und Kognition*, **3**, 52–54.

Jupp, J. J. (1989a) Neurolinguistic programming: An experimental test of the effectiveness of 'leading' in hypnotic inductions. *British Journal of Experimental and Clinical Hypnosis*, **6**, 91–97.

Jupp, J. J. (1989b) A further empirical evaluation of neurolinguistic primary representational systems (PRS). *Counselling Psychology Quarterly*, **2**, 441–450.

Karasu, T. B. (1986) The specificity versus non-specificity dilemma: Toward identifying therapeutic change agents. *American Journal of Psychiatry*, **143**, 687–695.

Kleinke, C. L. (1994) *Common Principles of Psychotherapy*. Pacific Grove: Brooks/Cole.

Konefal, J., Duncan, R. C. & Reese, M. A. (1992) Neurolinguistic programming training, trait anxiety, and locus of control. *Psychological Reports*, **70**, 819–832.

Korchin, S. J. & Sands, S. H. (1983) Principles common to all psychotherapies. In *The Handbook of Clinical Psychology: Theory, Research and Practice*, vol. 1, edited by C. E. Walker. Chicago: Dorsey.

Krishna, P. G. (1976) *Kundalini. Path to Higher Consciousness.* Delhi, India: Orient.

Lama Chime Rinpoche (1992) Personal communication.

Lang, P. (1984) Cognition in emotion: Concept and action. In *Emotion, Cognition and Behavior,* edited by C. Izard, J. Kagan & R. Zajonc, pp. 192–226. Cambrige: Cambridge University Press.

Lazarus, R. S. (1984) On the primacy of cognition. *American Psychologist*, **39**, 124, 129.

Lehrer, P. M. & Woolfolk, R. L. (eds.) (1993) *Principles and Practice of Stress Management,* (2nd Edn). New York: Bantam.

Lipke, H. & Botkin, A. (1992) Brief case studies of eye movement desensitization and reprocessing with chronic post-traumatic stress disorder. *Psychotherapy*, **29**, 591–595.

Linden, W. (1990) *Autogenic Training: A Clinical Guide.* New York: Guilford.

Linden, W. (1994) Autogenic training: A narrative and quantitative review of clinical outcome. *Biofeedback and Self Regulation*, **19**, 227–264.

Linden, W. & Lenz, J. W. (1997) Autogenic training. In *Treating Anxiety Disorders*, edited by W. T. Roth & I. D. Yalom, pp. 117–150. San Francisco: Jossey-Bass.

Linville, P. W. (1985) Self-complexity and affective extremity: Don't put all your eggs in one cognitive basket. *Social Cognition*, **3**, 94–120.

Linville, P. W. (1987) Self-complexity as a cognitive buffer against stress-related illness and depression. *Journal of Personality and Social Psychology*, **52**, 663–676.

Lohr, J. M., Kleinknecht, R. A., Tolin, D. F. & Barrett, R. H. (1995) The empiricial status of the clinical application of eye movement desensitization and reprocessing. *Journal of Behavior Therapy and Exxperimental Psychiatry*, **26**, 285–302.

Luthe, W. (ed.) (1969) *Autogenic Therapy.* 6 vols. New York: Grune & Stratton.

Macdonald, L. (1997) Neuro Linguistic Programming as an experiential constructivist therapy for semantic pragmatic disorder. In *Communication and the Mentally Ill Patient: Developmental and Linguistic Approaches to Schizophrenia*, edited by J. France & N. Muir, pp. 139–152. London: Jessica Kingsley.

Mahaniranonda, A. N. (undated). *Vipassana Bhavana.* Pattaya: Boonkanjanaram Meditation Center.

Marmor, J. (1985) *The Nature of the Psychotherapeutic Process.* Audiotape (L330-19) from The Evolution of Psychotherapy Conference, Phoenix, AZ. Phoenix, AZ: Milton Erickson Foundation.

Marmor, J. (1990) *The Essence of Dynamic Psychotherapy: What Makes it Work?.* Audiotape (C289-27) from The Evolution of Psychotherapy Conference, Anaheim, CA. Phoenix, AZ: Milton Erickson Foundation.

Masters, B. J., Rawlins, M. E., Rawlins, L. D. & Weidner, J. (1991) The NLP swish pattern: An innovativve visualizing technique. *Journal of Mental Health Counseling*, **13**, 79–90.

Mayers, K. S. (1993) Enhancement of psychological testimony with the use of neurolinguistic programming techniques. *American Journal of Forensic Psychology*, **11**, 53–60.

McGuigan, F. J. (ed.) (1975) *Tension Control.* Blackburg, VA: University Publications.

McGuigan, F. J. (1991) Control of normal and pathologic cognitive functions through neuromuscular circuits. Applications of principles of progressive relaxation. In *International Perspectives on Self-Regulation and Health*, edited by J. G. Carlson & A. R. Seifert, pp. 121–132. New York: Plenum.

Maslow, A. H. (1970) *Motivation and Personality,* (2nd edn). New York: Harper & Row.

Metter, J. & Michelson, L. K. (1993) Theoretical, clinical, research and ethical constraints of the Eye Movement Desensitization Reprocessing technique. *Journal of Traumatic Stress*, **6**, 413–415.

Monguio-Vecino, I. & Lippman, L. G. (1987) Image formation as related to visual fixation point. *Journal of Mental Imagery*, **11**, 87–96.

Nanasamvara, S. P. (1984) *The Rudiments of Mental-collectedness.* Bangkok: Wat Bovoranives Vihara, Royal Academy Foundation, Wat Nyanasamvaaram, Foundation for the Promotion of Buddhist Meditation.

Nicosia, G. J. (1995) Eye movement desensitization and reprocessing is not hypnosis. *Dissociation: Progress in the Dissociative Disorders*, **8**, 69.

Ochs, L. (1992) EEG treatment of addictions. *Biofeedback*, **20**, 8–16.

O'Connor, P. (1981) *Understanding the Mid-life Crisis*. Melbourne: Sun.

Ossoff, J. (1993) Reflections of *Shaktipat*: Psychosis or the rise of kundalini? A case study. *The Journal of Transpersonal Psychology*, **25**, 29–42.

Patterson, C. H. (1966) *Theories of Counselling and Psychotherapy*. New York: Harper & Row.

Patterson, C. H. (1977) New approaches in counselling: Healthy diversity or anti-therapeutic? *British Journal of Guidance and Counselling*, **5**, 19–25.

Paulsen, S. (1995) Eye movement desensitization and reprocessing: Its cautious use in the dissociative disorders. *Disssociation: Progress in the Disssociative Disorders*, **8**, 32–44.

Peniston, E. (1990) EEG brainwave training as a bio-behavior intervention for Vietnam combat-related PTSD. *The Medical Psychotherapist*, **6**, 2.

Peniston, E. (1992) *EEG Training for Alcohol and Post-traumatic Stress Disorders: A Three-year Follow-up*. Paper presented at the 23rd Annual Conference of the Association for Applied Psychophysiology and Biofeedback, Colorado Springs, USA.

Peniston, E. (1994a) *EEG Section: Invited Address*. Paper presented at the 25th Annual Conference of the Association for Applied Psychophysiology and Biofeedback, Atlanta, USA.

Peniston, E. (1994b) Personal communication.

Peniston, E. (1996) EMG biofeedback-assisted desensitization treatment for Vietnam combat veterans post-traumatic stress disorder. *Clinical Biofeedback and Health*, **9**, 35–41.

Peniston, E. G. & Kulkosky, P. J. (1989) Alpha-theta brainwave training and B-endorphin levels in alcoholics. *Alcoholism: Clinical and Experimental Research*, **13**, 271–279.

Peniston, E. G. & Kulkosky, P. J. (1990) Alcoholic personality and alpha-theta brainwave training. *Medical Psychotherapy*, **3**, 37–55.

Peniston, E. G. & Kulkosky, P. J. (1991a) Alpha-theta brain wave neurofeedback therapy for Vietnam veterans with combat-related post-traumatic stress disorder. *Medical Psychotherapy*, **4**, 47–60.

Peniston, E. G. & Kulkosky, P. J. (1991b) Alpha-theta EEG biofeedback training in alcoholism and post-traumatic stress disorder. *Newsletter, The International Society for the Study of Subtle Energies and Energy Medicine*, **2**, 5–7.

Penzel, F., Ricciardi, J. & Baer, L. (1992) Letters to the Editor. EMDR workshop: Disturbing issues. *The Behavior Therapist*, May.

Phares, E. J. (1988) *Clinical Psychology. Concepts, Methods and Profession, 3rd edition*. Chicago: Dorsey.

Pinkerton, S., Hughes, H. & Wenrich, W. W. (1982) *Behavioral Medicine: Clinical Applications*. New York: Wiley-Interscience.

Puk, G. (1991) Treating traumatic memories: A case report on the eye movement desensitization procedure. *Journal of Behavior Therapy and Experimental Psychiatry*, **22**, 149–151.

Rachman, S. J. (1981) The primacy of affect: Some theoretical implications. *Behavior Research and Therapy*, **19**, 279–290.

Rickman, J. (ed.) (1953) *A General Selection from the Works of Sigmund Freud*. London: Hogarth/Institute of Psycho-Analysis.

Rogers, C. R. (1957) The necessary and sufficient conditions of therapeutic personality change. *Journal of Consulting Psychology*, **21**, 95–103.

Rosenfeld, J. P. (1992) 'EEG' treatment of addictions: Commentary on Ochs, Peniston, and Kukolsky. *Biofeedback*, **20**(2), 12–17.

Rothbaum, B. D. (1997) A controlled study of eye movement desensitization and reprocessing in the treatment of posttraumatic stress disordered sexval assault victims. *Bulletin of the Menninger Clinic*, **61**, 317–334.

Sannella, L. (1978) *Kundalini: Psychosis or Transcendence*. San Francisco: Dakin.

Saxby, E. & Peniston, E. (1995) Alpha-theta brainwave neurofeedback training: An effective treatment for male and female alcoholics with depressive symptoms. *Journal of Clinical Psychology*, **51**, 685–693.

Schultz, J. (1953) *Das Autogene Training*. Stuttgart: Geerg-Thieme Verlag.

Schultz, J. & Luthe., W. (1959) *Autogenic Training: A Psychophysiological Approach to Psychotherapy*. New York: Grune & Stratton.

Shapiro, F. (1989a) Efficacy of the Eye Movement Desensitization procedure in the treatment of traumatic memories. *Journal of Traumatic Stress*, **2**, 199–223.

Shapiro, F. (1989b) Eye Movement Desensitization: A new treatment for post-traumatic stress disorder. *Journal of Behavior Therapy and Experimental Psychiatry*, **20**, 211–217.

Shapiro, F. (1990) Eye Movement Desensitization: A new treatment for anxiety. *The California Psychologist*, **May**, 18–19.

Shapiro, F. (1991a) Eye Movement Desensitization and Reprocessing procedure: From EMD to EMD/R—A new treatment model for anxiety and related traumata. *The Behavior Therapist*, **14**, 133–135.

Shapiro, F. (1991b) Eye Movement Desensitization and Reprocessing: A cautionary note. *The Behavior Therapist*, **14**, 188.

Shapiro, F. (1992a) Dr. Francine Shapiro responds. *The Behavior Therapist*, May.

Shapiro, F. (1992b) Personal communication.

Shapiro, F. (1993) Eye Movement Desensitization and Reprocessing (EMDR) in 1992. *Journal of Traumatic Stress*, **6**, 411–417.

Shapiro, F. (1995) *Eye Movement Desensitization and Reprocessing: Basic Principles, Protocols and Procedures*. New York: Guilford.

Shapiro, F. (1996a) Eye movement desensitization and reprocessing (EMDR): Evaluation of controlled PTSD research. *Journal of Behavior Therapy and Experimental Psychiatry*, **27**, 209–218.

Shapiro, F. (1996b) Errors of context and review of eye movement desensitization and reprocessing research. *Journal of Behavior Therapy and Experimental Psychiatry*, **27**, 313–317.

Shapiro, F. (1997) Eye Movement Desensitization and Reprocessing: Research and clinical significance. In *Current Thinking and Research in Brief Therapy: Solutions, Strategies, Narratives*, vol. 1, edited by W. J. Matthews & J. H. Edgette, pp. 239–260. New York: Brunner/Mazel.

Shapiro, F. & Forrest, M. S. (1997) *EMDR: The Breakthrough Therapy for Overcoming Anxiety, Stress and Trauma*. New York: Basic.

Shapiro, F., Solomon, R. & Kaufman, T. (1991) *Origins and Update: Use of EMDR with Critical Incident: Preliminary Research Results*. Paper presented at the International Society for Traumatic Stress Studies Conference, Washington, DC.

Shapiro, F., Vogelman-Sine, S. & Sine, L. F. (1994) Eye movement desensitization and reprocessing: Treating trauma and substance abuse. *Journal of Proactive Drug*, **26**, 379–391.

Sheldon, V. E. & Shelden, R. G. (1989) Sexval abuse of males by females: The problem, treatment modality and case example. *Family Therapy*, **16**, 249–258.

Sheppard, J. L. (1989) Relaxation and meditation as techniques for stress reduction. In *Advances in Behavioural Medicine, Vol. 6*, edited by J. L. Sheppard, pp. 137–157. Sydney: Cumberland College of Health Sciences.

Solomon, R. M. & Shapiro, F. (1997) Eye Movement Desensitization and Reprocessing: A therapeutic tool for trauma and grief. In *Death and Trauma: The Traumatology of Grieving. The Series in Trauma and Loss*, edited by C. R. Figley, B. E. Bride & N. Mazza, pp. 231–247. Washington, DC: Taylor & Francis.

Stanton, H. E. (1989) Using rapid change techniques to improve sporting performance. *Australian Journal of Clinical and Experimental Hypnosis*, **17**, 153–161.

Starker, S. & Pankratz, L. (1996) Soundness of treatment: A survey of psychologists' opinions. *Psychological Reports*, **78**, 288–290.

Sterman, C. M. (1991) Neuro-linguistic programming as psychotherapeutic treatment in working with alcohol and other drug addicted families. Special Issue: Chemical dependency: theoretical approaches and strategies working with individuals and families. *Journal of Chemical Dependency Treatment*, **4**, 73–85.

Stiles, W. B., Shapiro, D. A. & Elliott, R. (1986) 'Are all psychotherapies equivalent?' *American Psychologist*, **41**, 165–180.

Strupp, H. H. (1986) Psychotherapy: Research, practice, and public policy (how to avoid dead ends). *American Psychologist*, **41**, 120–130.

Suinn, R. (1990) *Anxiety Management Training*. New York: Plenum.

Suinn, R. (1992) Personal communication.

Suinn, R. & Richardson, F. (1971) Anxiety management training: A non-specific behavior therapy program for anxiety control. *Behavior Therapy*, **2**, 498.

Sullivan, H. S. (1953) *The Interpersonal Theory of Psychiatry*. New York: Norton.

Swami Muktananda (1978) *Play of Consciousness*. San Francisco: Harper & Row.

Swami Muktananda (1979) *Kundalini: The Secret of Life*. S. Fallsburg, N.Y.: SYDA Foundation.

Swami Satyanananda Saraswati (1982) *Taming the Kundalini*, (4th edn). Munger, India: Bihar School of Yoga.

Swami Vishnu Tirtha (1962) *Devatma Shakti (Kundalini) Divine Power*. Rishikresh, India: Yoga Shri Peeth Trust.

ten Broeke, E. & de Jongh, A. (1995) Eye movement desensitization and reprocessing: 'Ordinary' imaginal exposure? *Psycholoog*, **30**, 459–464.

Thalbourne, M. A. & Fox, B. (1993) *The Kundalini Experience: Its Measurement and Relationship to Panic Attacks and other Variables*. Unpublished manuscript, University of Adelaide, Department of Psychology, Adelaide, South Australia.

Tierney, M. J. (1990) Neuro-linguistics as a treatment modality for alcoholism and substance abuse. In *Neuro-linguistic Programming in Alcoholism Treatment. Haworth Series in Addictions Treatment*, vol. 3, edited by C. M. Sterman, pp. 141–154. New York: Haworth.

Tolin, D. F., Montgomery, R. W., Kleinknecht, R. S. & Lohr, J. M. (1995) An evaluation of Eye Movement Desensitization and Reprocessing (EMDR). In *Innovations in Clinical Practice: A Source Book*, vol. 14, edited by L. VanDeCreek, S. Knapp & T. L. Jackson, pp. 423–437. Sarasota: Professional Resource.

Trungpa, C. (1976) *The Myth of Freedom and The Way of Meditation*. Berkeley & London: Shambala.

Van Ommeren, M. (1996) Comment on Greenwald (1996): The assessment of fidelity to the EMDR treatment protocol. *Professional Psychology—Research and Practice*, **27**, 529

Waters, L. (1997) 'Eye movement desensitization and reprocessing treatment for combat PTSD': Commentary. *Psychotherapy*, **34**, 99.

Wertheim, E. H., Habib, C. & Cumming, G. (1986) Test of the neurolinguistic programming hypothesis that eye-movements relate to processing imagery. *Perceptual and Motor Skills*, **62**, 523–529.

Wickramasekera, I. (1993) Observations, speculations and an experimentally testable hypothesis. *Biofeedback*, **21**, 17–20.

Wilbur, M. P. & Roberts-Wilbur, J. (1987) Categorizing sensory reception in four modes: Support for representational systems. *Perceptual and Motor Skills*, **64**, 875–886.

Wilson, J. P. & Raphael, B. (1993) *International Handbook of Traumatic Stress Syndromes*. New York: Plenum.

Wilson, S. A, Becker, L. A. & Tinker, R. H. (1995) Eye movement desensitization and reprocessing (EMDR) treatment for psychologically traumatized individuals. *Journal of Consulting and Clinical Psychology*, **63**, 928–937.

Wilson, S. A, Becker, L. A. & Tinker, R. H. (1997) Fifteen-month follow-up of eye movement desensitization and reprocessing (EMDR) treatment for posttraumatic stress disorder and psychological traumas. *Journal of Consulting and Clinical Psychology*, **65**, 1047–1056.

Wolpe, J. (1958) *Psychotherapy by Reciprocal Inhibition*. Stanford, CA: Stanford University Press.

Wolpe, J. (1969) *The Practice of Behavior Therapy*. 2nd Edition 1973. New York: Pergamon, 2nd Edition 1973.

Wolpe, J. & Lazarus, A. (1966) *Behavior Therapy Techniques*. Oxford: Pergamon.

Woodroffe, J. (1973) *The Serpent Power*. Madras, India: Ganesh.

Wuttke, M. (1992) Addiction, awakening, and EEG biofeedback. *Biofeedback*, **20**, 18–22.

Yalom, I. D. (1980) *Existential Psychotherapy*. New York: Basic.

Yupho, D. (1984) *Self-study Practical Insight Meditation*. Bangkok: Dharmanoon Singgaravanij Foundation.

Zajonc, R. (1984) On the primacy of affect. *American Psyhologist*, **39**, 117–123.

Zastrow, C., Dotson, V. & Koch, M. (1986) The Neuro-Linguistic Programming treatment approach. *Journal of Independent Social Work*, **1**, 29–38.

Chapter 12

STRESS MANAGEMENT IN HEALTH EDUCATION

J. Macdonald Wallace

For 40 years I have approached the subject of stress management from the perspective of a health educator—a trainer of teachers in health and physical education. When teaching physical skills that had an element of danger, such as somersaulting or high diving, I noticed that adults, as well as children, tended to become unduly muscularly tense as they attempted to perform. So I spent much of my time teaching them to be more relaxed in order to enhance performance.

It was not until 1950 when I encountered Jacobson's (1929) seminal book, *Progressive Relaxation*, that I found a sound theoretical basis for teaching relaxation skills. In 1956 I came across Hans Selye's (1956) book, *The Stress of Life*, when I was introducing a new extramural course in health education for adult students at the University of Otago in New Zealand. Selye's General Adaptation Syndrome, which defined biological stress as the state within a biologic system consisting of all nonspecific changes in response to a stimulus, seemed to parallel the various descriptions of the effects of excessive or chronic muscular tension in Jacobson's writings. Undoubtedly Selye can be named as the progenitor of biologic stress research; but I think it safe to say that Jacobson was the progenitor of scientific stress management, although he never used the term.

STRESS MANAGEMENT IN HIGHER EDUCATION

As a result of my reading, in 1956 sessions on understanding stress, stress control and relaxation were included in my health education course along with sessions on exercise, diet, alcohol, smoking, and drug abuse. This was, perhaps, the first university course ever offered on stress management for education rather than for therapy. After offering the course for a few academic terms, I became increasingly convinced by the evaluations of my students that, indeed, the most effective parts of the health education course were those sessions dealing with understanding stress through Jacobson's differential relaxation during everyday activities. So I increased the amount of time devoted to stress management topics, presented more biological and psychological information and decreased the time spent on other aspects of health education.

There was very little published relating to management of stress during those years—the early 1950s and 1960s—although significant literature was accumulating. The concept of biologic stress had not yet entered into dictionaries of psychology (e.g. Drever, 1971), and apparently no other institution of higher education taught the subject of stress management. My work was orthodox enough—based mainly on the work of Selye and Jacobson, following sound educational theory and practice—but it was barely tolerated by some academics and regarded with some amusement as a form of esoteric cult, unworthy for use in higher education.

I established a course during the late 1960s in the Extra-Mural Department of London University in England that I wanted to call simply 'Stress Management'. This was not an academically acceptable term to the department. Finally I agreed to title the course 'Health Education: Stress and the Individual'. Stress management did not become accepted in any British university until the early 1970s when I introduced it as a subject of study for the Bachelor of Education Degree at London University. Now nearly all universities have units or courses in stress management that are usually, but not always, offered in the department of psychology. Most medical graduates still remain ill-informed about stress and stress management.

Once psychologists entered the field of stress and stress management, research studies, theses and methods quickly proliferated, sowing confusion through the coinage of doubtful or ill-defined terms, such as occupational stress, executive stress, emotional stress, replacing the term biologic stress. Such terms may well have been useful contributions to creative marketing strategy, but I am less sure that they have been helpful in promoting the realities of stress management nor am I persuaded that many who have parachuted into the stress management field recently have made significant contributions to its development.

STRESS AND THERAPY

Therapists moved into the field of stress management when the concept of stress became popular through confusing articles that appeared in magazines and newspapers. Treatments for stress were offered by physical therapists, psychotherapists, music therapists, self-designated therapists who used exotic and homespun cures, etc. Such widespread use of unresearched 'stress therapy' techniques may have been the greatest stumbling block in the development of stress management. Biologic stress does not need therapy; it is not a condition requiring a cure. Biologic stress was later redefined by Selye (1976) as a nonspecific response of the body to any stimulus. In fact, Selye (1956) stated that he could not and should not be cured of his stress, merely taught to enjoy it. Stress is an expression of the primary instinct of all living things—the instinct of self-preservation. This instinct can run awry, but it can be controlled or managed. Research findings could be effectively synthesized with Jacobson's 'tension control' to manage this nonspecific response to any stimulus, which is biologic stress.

Curiously enough, although Jacobson and Selye were contemporaries publishing extensively in scientific journals for almost five decades, they completely ignored one another. In Jacobson's prolific publications, he mentioned Selye only once (1964, p. 43) in a half-sentence, somewhat dismissively. In turn, Selye (1976) in his encyclopaedic *Stress in Health and Disease* details a long list of potential 'treatments' including many unscientific approaches to controlling stress; but he does not mention Jacobson's scientifically-based 'tension control' or 'self-operations control'. As Lennart Levi (1991) pointed out, it is quite possible to be an expert in stress and know nothing about stress management. The reverse is unlikely.

There are many methods for managing stress as a biologic response, but the final common pathway is through relaxation—there is no other gateway. There may be several valid and reliable methods of stress management, but progressive relaxation is the original and most effective one.

QUIETING AND THE RESTLESS MIND

Frequently during my courses some student would say I can relax my body all right, but it is my mind that is the trouble. It just keeps going on and on, even keeping me awake at night. What am I to do? At first I had no answer, not understanding the mind. I tried various mantras— 'om' and 'um' sounds used in Oriental philosophies—and fruitless, high-sounding phrases, such as the 'inner depths of mind' or 'your innermost being' but they led nowhere. During the 1930s Jacobson (1930–31) published a series of laboratory studies concerning covert muscular processes in mental activity. These studies were incorporated into his revised edition of *Progressive Relaxation* (1938). I turned to this book in my attempt to answer my students' questions about quieting the restless mind.

There have been long arguments concerning theories of the mind by philosophers from ancient Greek times through to the present. 'Monism', where the mind and body are regarded as the same, or 'dualism', where the mind and body are unsidered separate and distinct entities. There is considerable confusion about what comprises the mind and the body.

Jacobson's studies rejected all these speculative theories. In his last book *The Human Mind*, Jacobson (1982) reviewed these long-standing theoretical conflicts about the mind and demonstrated that *there can be no mental activity without contraction of striated muscle*. A detailed account of Jacobson's proven research (confirmed by many others) can be found in McGuigan's (1978) book, *Cognitive Psychophysiology: Principles of Covert Behaviour*. Jacobson defined the human mind in part as the components of the body that engage in external and internal representation of matters; furthermore, the mind responds for the organism's welfare. That is, the mind includes functions performed by the organism's nervous and muscular systems in response to internal and external stimulation.

I was inspired by Jacobson's writings to teach my students that relaxation of the speech and visual muscles was an essential part of the management of stress long before Jacobson's definition of mind was published. I did not have access to electromyographic instruments available in Jacobson's laboratory, so I had to devise other methods to raise awareness—particularly since between 15 and 30 students attended each of my classes. I used various cognitive devices to help the students become aware of covert, internal events, develop awareness of tension in these muscles (called 't' signals by Steinhaus in 1963), and then to relax the muscles. My students became aware of the inner (covert) speech or sub-vocalisation aspect of thinking by loudly reciting some well-known song, such as 'Humpty Dumpty sat on a wall', or in other ways quieting covert speech. The students learned to control covert speech by letting the muscles of speech relax.

I found that control of eye muscles is a more difficult task. Most people are unaware that their eyes move while they think, so I paired students in the classes—one student acted as a subject and one acted as the experimenter. The subject talked for one minute on a given topic and the experimenter tried to count the eye movements while the subject was talking. Then the students exchanged roles. Results from scores of groups showed that the individual's eye movements ranged from zero to over 100 movements per minute. Within groups, the mean number of eye movements was between 30 and 40 per minute. In this way students could observe and accept that eye muscles are involved in thinking. They then had to learn how to control these tensions and how this influences the management of stress.

Recently I had the opportunity of working with a group of seven veterans blinded during the war. I asked them whether their eyes moved when they were thinking, and they did not know. Then I asked each one to speak to me for exactly one minute on a descriptive topic. I found that the number of eye movements ranged from 24 to 74, with a mean of 41. Thus, noncongenitally blind people also use eye muscles during mental activity, perhaps even more than sighted persons.

It is difficult to relax specific eye and speech muscles—for some people it is extremely difficult— and this is a major cause of insomnia. Many individuals lie in bed going over the day's problems verbally, often aloud, and visualizing past, present and future events. The feedback to and from the brain from these muscles, richly endowed with proprioceptors, maintains bodily arousal, which takes a long time to fall below the level necessary for sleep to prevail. The ability to quieten the mind, based on Jacobson's research, has proved invaluable to thousands of people.

WHO TEACHES?

Edmund Jacobson was a psychologist, physiologist and physician, who was the leader in the stress management field during the Twentieth Century. Jacobson almost invariably dealt with patients and experimental subjects— on a one-to-one basis. Therefore, he realized by this method it would take a very long time for the world to learn how to relax. In a paper presented at Strasbourg University in France, Jacobson (1962) stated that the popularization of tension control methods lies within the schools—from elementary schools to universities. The task is too great for teaching on a one-to-one basis so that reorganisation of public education is necessary. Some years before, I had already come to that conclusion and acted upon it. It remains my opinion that really large numbers of people can only be effectively helped to understand stress, how excessive stress affects health, and how to manage their stress through sound knowledge and practice spread through the vector of public education—not through research or therapists' clinics. This has already been accomplished in several countries (Frederick, 1979; Masson, 1984; McGuigan, 1992; Setterlind & Patriksson, 1984; Wallace, 1965, 1974, 1980). I leave it to you to help implement Edmund Jacobson's proposal to teach the whole world to relax.

References

Drever, J. (1971) *A Dictionary of Psychology*. London: Pelican Press.
Frederick, A. B. (1979) *Relaxation—Education's Fourth 'R'*. Washington, D.C: ERIC Clearing House on Teacher Education.
Jacobson, E. (1929, rev. ed. 1938) *Progressive Relaxation*. Chicago: University Press.
Jacobson, E. (1930–31) Electrical measurements of neuromuscular states during mental activities. *American Journal of Physiology*, **91**, 67; **94**, 92: **703**, 96, 115.
Jacobson, E. (1962) *Le Controle de la Tension*, Cahiers de Psychatrie. Strasbourg: University Press.
Jacobson, E. (1964) *Anxiety and Tension Control*. Philadelphia: J. B. Lippincott.
Jacobson, E. (1982) *The Human Mind*. Springfield, Illinois: Chas C. Thomas.
Levi, L. (1991) Personal Communication.
McGuigan, F. J. (1992) *Calm Down: A Guide for Stress and Tension Control* (2nd edn). Duburque, IA: Kendall/Hunt.
McGuigan, F. J. (1978) *Cognitive Psychophysiology: Principles of Covert Behaviour*. Englewood Cliffs, New Jersey: Prentice Hall.

Masson, S. (1984) Teaching dynamic relaxation at the University of the Third Age. In *Stress and Tension Control 2*, edited by F. J. McGuigan, W. E. Sime & J. M. Wallace. New York: Plenum Press.

Selye, H. (1956) *The Stress of Life*. New York: McGraw-Hill.

Selye, H. (1976) *Stress in Health and Disease*. Boston and London: Butterworth.

Setterlind, S. & Patriksson, G. (1984) An experimental study of relaxation in Swedish schools. In *Stress and Tension Control 2*, edited by F. J. McGuigan, W. E. Sime & J. M. Wallace. New York: Plenum Press.

Steinhaus, A. S. (1963) *Towards an Understanding of Health for Adults*. Dubuque, Iowa: W. C. Brown Co.

Wallace, J. M. (1980) Behavioural health changes through tension control learning in adult education classes. In *Stress and Tension Control*, edited by F. J. McGuigan, W. E. Sime & J. M. Wallace. New York: Plenum Press.

Wallace, J. M. (1974) Health education and the control of stress. *Health Education Journal*, **35**, 199.

Wallace, J. M. (1965) *Health Education Journal*, **24**, 200.

Chapter 13

STRESS MANAGEMENT AND PREVENTION ON A EUROPEAN COMMUNITY LEVEL: Options and Obstacles

Lennart Levi, MD, PhD

In a major study of conditions of work in the 12 Member States of the European Union at that time (1991–1992), the European Foundation for the Improvement of Living and Working Conditions (Paoli, 1992) found that 23 million workers had night work representing more than 25% of their total hours worked; every third worker reported repetitive work and every fifth male and every sixth female worked under continuous time pressure. 30% of the European workforce regarded their health at risk from work.

INCREASING AWARENESS

The awareness that such stressors and the resulting stress and stress-related ill health constitute a great and growing threat to all parties on the labour market has developed gradually during the 1970s and 1980s. In 1974, the 27th World Health Assembly requested the Director-General of the World Health Organization (WHO) to organize multidisciplinary programmes that would explore the role of psychosocial factors in relation to health and human development and to prepare proposals for strengthening WHO's activities in this field. In its ninth session in 1984, the joint ILO/WHO Committee on Occupational Health issued a report entitled 'Psychosocial factors at work: recognition and control'.

The report defined the concept of psychosocial factors at work and their impact on workers' health and well-being, specifically addressing physical work environments able to influence health through psychosocial mechanisms, as well as factors intrinsic to the job, work time arrangements, management and operating practices in the enterprises, and technological changes. Their potential consequences were described in terms of physiological, psychological, behavioural and health outcomes. A separate chapter was devoted to methods of measurement for both situational factors and outcomes, as well as to the need further to develop some of these measures.

The document also spelled out a number of actions to be taken at the establishment, national, and international levels.

The former should be comprehensive and geared to major occupational health problems, but also to situational and individual determinants of such problems. Monitoring methods should be reliable and valid, simple to administer, inexpensive and broadly available. Examples of such methods were given. Interventions based on findings obtained in such a manner should include job redesign, a wide range of organizational and ergonomic measures, and adjustments of working space and working time, with an emphasis on workers' participation, access to appropriate training and education, and ways of helping workers to cope.

Because of the multi-cause/multi-effect nature of health problems related to psychosocial factors, a multidisciplinary approach was advocated.

Action at the national level should promote tripartite and public awareness, include information and training, make better use of existing knowledge, provide more support for research, adapt the texts of laws and regulations to include psychosocial occupational aspects, strengthen labour inspection services, and monitor regularly psychosocial factors at work and workers' health.

At the international level, WHO and ILO should encourage and assist Member States to promote psychosocial occupational health, establish institutions and relationships between institutions, and, if there is no adequate infrastructure for occupational environment and health, integrate psychosocial occupational factors into the primary health care system.

This report by the joint ILO/WHO Committee was endorsed by the Governing Body of ILO as well as by the Executive Board of WHO and thereby became a policy document for such activities in this field worldwide (ILO, 1986).

A number of subsequent consultations and working group meetings organized by WHO resulted in a report entitled 'Psychosocial factors at work and their relations to health' (Kalimo et al., 1987). In 1992, based on a series of subsequent consultations, ILO published another major report: 'Preventing Stress at Work' (ILO, 1992). In its opening chapter, the ILO programme director for this field (Di Martino, 1992) concluded that:

> Stress is becoming an increasingly global phenomenon affecting all countries, all professions and all categories of workers, families and society in general. In short, the data and the studies ... clearly show why occupational stress is an important concern for workers, enterprises and society. It has detrimental effects on workers' health (cardio-vascular, gastro-intestinal, allergy, respiratory reactions; increased accident risks; emotional distress) and on the

performance of enterprises (absenteeism, demotivation, turnover, low productivity, interpersonal tensions). The economic impact of stress on society is also large and growing.

A EUROPEAN CALL FOR ACTION

Recognizing the urgency to deal with the root causes of stress-related ill health, the European Foundation for the Improvement of Living and Working Conditions held an international conference entitled 'Stress at Work: A Call for Action' in Brussels in 1993. Co-hosted by the Belgian Presidency and the EC Commission, the conference underlined 'stress as the leading illness among workers' (European Foundation, 1994).

The evidence for this is further reviewed by Kompier and Levi (1994). In this guide for small and medium-sized enterprises, commissioned by the European Foundation, the authors define the concepts and terms, discuss the causes and consequences of stress at work and those at risk of developing work-related stress and ill health. They further provide five reasons for monitoring occupational stress by small and medium-sized enterprises:

- stress is a problem for the worker and the company;
- work stress problems are on the increase;
- it is a legal obligation (in EU Member States);
- harmful stress can be avoided, since it is to a large extent work-related and work can be adjusted;
- stress prevention contributes to creating a workforce which is willing to change and innovate, which is customer-oriented and highly motivated,

thereby increasing the EU potential to compete with other markets such as the United States of America, Japan and South-East Asia. The booklet provides instruments for monitoring stress at company levels, discusses who should carry out such monitoring, and reviews preventive approaches targeted both at the working situations and at the workers exposed to it.

In two subsequent reports, also commissioned by the European Foundation, the socio-economic costs at both enterprise and community level have been analysed (Cooper et al., 1996; Levi and Lunde-Jensen, 1996).

Based on three European case studies at the *enterprise* level, Cooper et al. (1996) describe costs caused by occupational stress, interventions chosen by the enterprises to reduce stressors, stress and stress-related ill health, and resulting cost benefits. Interventions included job enlargement and enrichment and the creation of autonomous work teams (Sweden), improvement of communication and consultative structure, provision of individual skills training for managers (the Netherlands), and improvement of individuals' skills and resources and creation of organizational awareness and support (United Kingdom).

Observed *benefits* due to such interventions could be due to: productivity improvements, reduced employee health and insurance costs, reduced human resource development costs, and organizational image, whereas potential *costs* could be categorized into organizational, administrative, intervention, and participant costs. The authors conclude that stress prevention would seem to present a means whereby an organization can not only reduce or contain the costs of employee ill health, but can also positively maintain and improve organizational health and productivity. Their report may be a useful first step towards the future development of a practical methodology for organizations to enable them to do so.

The second report (Levi & Lunde-Jensen, 1996) concerns itself with corresponding costs and benefits at *national* level. The authors conclude that stress has clear implications for society as a whole. The first chapter spells out the possibilities of a national prevention strategy. The second chapter deals with basic concepts such as stress reactions, health effects and high-risk groups. The third chapter introduces the socio-economic model used to evaluate stress costs at national level and presents results for two European countries, Denmark and Sweden. The report includes a technical annex on the socio-economic model utilized by the authors and a glossary to facilitate the reading.

RECENT EUROPEAN DATA

The most recent European data come from the Second European Survey of Working Conditions, conducted by the European Foundation in early 1996.

Its recent report (Paoli, 1997) calls attention to the pronounced transformation of European working life from the industrial to the service sector, with a consequent change in job profile: introduction of new technology (one third of the workforce uses computers) and more client-oriented jobs (49% of the workers indicate permanent and direct contact with clients or patients). Work organization has also changed, with new management models, teamwork, just-in-time and TQM.

At the same time, the workforce profile has changed. European workers are getting older; they are more often working on fixed term or temporary contracts; there is a rapid growth in the proportion of female workers; the traditional employee-employer relationship is slowly disappearing; and the unemployment rate remains very high (Paoli, 1997).

According to this survey (Paoli, 1997), 45% of the 147 million workers in the EU Member States report having monotonous tasks; 44% no task rotation; 50% short, repetitive tasks; 35% no influence on task order; and 28% no influence on work rythm; while 54% work at a very high speed, and 56% to tight deadlines. Furthermore, 30% complain of backache, 28% of stress, 20% of fatigue, 17% of muscular pains and 13% of headaches.

THE EU FRAMEWORK DIRECTIVE

Under the European Union Framework Directive (89/391/EEC), employers have a 'duty to ensure the safety and health of workers in every aspect related to the work, on basis of the following general principles of prevention:

- avoiding risks;
- evaluating the risks which cannot be avoided;
- combating the risks at source;
- adapting the work to the individual, especially as regards the design of workplaces, the choices of work equipment and the choice of working and production methods, with a view, in particular, to alleviating monotonous work and work at a predetermined work rate and to reducing their effects on health;
- developing a coherent overall prevention policy which covers technology, organization of work, working conditions, social relation-ships and the influence of factors related to the working environment.'

EUROPEAN *AD HOC* GROUP ON WORK-RELATED STRESS

Against this background, the European Commission issued an Orientation Document for its Ad Hoc Group (AHG) on 'Work-Related Stress', providing the following reasons for its endeavours:

- stress at work may lead to mental or physical ill-health;
- also stress that is not work-related can manifest itself in the workplace;
- the human and economic costs of such stress are very high to all concerned;
- such costs should therefore be reduced by preventing work related stress.

The AHG has recently issued its Draft Opinion (Doc. 5501/2/96). The latter was discussed at the Plenary Meeting of the EU Advisory Committee for Safety, Hygiene and Health Protection at Work in late November, 1996, and accepted unanimously (European Commission, 1997).

Its Recommendations include support for:

- *Research* on work, stress and health;
- *Guidance* for National Guidelines;
- *Exchange of information* on Work-Related Stress; and
- *Education and training*.

The key paragraph of the current (Fourth) EU Framework Programme (for research) indicates that 'the Union is giving priority to projects which are likely to have a direct impact in terms of competitiveness and quality of life and will therefore respond to the concerns of European enterprises and citzens'. A related approach seems to be well founded also in the area of prevention and management of work-related stress in European enterprises.

CONTEXT

Stress management and prevention have traditionally focused on individual approaches, usually by counselling individuals or small groups of employees on ways to adapt to, or cope with, various occupational stressors and/or their consequences. More recently, approaches have started to include encouraging employees to adjust their work environment to their abilities and needs, thereby improving the 'person-environment fit', and advising management and supervisors to allow or even promote such adjustments.

An *example* of such an approach has been reported by Kvarnström (1992) from the multinational Asea Brown Boveri (ABB) Company. In one of its Swedish departments, plagued by high sick leave absence rates, low productivity and high personnel turnover, an intervention was carried out aiming at increasing the variety of the work tasks, increasing understanding of the various links of the production chain, as well as job enlargement and job enrichment.

This was facilitated by a step-by-step increase of workers' competence through education and training, enabling the workers to rotate among various assembly and operation tasks in an autonomous group. When this had been achieved, workers were further trained also to be in charge of product control and packaging.

These steps in employee development were followed by three additional steps aimed at job enrichment, namely planning of materials, securing quality and coordinating production.

Most of the employees attained a developmental level beyond the three first mandatory steps, but not all considered themselves sufficiently competent to take responsibility of overall planning and coordination of the work for the entire group. This latter task was allowed to rotate among the members of the group who had advanced to the highest level of this competence staircase.

This training process was not conducted in the traditional way, which usually consists of trainees passively attending formal lectures. Instead, the trainees accompanied a trained worker or salaried employee to 'learn by doing'.

No professional lecturers were used in this training programme. Instead, skilled workers and salaried employees were encouraged to take on one apprentice each and to train him or her for the new tasks. Care was taken not to place new work demands upon an employee who had not yet received adequate training. By harmonizing job demands and corresponding competence through step-by-step education and training, employees were able to succeed in their new roles, with positive effects on their self-esteem resulting.

A final component in this programme was to designate a special production officer to implement the day-to-day improvements in working life proposed by members of the group. In this way, workers suggesting improvements were allowed to implement their own proposals and to see the results with very rapid feedback. Thus, new ideas were promoted much more efficiently than with the old system, which required expert review of each proposal and resulted in late, or no, implementation.

The author discusses some of the inevitable difficulties encountered but concludes that this package of interventions did result in a pronounced decrease in personnel turnover and sick leave absence rates, and a dramatic increase in productivity.

It should be noted that this type of approach, usually combined with the other approaches, has been pursued not only on an individual or company level (cf. ILO, 1992; Murphy et al., 1995), but at a *national* level as well (Levi, 1992).

TARGETS FOR NATIONAL ACTION

It is instructive to see how the Swedish Government has approached this task in a step-by-step manner. Following a decade of intensive interactions with the scientific community, in which available information on the interrelationships between living conditions, lifestyles, and health was reviewed, the Swedish Government presented its Public Health Service Act (Act No. 560, 1985) which states the following:

- 'Our health is determined in large measure by our living conditions and lifestyle'.
- 'The health risks in contemporary society take the form of, for instance, work, traffic and living environments that are physically and socially deficient, unemployment, abuse of alcohol and illicit drugs, consumption of tobacco, unsuitable dietary habits, as well as psychological and social strains associated with our relationship—and lack of relationship—with our fellow beings'.
- 'These health risks ... are now a major determinant of our possibilities of living a healthy life. This is true of practically all the health risks which give rise to today's most common diseases, e.g. cardiovascular disorders, mental ill health, tumours and allergies, as well as accidents'.
- 'Care must (therefore) start from a holistic approach ... By a holistic approach we mean that people's symptoms and illnesses, their causes

and consequences, are appraised in both a medical and a psychological and social perspective'.

Three years later, the Swedish Government focused in on one of the key components of the 'living conditions' mentioned in its Public Health Service Act, namely the work environment. It appointed and issued its terms of reference for a Swedish Commission on the Work Environment, against a background of the Government's concern about recent trends in work-related morbidity, long-term absence due to sickness and premature retirement.

The Swedish Commission on the Work Environment presented its final report in 1990. The report proposed a number of amendments to the Work Environment Act of 1977.

Based on these proposed amendments, the resulting amended Swedish Work Environment Act (Act No. 677, 1991) now states the following concerning the characteristics of the work environment:

- 'Working conditions shall be adapted to people's differing physical and psychological circumstances.
- Employees shall be enabled to participate in the arrangement of their own job situations as well as in work changes and development that affect their jobs.
- Technology, work organization and job content shall be arranged so that the employee is not exposed to physical or mental loads that may cause ill health or accidents.
- The matters to be considered in this context shall include forms of remuneration and the scheduling of working hours.
- Rigorously controlled or tied work shall be avoided or restricted.
- It shall be the aim of work to afford opportunities for variety, social contacts and cooperation as well as continuity between individual tasks.
- It shall further be the aim for working conditions to afford opportunities for personal and occupational development as well as for self-determination and occupational responsibility.'

Theoretically, work-related disease may be prevented at any of several links of the pathogenetic chain. Thus, work environment stressors might be removed, modified or avoided by adjusting the work environment, organization and content. Salutogenic variables might be increased (e.g. by improving social networks or expanding the workers' coping abilities). Physiological, behavioural and emotional pathogenic mechanisms might be interrupted (e.g. by blocking adrenergic beta-receptors, anti-smoking campaigns, psychotherapeutic conselling, tranquilizers). Precursors of disease might be treated so that they do not progress to overt disease (cf. Levi, 1981, 1992).

In order to safeguard individual rights, prevent the perpetuation of harmful or useless measures, limit losses to the community's purse and advance knowledge of the future, any of these, or other, actions must be evaluated when implemented. Such evaluation is the modern, humane substitute for nature's slow, cruel 'survival of the fittest', and is a means of enabling people to adapt with minimal trauma to a rapidly changing work environment and to control this change (Kagan & Levi, 1975; Levi, 1979).

One of the very few large-scale interventions that has been evaluated, although in a somewhat simplistic manner, is the Swedish initiative to promote both humanization of working life and increased productivity by applying what is essentially the principles of the Swedish Work Environment Act (and the European Union's Framework Directive). To promote practical work along these lines, the Swedish Working Life Fund was set up by a decree of the Swedish Parliament. It has distributed a total of 15 billion Swedish kronor over a six-year period aimed at a radical renewal of Swedish working life. The amount corresponded at that time to nearly US\$ 3 billion for a total labour force of 4 million employees. The money has been collected from Swedish employers through a special charge. Through financial grants to the employers, the Fund tried to promote a healthy work environment and work organization and productivity, as well as active rehabilitation programmes in the workplace.

It was used for some 25,000 work life programmes covering approximately 3 million out of Sweden's 4 million employees. Evaluation was carried out by a survey to 20% of a random sample of 7,500 of the major programmes. The survey was addressed to key persons in each programme, both management and labour.

According to Brulin and Nilsson (1995) it was found in service sector programmes that waiting time for customers decreased by > 10% in 34% of the cases. Performance time decreased by > 10% in 33% of the cases. Costs went down by > 10% in 23% of the cases because of better understanding of customer needs. And performed work per employee went up by > 10% in 42% of the cases. In industrial programmes included in the sample it was found that production errors went down by > 10% in 45% of the cases. Time for delivery decreased by > 10% in 52% of the cases, and readjustment time by > 10% in 34% of the cases. Productivity increased by > 10% in 45% of the cases.

Across sectors, physical job strain decreased by > 10% in 59%, employee co-determination (decision latitude) increased in 64% of all cases, and employee work satisfaction and motivation increased in 71% of the cases. Virtually no negative effects were reported.

It was found that rating by management and labour union representatives, respectively, were almost equal (Brulin and Nilsson, 1995).

CRITERIA FOR ACTION

Six criteria have been proposed which should be considered before setting specific goals for action against psychosocially-induced occupational and other health problems and their causes (WHO, 1976):

- Public health significance of the problem, reflected in number of people affected, severity of its consequences and implications for other spheres of community life.
- Level of public awareness of the problem and priority assigned to it. A problem of demonstrable public health importance may not be perceived as such by the community and rank low in the order of priorities (and vice versa).
- Modifiability of the problem by the available means.
- Societal (and enterprise) cost of action (or of inaction), including not just economic costs but also social and ethical considerations, evaluated against projected costs of inaction.
- Possibility to identify target population for action. The group which manifests a psychosocially-induced disturbance may not necessarily be the group to which action should be directed to prevent the disturbance (supervisors or management may be the primary target population for preventing psychosocially-induced work-related disorders in workers, for example).
- Availability of an appropriate agent of change. In some instances, the agent would be personnel of the occupational health services, but in others there may be people who are better placed to reach and influence the target population (e.g. legislators, management, unions, supervisors).

After applying these criteria, occupational health services should function in the following two different ways: (a) by designing psychosocial remedial measures based on sound situational analysis (for example, making the occupational health service more responsive to the psychosocial needs of employees, strengthening health education and coping skills); (b) by working together with all three parties on the labour market to combat high risk situations, specifically on the structural level, as requested in the amended Work Environment Act and the EU Framework Directive quoted above.

Whereas in each community the choice of a particular approach or strategy aimed at influencing psychosocial factors that affect occupational health and health care will be determined by a range of situation-specific considerations, four general categories of approaches and strategies proposed by the US National Institute for Occupational Safety and Health (NIOSH, 1988) can be applied in any community:

1. Improve job content and organization (in accordance with, for example, the amended Work Environment Act) for controlling psychosocial and other risk factors at work.

2. Monitor changes in work situations, workers' health and their interrelationship.
3. Increase awareness, inform, train, educate.
4. Broaden goals and strategies of occupational health services.

CONSTRAINTS TO PREVENTIVE ACTION

Applying these strategies will sometimes be difficult owing to a large number of constraints (cf. Kagan & Levi, 1975). First, there are constraints common to the health services in general: lack of manpower, funds, facilities, treatment and prevention technology, and the uncoordinated and wasteful use of such resources. Secondly, there are constraints to the field of health, including difficult ethical issues, ambiguities and vagueness of many of the concepts used, and the lack of operational content in many of the proposals made by experts. There is also the harmful separation of psychiatry from general medicine, and of the medical disciplines from psychological, social and economic fields of study. The medical profession as a whole has, in the past, shown a preference for the specialist approach rather than generalization, and has favoured disease treatment rather than health promotion. Furthermore, the medical profession has traditionally regarded health services as a goal rather than a tool to make life more satisfactory for the largest number of people. In order to counteract the above-mentioned constraints, initiative is needed in several directions.

An in-depth discussion of goals, mechanisms, options and obstacles for primary prevention practices is provided by Bloom (1996).

MONITORING

We need to monitor the physical and psychosocial conditions of work (and outside work), and workers' health, well-being and performance. This will inform us of relevant trends and, most importantly, help elucidate the relationships between these work and non-work sectors (Kagan & Levi, 1975). We use the term monitoring for several purposes. The first and most important, although most difficult to achieve, is as an early warning system. In this capacity, monitoring can indicate impending trouble in the occupational ecosystem in terms of working conditions, health and quality of life at a time when something can still be done to prevent the problems. If the entire flow of events that translates this warning into a decision to act (or not act) functions optimally, the threatened trouble can be avoided through social action, particularly participation at tripartite level, i.e., involving government, management, and labour. But even when early warning can be given, in reality there is often little avoiding action to take.

However, the warning may still be useful in that it gives time to prepare for the problems envisaged. Another equally important use of monitoring is to assess whether action to increase the quality of working life is effective or not (cf. Swedish Statistical Bulletin, 1996). Since 1989, the National Swedish Board of Occupational Safety and Health, in collaboration with Statistics Sweden, undertakes surveys of the working conditions in Sweden by questioning 10,000 to 15,000 persons of the working population (employees, self-employed persons and family workers) every other year. The Labour Force Survey is used as a foundation for this Working Environment Survey. The investigation is partly carried out by interviews, partly by questionnaires. In 1995 the questionnaire consisted of around 130 items. These studies are very extensive, and by combining the results from several studies it is possible to create extremely thorough statistical material which, in turn, makes it possible to subdivide and report on the labour market in many different categories.

By comparing the outcomes of these surveys from different years, the reader gets a very detailed picture of the present situation in terms of work environment and workers' subjective health, as well as of the interrelations between these sets of measures and of secular trends, for females and males, different age groups, occupations, economic activities and socio-economic classification.

Information that relates to many disciplines is collected for monitoring. The collected information is longitudinal and standardized in order to make data comparable over time. Although not likely to be conclusive in any way, high and/or rapidly increasing rates for suicide, neuroses, cardiovascular disorders, substance abuse and/or distress, dissatisfaction and alienation would indicate a need for more detailed inquiry and subsequent action.

Monitoring occupational and other environmental stimuli, level of living and quality of life also serves as a useful basis for epidemiological research and social action. If properly conducted and evaluated, the monitoring of these factors can be regarded as part of a national, or even international, experiment.

Tripartite decision-making, social action and research, therefore, should be closely integrated (Levi, 1979; 1998).

SUPPORTING ACTIVITIES

Besides applying existing information and acquiring new knowledge (i.e. research) to reduce the impact of negative psychosocial occupational and other factors on workers' health, a number of supporting activities are needed (cf. Shimomitsu, Sauter, Levi et al., 1998):

- to motivate and train occupational health workers and investigators for

cooperation in planning, administration and evaluation of occupational health and/or social actions, and for testing key hypotheses;
- to develop terminology and methods;
- to coordinate activities and cooperate with international, regional and national organizations;
- to collect, store and retrieve information on published and on-going activities (documentation); and
- to formulate and disseminate information on occupational health/social actions in an appropriate manner.

Although much of the above remains to be implemented, I have the impression that international and national authorities alike are moving in the direction indicated above. This is true for the 15 EU Member States in line to implement the most recent of these recommendations (European Commission, 1997). Similar trends can also be seen in the United States (cf. Murphy et al., 1995) and in Japan (Shimomitsu et al., 1998).

References

Bloom M. (1996) *Primary Prevention Practices*. London, New Delhi: Sage, Thousand Oaks.

Brulin, G. & Nilsson, T. (1995) *Arbetsutveckling Och Förbättrad Produktivitet. (Work Development and Improved Productivity.)* Stockholm: School of Business Research.

Cooper, C. L., Liukkonen, P. & Cartwright, S. (1996) *Assessing the Benefits of Stress Prevention at Company Level*. Dublin: European Foundation for the Improvement of Living and Working Conditions.

Di Martino, V. (1992) Occupational Stress: A Preventive Approach. *Conditions of Work Digest*, **11**, 2, 3–21.

E. U. (in press) *Ad Hoc Group on 'Work Related Stress': Draft Opinion*. Doc. 5501/2/96. European Commission. Luxembourg: Office for official publications of the European Communities.

European Foundation for the Improvement of Living and Working Conditions (1994) *European Conference on Stress at Work—A Call for Action Proceedings*. Luxembourg: Office for Official Publications of the European Communities.

International Labour Office (ILO) (1986) *Psychosocial Factors at Work: Recognition and Control*. Report of the Joint ILO/WHO Committee on Occupational Health, Ninth Session, Geneva, ILO.

International Labour Office (ILO) (1992) Preventing Stress at Work. *Conditions of Work Digest*, **11**.

Kagan, A. R. & Levi, L. (1975) Health and Environment—Psychosocial Stimuli. A Review. In *Society, Stress and Disease—Childhood and Adolescence*, edited by L. Levi, Vol. II. Oxford University Press.

Kalimo, R., El-Batawi, M. A. & Cooper, C. L. (eds.) (1987) *Psychosocial Factors at Work and Their Relation to Health*. Geneva: World Health Organization.

Kompier, M. & Levi, L. (1994) *Stress at Work: Causes, Effects and Prevention*. Dublin: European Foundation for the Improvement of Living and Working Conditions.

Kvarnström, S. (1992) Organizational approaches to reducing stress and health problems in an industrial setting in Sweden. *Conditions of Work Digest*, **11**(2), 227–232.

Levi, L. (1979) Psychosocial Factors in Preventive Medicine. In *Healthy People. The Surgeons General's Report on Health Promotion and Disease Prevention*, edited by D. A. Hamburg, E. O. Nightingale & V. Kalmar. Background Papers. Washington DC: Government Printing Office, 207–252.

Levi, L. (ed.) (1981) *Society, Stress and Disease—Working Life*, Vol. IV. Oxford, New York, Toronto: Oxford University Press.

Levi, L. (1992) Managing Stress in Work Settings at the National Level in Sweden. *Conditions of Work Digest*, **11**, 139–143.

Levi, L. & Lunde-Jensen, P. (1996) *Socio-Economic Costs of Work Stress in Two EU Member States—A Model for Assessing the Costs of Stressors at National Level*. Dublin: European Foundation for the Improvement of Living and Working Conditions.

Levi, L. (1998) The Welfare of the Future. A Swedish Case Study. Technical Input for the Verona Initiative. World Health Organization, Copenhagen.

Murphy, L. R., Hurrell, J. J., Jr., Sauter, S. L. & Keita, G. P. (1995) *Job Stress Interventions*. Washington: American Psychological Association.

National Institute for Occupational Safety and Health (NIOSH) (1988) *Prevention of Occupational Generated Illnesses: A proposed Synoptic National Strategy to Reduce Neurotoxic Disorders in the U.S. Workplace*. Cincinnati, Ohio: NIOSH (NTIS No. PB89-130348, pp. 31–50).

Paoli, P. (1992) *First European Survey on the Working Environment 1991–1992*. Dublin: European Foundation for the Improvement of Living and Working Conditions.

Paoli, P. (1997) *Second European Survey on Working Conditions 1996*. Dublin: European Foundation for the Improvement of Living and Working Conditions.

Shimomitsu, T., Sauter, S., Levi, L. et al. (1998) The Tokyo Declaration on Work-Related Stress and Health in Three Post-Industrial Settings. Tokyo Medical University, Tokyo.

Statistical Bulletin: The Working Environment 1995 (1996). *Statistical Bulletin No. Am 68 SM 9601*. Stockholm: National Board of Statistics, and National Board of Occupational Safety and Health.

World Health Organization (WHO) (1976) *Report of the First WHO Interdisciplinary Workshop on Psychosocial Factors and Health*. Geneva: WHO.

Chapter 14

COGNITIVE-BEHAVIORAL TREATMENT OF INSOMNIA:
Knitting Up the Ravell'd Sleave of Care

Richard R. Bootzin, PhD

> MACBETH: Methought I heard a voice cry, Sleep no more!
> Macbeth does murder sleep,—the innocent sleep;
> Sleep that knits up the ravell'd sleave of care,
> The death of each day's life, sore labour's bath,
> Balm of hurt minds, great nature's second course,
> Chief nourisher in life's feast. (Macbeth, Act II, Scene I)

As Shakespeare recognized, being unable to sleep is a dire personal consequence. Although there are multiple theories of the function of sleep, one important aspect of sleep, recognized for centuries, is that sleep helps restore the mind and body from the stresses of the day. The lack of sleep, insomnia, is a widespread problem. Surveys indicate that about 15% of adults report severe or frequent insomnia and another 15% report mild or occasional insomnia (Ford & Kamerow, 1989; Mellinger, Balter & Uhlenhuth, 1985). The diagnosis of primary insomnia is characterized by difficulty in initiating or maintaining sleep or of nonrestorative sleep that lasts for at least one month and is accompanied by marked distress or impairment in social, occupational, or other important areas of functioning (American Psychiatric Association, 1994).

Persistent insomnia has a significant impact on health, mood, and daytime functioning. Thus, in comparison to noninsomniacs, insomniacs more frequently report feeling less physically well, more often visit their physicians, have more absences from work due to illness, have more trouble with memory, concentration, and performance, and have more work-related accidents and injuries (Balter & Uhlenhuth, 1992; Leger et al., 1997; Silva, Chase, Sartorius & Roth, 1996).

During the past twenty-five years, a number of short-term psychological interventions for insomnia have been developed and evaluated (for reviews see Bootzin & Nicassio, 1978; Lacks & Morin, 1992; Lichstein & Riedel, 1994). Two separate meta-analyses of over 50 outcome studies have been published (Morin, Culbert & Schwartz, 1994; Murtagh & Greenwood, 1995). Both meta-analyses concluded that short-term psychological treatments have been found to improve the sleep of insomniacs over control conditions, and improvements were maintained at six month follow-ups.

This is in sharp contrast to the effects of general psychotherapy on sleep disturbance. Sleep complaints are among the least likely symptoms to change when patients receive as much as a year of psychodynamic or eclectic outpatient psychotherapy (Kopta, Howard, Lowry & Beutler, 1994). Consequently, to effectively treat sleep disturbance and to allow sleep once again to knit up 'the ravell'd sleave of care', therapists must focus directly on the assessment and treatment of the sleep complaint itself and not depend on change in sleep as the result of general psychotherapy.

CAUSES OF SLEEP DISTURBANCE

There are many causes of sleep disturbance including substances, biological rhythm disorders, physical disorders, psychological factors, poor sleep environments, and poor sleep habits. Sleep disturbance encompasses many specific sleep disorders. More detailed information about the diagnosis of sleep disorders can be found in the *International Classification of Sleep Disorders: Diagnostic and Coding Manual, Revised* (ASDA, 1997).

Substances

Both prescription and nonprescription substances can cause sleep disturbances. The use of drugs to induce or to suppress sleepiness may cause adverse effects with chronic use.

Hypnotics. The prescription of sedative/hypnotics is the most frequently-used treatment for insomnia. About 4.3% of adults in the U.S. use medically prescribed psychoactive medication to promote sleep (i.e., hypnotics, anxiolitics and antidepressants; Mellinger, Balter & Uhlenhuth, 1985). Of the sedative/hypnotics, benzodiazepines are the most frequently prescribed, having almost completely replaced barbiturates. As high as the prevalence rates for hypnotic medication are in the U.S., they are even higher in other countries. In France, the figures of habitual use range between 3.8%–6.2% (Quera-Salva, Orluc, Goldenberg & Guilleminault, 1991). In Israel, the percent of individuals who had four or more monthly prescriptions within a six month period was estimated as 6.5% (Matalon, Yinnon & Hurwitz 1990).

Five principles for pharmacotherapy for persistent insomnia have been summarized by Kupfer and Reynolds (1997): use the lowest effective dose; use intermittent dosing to delay tolerance (two to four times weekly);

prescribe medication for short-term use; discontinue medication gradually; and be alert for rebound insomnia following discontinuation.

The use of sedative/hypnotics to induce sleep is effective for short-term use, with effects that last 2 to 4 weeks. However, there have been no published randomized clinical trials of hypnotics for longer than 35 days (Kupfer & Reynolds, 1997). Thus, long-term effectiveness is unknown. The magnitude of improvement in sleep produced by hypnotics is modest. The average reduction in sleep onset latency in sleep laboratory studies is about 15 minutes and the average increase in total sleep is about an hour (e.g., Mendelson, 1995). Hypnotics also change the perception of being asleep. Insomniacs are more likely to report being asleep on nights they took a hypnotic than on nights they took a placebo, even when awakened from the same sleep stage. For example, insomniacs, awakened from stage 2 sleep, reported being asleep 50% of the time after taking a hypnotic as compared to 10% of the time after taking a placebo (Mendelson, 1995). The primary effect of hypnotics may be on the perception of sleep, and not directly on sleep itself (Mendelson, 1993).

Despite their frequent use, hypnotics are not the treatment of choice for persistent insomnia. Several problems are likely to occur with chronic use or attempted withdrawal. These include alterations of sleep stages, daytime sedation, impaired motor and cognitive functioning, dysphoric mood, dependence, and rebound insomnia (Shader & Greenblatt, 1993). The pharmacological effects of hypnotics depend upon dose, absorption rate, and serum half-life (Nicholson, 1994). Hypnotics with long half-lives (such as flurazepam) are likely to produce drug hangover and daytime sedation. Hypnotics with short half-lives (such as triazolam) may produce rebound insomnia the very same night the medication was taken and daytime anxiety.

Once benzodiazepine hypnotics or tranquilizers are begun, it is often difficult for individuals to withdraw. In a study of abrupt discontinuation of individuals who had been taking benzodiazepines for one year or longer, 56% taking long half-life and 62% taking short half-life benzodiazepines failed to remain free of drugs during a 5-week follow-up (Rickels et al. 1990). In a companion study of gradual taper, 32% of long half-life and 42% of short-half life benzodiazepine treated patients failed to achieve a drug-free state (Schweizer et al., 1990).

For the past several years, a new nonbenzodiazepine hypnotic, zolpidem, has been widely prescribed. Zolpidem is an imidazopyridine which is related to benzodiazepines but so far has not been shown to produce rebound insomnia or daytime residual effects (Monti, et al., 1994; Nicholson, 1994). Zolpidem is a very short half-life medication and is primarily useful for sleep onset problems. However, zolpidem, like all hypnotics, is a central nervous system depressant and may exacerbate other health problems.

Alcohol. The problems associated with benzodiazepine hypnotics and tranquilizers are true for alcohol as well. Continued use results in tolerance and sleep fragmentation becomes more frequent. Alcohol is REM-sleep depriving and withdrawal from heavy drinking produces REM rebound which is often accompanied by restless sleep and nightmares. Alcohol and hypnotics also exacerbate sleep apnea (see section on physical disorders). An important additional danger is that alcohol potentiates the effects of hypnotics and other depressants. Thus, the combination of alcohol and hypnotics may intensify and prolong deleterious side effects.

Antidepressants. Tricyclic antidepressants suppress REM sleep and can exacerbate periodic limb movements during sleep (see section on physical disorders). Many, but not all, of the new generation of antidepressants, selective serotonin reuptake inhibitors (SSRIs), produce increased physiological arousal during sleep resulting in reduced slow-wave sleep and decreased sleep efficiency (Armitage, Trivedi, Rush & Hoffmann, 1995). On the other hand, serotonin receptor modulators, such as trazodone and nefazodone, increase sleep continuity and do not reduce slow-wave sleep (Reynolds, Buysse, Nofzinger & Kupfer, 1995). In recent years, there has been a 100 percent increase in the use of antidepressant medication for insomnia (Kupfer & Reynolds, 1997). This increase, however, is not based on data from controlled clinical trials. There have been few controlled clinical trials on the use of antidepressants for insomnia.

Melatonin. There is substantial current interest in the use of melatonin for sleep, particularly in the elderly, and the regulation of the sleep/ wake circadian rhythm. The release of melatonin is suppressed by light during the day. Therefore, melatonin release serves as a circadian time-keeper. Taking exogenous melatonin can be effective as a means of resetting the sleep/wake circadian rhythm; e.g., to reduce jet lag. However, exposure to bright light accomplishes the same effect, as discussed in the section on biological rhythm problems. The use of exogenous melatonin for persistent insomnia is premature. While there are some promising research results for elderly insomniacs who were shown to be deficient in endogenous melatonin (e.g., Haimov, et al., 1995), important questions about dose size and long-term effects have yet to be answered.

Stimulants. Many drugs such as cocaine, amphetamines, and caffeine are used primarily for their sleep suppressing effects. Caffeine is contained in many foods and beverages, including coffee, tea, soft drinks, and chocolate. Other medications including analgesics (those that contain caffeine), bronchodilators, decongestants, and appetite suppressants are or contain stimulants that produce an increase in sleep latency, decrease in total sleep time, and an increase in spontaneous awakenings (ASDA, 1997; Brown et al., 1995). Nicotine is also a central nervous system stimulant and produces lighter and more fragmented sleep. Cessation of these substances may be associated with withdrawal symptoms such as sleepiness, irritability, and lassitude (ASDA, 1997).

Complaints of insomnia and/or anxiety may be due to excessive ingestion of caffeine, nicotine, or other stimulants. Since caffeine has a plasma half-life of approximately 6 hours, individuals continue to experience its effects long after it has been ingested. Reducing or eliminating the intake of caffeine, particularly in the afternoon and evening, and quitting smoking can lead to substantial improvement in sleep. However, an increase in disturbed sleep can be expected during the initial period of smoking withdrawal (Wetter, Fiore, Baker & Young, 1995).

Biological Rhythm Problems

Circadian rhythms refer to daily biological rhythms such as the daily sleep-wake rhythm. Circadian rhythm disorders occur when individuals attempt to sleep at times that are inconsistent with their underlying biological clocks. In *delayed sleep phase syndrome (DSPS)*, the sleep-wake circadian rhythm is delayed compared to when the individual attempts to sleep. Individuals with this problem report difficulty falling asleep at a desired bedtime, but have normal sleep if they attempt to sleep a few hours later. Delayed sleep phase individuals commonly identify themselves as 'night people' and report being most alert during the late evening and night hours. This problem is often seen in adolescents and young adults. In contrast, in *advanced sleep phase syndrome (ASPS)*, sleep occurs at an earlier than desired time and the individual awakens earlier than desired. Normal aging in older adults is often associated with a phase advance.

Evaluations of patients with insomnia have found that the sleep-wake circadian rhythm is shifted depending on the nature of the insomnia. Patients with sleep-onset insomnia, who have difficult falling asleep and difficulty waking up in the morning, have been found to have a delayed sleep-wake circadian rhythm as measured by core body temperature (Morris, Lack & Dawson, 1990). In contrast, patients with sleep-maintenance insomnia, who are sleepy in the early evening and have difficulty sustaining sleep, have been found to have an advanced sleep-wake circadian rhythm (Lack & Wright, 1993). Appropriately timed bright light exposure has been found to shift the sleep-wake rhythm; that is, bright light in the morning advances and bright light in the evening delays the sleep-wake rhythm.

Two common environmentally caused circadian rhythm problems are shift work and time-zone changes. Because of family and social demands, night shift workers usually attempt to live their days off on a different schedule than their work days. A disrupted sleep-wake schedule often results in disturbed and shortened sleep, sleepiness on the job, reduced performance levels, and psychological distress due to disruptions in family and social life. Workers on rotating shift schedules have greater difficulty than those on permanent night shifts. The severity of the problem increases with age.

Many researchers recommend that rotating shift schedules should be designed to be consistent with a natural underlying tendency of humans to phase delay. That is, the direction of rotation should be progressively later and the duration of the shift should be long enough to allow for adaptation. A variety of methods for enhancing alertness and performance among shift workers has been suggested (Penn & Bootzin, 1990). The optimal timing of work breaks, social activity during breaks, bright light and other sensory stimulation have the most potential for short-term alerting effects. Stress coping techniques, sleep hygiene information, and family counseling have the most potential for addressing the long-term effects of shift work.

Disturbed sleep associated with rapid time-zone change ('jet lag') is due to a desynchrony between the endogenous sleep-wake rhythm and the light/dark cycle. For most people disturbed sleep and daytime sleepiness subside after a few days, depending on the number of time-zones crossed. Westward travel is associated with disturbed sleep at the end of the sleep period, which coincides with habitual wake-up time, and eastward travel is associated with sleep onset insomnia. Due to the natural tendency to phase delay, travel westbound is easier to adjust to than travel eastbound. Frequent travelers, such as transatlantic airline crews, may experience more persistent difficulties.

Longer biological rhythms also affect sleep. Seasonal and monthly biological rhythms are called infradian rhythms. Individuals who live in the extreme northern and southern latitudes experience disrupted sleep during seasonal periods of 24-hour darkness and 24-hour sunlight. Individuals with seasonal affective disorder (SAD) also report changes in sleep need and sleep quality with changes in the seasons. The biological clock that regulates menstruation is another infradian rhythm and interacts with the sleep-wake system. Both subjective and objective data indicate that sleep is more disturbed and more fragmented premenstrually compared to the more hormonally quiescent pre-ovulatory phase (Manber & Bootzin, 1997).

Preliminary results indicate that bright light therapy may be effective for a number of biological rhythm sleep disorders (Terman, 1994). Bright light treatment during night shift work resulted in increased duration of daytime sleep and improved alertness on the job. Bright light has also been shown to benefit jet lag sufferers, those with sleep phase disorders, and those with SAD.

Physical Disorders

The most common physical disorders that affect sleep are sleep-related respiratory disturbances, including sleep containing *sleep apneas* (a cessation of airflow for 10 seconds or longer) and *hypopneas* (50% or greater reduction of airflow for 10 seconds or longer). These may occur repeatedly throughout the night's sleep producing frequent brief arousals during sleep leading to excessive daytime sleepiness. Three types of sleep apnea have been defined: (a) obstructive—cessation of airflow despite thoracic and abdominal respiratory effort, (b) central—cessation of airflow characterized by cessation of respiratory movements due to disordered central regulation of respiration, and (c) mixed—cessation of airflow without respiratory movement initially and then followed by respiratory effort. Most patients have a predominance of obstructive and mixed events and these patients are considered to have *obstructive sleep apnea* (OSA).

The most common symptoms of OSA are excessive daytime sleepiness and loud snoring (see Bootzin, Quan, Bamford & Wyatt, 1995). The prevalence of OSA has been estimated to be 4 percent in middle-aged men and 2 percent in middle-aged women. Respiratory pauses and sleep apneas increase with age. Women with OSA are generally postmenopausal. Obesity is often associated with obstructive sleep apnea, although not all patients are overweight. The course of treatment is dependent on the severity of the condition and the prominent symptoms associated with it. Initial treatment may consist of dietary control of weight, avoiding the use of alcohol at bedtime, keeping the individual from sleeping on his/her back, and avoiding the use of sedative hypnotics which, as depressants, may exacerbate the respiratory problems and reduce the patient's ability to wake up and breathe. Continuous positive air pressure (CPAP) which is administered by means of a nasal mask is an effective treatment for severe OSA. There are also a number of surgical procedures, such as uvulopharyngopalatoplasty (UPPP) which is intended to surgically widen air passageways, but they have had mixed success.

Patients with *central sleep apnea* (CSA), in contrast to those with OSA), often have insomnia (Bootzin, Quan, Bamford & Wyatt, 1995). Central apneas may occur at sleep onset reawakening the patient and contributing to an inability to fall asleep. Excessive daytime sleepiness, snoring, and obesity are not prominent clinical characteristics of CSA. Patients with CSA have many fewer apneas, and fewer disruptions during sleep, than patients with OSA. The treatment for CSA is pharmacological and usually involves respiratory stimulants.

Two muscular disorders—*periodic limb movement (PLM) disorder* and *restless legs syndrome* (RLS)—can also impair sleep. PLM disorder is characterized by periodic episodes of repetitive and stereotypic limb movements during sleep. The most common sleep characteristics associated with PLMs are frequent arousals and complaints of nonrestorative sleep. Patients are often unaware of PLMs and may report problems with insomnia or excessive daytime sleepiness.

RLS is a disorder characterized by irresistible leg movements usually prior to sleep onset (ASDA, 1997) and often described as a 'creeping' sensation. The most prominent characteristic of this disorder is the partial or complete relief of the sensation with leg motion and return of the symptom with cessation of movement. Symptoms often appear soon after getting into bed and tend to cease long enough for the patient to fall asleep, but may reappear later in the night. RLS may occur at times during the day after prolonged periods of sitting. Treatment for PLMs and RLS is pharmacological. The most effective drugs are benzodiazepines, dopamine agonists, and opioids (Bootzin, Quan, Bamford & Wyatt, 1995).

A number of other physical disorders can interfere with sleep. These include painful conditions such as arthritis, low back pain, fibromyalgia, and headaches, as well as chronic illnesses associated with pain including cancer, diabetes, and cardiovascular, gastrointestinal, and chronic obstructive pulmonary disease.

There are also striking sleep changes in persons with *Alzheimer's Disease* and other forms of dementia (see Bootzin, Epstein, Engle-Friedman & Salvio, 1996). Decreased sleep efficiency, increased percentage of stage 1 sleep and higher rate of arousals and awakenings have been confirmed by meta-analysis (Benca, Obermeyer, Thisted & Gillin, 1992). The aspect of sleep disturbance most likely to be brought to the attention of the clinician is what has been called *sundowning*. This describes late afternoon or early evening exacerbation of behavioral disruption and agitation. Sundowning is a complex and poorly defined syndrome. Several treatment approaches have been suggested (Bliwise, 1993). Pharmacological treatment has not been promising since hypnotics have minimal effect and neuroleptics have strong risks for side-effects in older persons. Behavioral treatments include regularly scheduled activities both in the day and during the usual night time awakenings, exposure to bright outdoor light, and sleep restriction (Bliwise, 1993). Family caretakers may also suffer sleep disturbances and benefit from respite breaks.

Psychological Factors

Many important life events occur that may be difficult to adjust to and thus may affect sleep. Individuals who ordinarily have little trouble sleeping often develop insomnia during periods of stress. Important life changes associated with aging such as retirement and the illness and death of loved ones can produce insomnia (see Bootzin, Epstein, Engle-Friedman & Salvio, 1996).

There is a large literature on the relationship between psychopathology and sleep disturbance (see Bootzin, Manber, Perlis, Salvio & Wyatt, 1993). Sleep problems are one of the primary symptoms of a major depressive episode (American Psychiatric Association, 1994). Difficulty initiating and maintaining sleep is common in depression. Early morning awakenings are seen more frequently in older than younger depressives. Sleep complaints appear to precede other symptoms in individuals vulnerable to depression. In a follow-up study of patients who had previously been depressed, complaints of sleep disturbance preceded and predicted the recurrence of depression (Perlis et al., 1997).

It is estimated that approximately 90 percent of all individuals with depression will have at least a mild degree of sleep architecture abnormality (Reynolds, 1989). The sleep of depressed individuals is characterized by an earlier-than-normal first rapid-eye-movement (REM) sleep period (the sleep period during which dreams typically occur), increased REM sleep during the first half of the night, and increased density of eye movement during REM sleep (Reynolds & Kupfer, 1987). Interestingly, one of the most reliable effects of programs of exercise is to increase REM latency and decrease the amount of REM sleep (Youngstedt, O'Connor & Dishman, 1997). This suggests that exercise might have an antidepressant effect.

It is commonly recommended that antidepressant medication be prescribed for patients whose insomnia is diagnosed as *resulting from* depression. It is difficult, if not impossible, however, to determine whether depression (or anxiety) is directly causing insomnia, because all that is observed is covariation (Bootzin & Nicassio, 1978). In cases in which psychological problems accompany sleep disturbance, separate therapeutic attention should be given to each. The therapist should not assume that improvement in one will automatically produce improvement in the other.

Poor Sleep Environment

Among the many environmental factors that affect sleep are sleeping surfaces, noise, temperature, room or bed sharing, and the need for vigilance during sleep such as occurs when an infant joins the household. There is no ideal room temperature or degree of mattress firmness. People can learn to sleep comfortably in a wide range of temperatures and on many different surfaces. Individuals may have developed strong preferences, however, so that sleep is disrupted if the sleep environment does not correspond to those preferences. This problem is frequently observed when people move to a new setting. The unfamiliarity of the setting and the lack of familiar personal belongings may cause a prolonged period of disrupted sleep.

Noise decreases both the amount of deep sleep and the continuity of sleep. There is an increase in body movements and sleep stage shifts. Even people who habitually sleep in noisy environments do not fully adapt to the noise. Unpredictable noise is especially disturbing (Sanchez & Bootzin, 1985). Thus, continuous white noise, such as from a fan or from the end of the dial of an FM radio, can be a useful means of dampening the effects of noisy environments.

Poor Sleep Habits

There are many daily living activities that have been found to be 'inconsistent with the maintenance of good quality sleep and full daytime alertness' (p. 73, ASDA, 1997). These include highly irregular sleep-wake schedules, extended time in bed, irregular naps and engaging in activities at bedtime that are incompatible with falling asleep.

The relation between biological rhythms and the sleep-wake cycle is the basis for the common recommendation to maintain a regular sleep schedule. Individuals who keep irregular schedules for long periods of time are at risk for developing sleep disturbances. Those with sleep disturbances frequently benefit from regularizing their sleep schedule. For example, to cope with insufficient sleep on school nights, high school and college students typically try to catch-up on the weekends leading to irregular sleep patterns and sleepiness during the day. In a study in which college students were required to regularize their sleep patterns in addition to scheduling adequate time for sleep, the students were more alert during the day than if they retained an irregular sleep- wake schedule, even if they had adequate time for sleep (Manber, Bootzin, Aceob & Carskadon, 1996).

Insomniacs may also engage in activities at bedtime that are incompatible with falling asleep (Bootzin & Nicassio, 1978). Insomniacs may, for example, use their bedrooms for reading, talking on the telephone, watch television, snacking, listening to music, and probably, most disturbing of all, worrying. The result is that the bed is no longer just a cue for sleeping; instead it becomes a cue for physiological arousal.

Cognitive intrusions may be particularly disruptive. Worries and concerns are often accompanied by emotional upset, yet they may appear in the absence of excessive physiological arousal. The content of the insomniac's concerns may shift from the general pressures of current and future problems to persevering worries regarding the inability to fall asleep or to get enough sleep during the night. The bedroom, then, can become a cue for the anxiety and frustration associated with trying to fall asleep. Insomniacs often sleep well any place other than in their own beds. For example, they may sleep better in a sleep laboratory than they do at home. In contrast, people who have no difficulty falling asleep in their own beds often have difficulty doing so in strange surroundings.

THERAPEUTIC APPROACHES

Because of the multifaceted etiology of insomnia, a thorough assessment is essential. Patients seen at the Insomnia Clinic at the University of Arizona Sleep Disorders Center provide medical and psychiatric histories, complete daily sleep diaries, have thorough insomnia intake interviews, and complete the following measures: the Beck Depression Inventory (Beck et al., 1961), the Brief Symptom Inventory (Derogatis & Melisaratos, 1983), the Sleep Anticipatory Anxiety Questionnaire (Bootzin, Shoham & Kuo, 1994), and the Beliefs and Attitudes about Sleep Scale (Morin, 1993). If it appears that other sleep disorders (e.g., PLMs, sleep apnea) may contribute to the problem, a one- or two-night polysomnographic study in a sleep laboratory would be done. In addition, interviews with family members are often a useful supplement.

Daily sleep diaries are a form of self-monitoring and are a critical component of the assessment and treatment process. Diaries typically include entries for naps, sleep latency, number and duration of awakenings, total sleep, quality of sleep, feelings upon awakening, and whether or not the night in question was a typical night. The patients fill out the diaries each morning.

Diaries are a practical, efficient means of obtaining information about the frequency of sleep problems in the patient's own environment. As a consequence of keeping daily diaries, patients often discover that their sleep problems are not as severe or as frequent as they thought. Daily diaries also provide a means of assessing whether or not interventions are having any effect. Without diaries, patients may become discouraged at the occurrence of even a single sleepless night. Keeping sleep diaries helps to keep the patients focused on whether or not the frequency of the sleep problem is changing.

A number of cognitive-behavioral treatments have been found to be effective for treating insomnia. These include sleep hygiene information, stimulus control instructions, sleep restriction, relaxation training, biofeedback, and cognitive therapy.

Sleep Hygiene Information

Basic information about sleep and sleep hygiene is usually provided as a core component of cognitive-behavioral treatments for insomnia. Inadequate sleep hygiene refers to daily living activities that are inconsistent with the maintenance of good quality sleep and daytime alertness (ASDA, 1997). Among the activities included in this category are the irregular use of daytime naps, extended amounts of time in bed, irregular sleep-wake schedules, the routine use of products that interfere with sleep such as caffeine, nicotine, or alcohol, scheduling of exercise close to bedtime, engaging in exciting or emotionally upsetting activities close to bedtime, having a poor sleep environment such as an uncomfortable bed or having the bedroom be too bright, stuffy, hot, cold, or noisy. In addition, emphasis is placed on the individual variability of sleep need and on changes in the nature and quality of sleep associated with aging.

In recent years, increased focus has been placed on the use of bright light to regularize the sleep/wake circadian rhythm. Encouraging results have been reported for the use of bright light with insomniacs. Morning light has been found to reduce sleep onset latency in sleep onset insomniacs (Lack, Wright & Paynter, 1995) and evening light has been found to delay wake-up time and increase total sleep (Lack & Wright, 1993) and increase sleep efficiency (Campbell, Dawson & Anderson, 1993) in sleep maintenance insomniacs.

The increasing literature on the effectiveness of bright light in resetting the sleep/wake circadian rhythm in a variety of settings has led many clinicians to add exposure to bright light as one of the sleep hygiene recommendations. In an evaluation of exercise and bright light recommendations, the strongest improvement was found for insomniacs who received morning bright light instructions along with other sleep hygiene recommendations (Guilleminault et al., 1995). Recommendations to exercise may not have been effective because of variability in compliance. A meta-analysis concluded that exercise must last for at least an hour in order to have reliable effects on sleep (Youngstedt, O'Connor & Dishman, 1997). Regular exercise programs in older men have been shown to produce increased continuous sleep, increased slow-wave sleep, and decreased nighttime awakenings (Edinger et al., 1993; Vitiello et al., 1992).

Sleep hygiene recommendations, as a sole intervention, is not as effective as other behavioral treatments (Morin, Culbert & Schwartz, 1994). Information about sleep and sleep hygiene is clearly important and is included in all multicomponent treatment packages. Caution should be exercised, however, in relying only on sleep hygiene recommendations since other behavioral treatments have been found to be more effective.

Stimulus Control Instructions

Stimulus control instructions are intended to help the insomniac relearn how to fall asleep quickly in bed. They consist of a set of instructions designed to (1) establish a consistent sleep-wake rhythm, (2) strengthen the bed and bedroom as cues for sleep, and (3) weaken them as cues for activities that might interfere or are incompatible with sleep.

The following rules constitute the stimulus control instructions (Bootzin, Epstein & Wood, 1991).

1. Lie down intending to go to sleep only when you are sleepy.
2. Do not use your bed for anything except sleep; that is, do not read, watch television, eat, or worry in bed. Sexual activity is the only exception to this rule. On such occasions, the instructions are to be followed afterward when you intend to go to sleep.
3. If you find yourself unable to fall asleep, get up and go into another room. Stay up as long as you wish and then return to the bedroom to sleep. Although we do not want you to watch the clock, we want you to get out of bed if you do not fall asleep immediately. Remember the goal is to associate your bed with falling asleep *quickly!* If you are in bed more than about 10 minutes without falling asleep and have not gotten up, you are not following this instruction.
4. If you still cannot fall asleep, repeat Step 3. Do this as often as is necessary throughout the night.
5. Set your alarm and get up at the same time every morning irrespective of

how much sleep you got during the night. This will help your body acquire a consistent sleep rhythm.
6. Do not nap during the day.

The focus of the instructions is primarily on sleep onset. For sleep maintenance problems, the instructions are to be followed after awakening when the patient has difficulty falling back to sleep. Although stimulus control instructions appear simple and straight-forward, compliance is better if the instructions are discussed individually and a rationale is provided for each rule (Bootzin, Epstein & Wood, 1991).

Rule 1. The goal of this rule is to help the patients become more sensitive to internal cues of sleepiness so that they will be more likely to fall asleep quickly when they go to bed.

Rule 2. The goals here are to have activities that are associated with arousal occur elsewhere and to break up patterns that are associated with disturbed sleep. If bedtime is the only time patients have for thinking about the day's events and planning the next day, they should spend some quiet time doing that in another room before they go to bed. Many people who do not have insomnia read or listen to music in bed without problem. This is not the case for insomniacs, however. This instruction is used to help those who have sleep problems establish new routines to facilitate sleep onset.

Rules 3 and 4. In order to associate the bed with sleep and disassociate it from the frustration and arousal of not being able to sleep, the patients are instructed to get out of bed after about 10 minutes (20 minutes for those over 60 years old). This is also a means of coping with insomnia. By getting out of bed and engaging in other activities, patients are taking control of their problem. Consequently, the problem becomes more manageable and the patient is likely to experience less distress.

Rule 5. Insomniacs often have irregular sleep rhythms because they try to make up for poor sleep by sleeping late or by napping the next day. Keeping consistent wake times helps patients develop consistent sleep rhythms. In addition, the set wake times mean that the patients will be somewhat sleep-deprived after a night of insomnia. This will make it more likely that they will fall asleep quickly the following night, strengthening the cues of the bed and bedroom for sleep. Often insomniacs will want to follow a different sleeping schedule on weekends or nights off than they do during the work week. It is important to have as consistent a schedule as possible, seven nights a week. In our experience, a deviation of no more than one hour in the wake time on days off does not produce problems in establishing a consistent rhythm.

Rule 6. The goals of this rule are to keep insomniacs from disrupting their sleep patterns by irregular napping and to prevent them from losing the advantage of the sleep loss of the previous night for increasing the likelihood of faster sleep onset the following night. A nap that takes place seven days a week at the same time would be permissible. For those elderly insomniacs who feel that they need to nap, a short daily afternoon nap of 30 to 45 minutes or the use of 20 to 30 minutes of relaxation as a nap substitute is recommended.

Cognitive-behavioral treatments for insomnia, including stimulus control instructions, are primarily self-management treatments. The treatments are carried out by the patients at home. Consequently, compliance may be a problem. Most compliance problems can be solved by direct discussion with the patients. A common problem is the disturbance of the spouses' sleep when the insomniacs get out of bed. Discussion with the spouses are often helpful in ensuring full cooperation. During the winter in cold climates, some patients may be reluctant to leave the warmth of their beds. Suggestions for keeping warm robes near the beds and keeping an additional room warm throughout the night, along with encouragement to try to follow instructions, are usually effective in promoting compliance (Bootzin, Engle-Friedman & Hazlewood, 1983).

There have been many studies from many different investigators evaluating the effectiveness of stimulus control instructions for insomnia. Reviews of those studies indicate that stimulus control instructions is one of the most effective, if not the most effective, single component therapy (Lacks & Morin, 1992; Morin, Culbert & Schwartz, 1994; Murtagh & Greenwood, 1995). It is useful, therefore, to have stimulus control instructions as a core treatment element, around which other elements can be added.

Sleep Restriction

Sleep restriction (Spielman, Saskin & Thorpy, 1987) is based on the observation that many insomniacs have low sleep efficiency; i.e., the proportion of time they are in bed that they are actually asleep is less than 85 percent. To help consolidate sleep, insomniacs are instructed to limit the time that they are in bed to the number of hours of sleep that they normally obtain. At first, patients experience partial sleep deprivation since they usually underestimate how much sleep they normally get. The sleep deprivation, however, helps to consolidate sleep. Patients are then instructed to follow a gradual schedule of increasing the amount of time spent in bed while maintaining the improved sleep efficiency.

In a meta-analysis, sleep restriction and stimulus control instructions were found to be the two most effective treatments (Morin, Culbert & Schwartz, 1994). Sleep restriction therapy has been included as a core component of treatment packages for patients with sleep maintenance insomnia. Significant reduction in time awake after sleep onset, increase in sleep efficiency and total sleep time, and less time in bed have been reported (e.g. Edinger et al., 1990; Friedman, Bliwise, Yesavage & Salom, 1991).

Relaxation Training, Meditation and Biofeedback

A commonly recommended treatment for insomnia is some type of relaxation training. This includes a variety of procedures such as progressive relaxation, diaphragmatic breathing, autogenic training, transcendental meditation, yoga, and hypnosis. Progressive relaxation, developed by Edmund Jacobson (1938) is the most widely researched single nonpharmacological treatment for insomnia (Lichstein & Riedel, 1994). Progressive relaxation involves sequentially tensing and releasing the body's major muscle groups while attending to the changing sensations of tension and relaxation.

There are a number of studies that indicate that relaxation procedures can produce improved sleep (e.g., Borkovec, Grayson, O'Brien & Weerts, 1979; Espie, Lindsay et al., 1989; Nicassio & Bootzin, 1974). The different types of relaxation and meditation procedures have all been found to be about equally effective as treatments for insomnia in controlled studies.

Studies investigating the relationship between physiological arousal and sleep onset latency have produced both positive (Bonnet & Arand, 1995; Freedman & Sattler, 1982) and negative (Good, 1975; Haynes, Follingstad & McGowan, 1974) results. Thus, not all insomniacs are hyperaroused. But those who are, are likely to be aroused both during the day and at night. Bonnet and Arand (1995) found that insomniacs had increased 24-hour metabolic rate when compared to age-matched controls. The insomniacs also had more disturbed sleep and took longer to fall asleep during the day on the Multiple Sleep Latency Test (MSLT).

Because many insomniacs are aroused and anxious during the day, relaxation training may provide a double benefit—first, as a general coping skill to reduce daytime arousal and deal more effectively with the stresses of the day and second, as a means of helping to induce sleep (Bootzin & Nicassio, 1978). Regardless of the type of relaxation method employed, it is important to teach relaxation as a 'portable' skill. The reliance on tapes may foster dependence on the machine and make it less likely that the insomniac will be able to use relaxation as a general coping skill for other life stressors.

Electromyogram (EMG) biofeedback is included as a relaxation procedure since it is best characterized as biofeedback-assisted relaxation. Patients are usually taught a relaxation procedure to practice at home when biofeedback is not available. EMG biofeedback has been found to be more effective than no treatment at relieving symptoms of insomnia, but it has not proven to be superior to relaxation training or other behavioral treatments (see Bootzin & Rider, 1997). A different type of biofeedback attempts to strengthen a 12–14 Hz rhythm from the sensory-motor cortex and is called sensory-motor rhythm (SMR) biofeedback. The different types of biofeedback have about equal overall effectiveness. However, EMG biofeedback has been found to be most effective for anxious insomniacs with sleep onset problems whereas SMR biofeedback has been found to be most effective for nonanxious insomniacs with sleep maintenance problems (Hauri, 1981; Hauri et al., 1982).

Cognitive Therapy

There are a number of cognitive symptoms that contribute to insomnia such as worry, cognitive intrusions, and dysfunctional beliefs about sleep and its consequences. Among the cognitive interventions are cognitive restructuring, paradoxical intention, thought-stopping, and articulatory suppression.

Cognitive restructuring. Insomniacs often subscribe to a number of irrational beliefs about sleep. Examples of these beliefs would be that the individual must get at least 8 hours of sleep to feel refreshed and function well the next day, or the worry that if the individual goes for one or two nights without sleep he or she will have a nervous breakdown, or the belief that the individual should avoid or cancel social, family, and work obligations after a poor night's sleep (Morin, 1993). Cognitive therapy directed at changing maladaptive attitudes and beliefs is called *cognitive restructuring.* Five types of dysfunctional cognitions are identified. These are (1) misconceptions about the causes of insomnia, (2) misattributions or amplifications of the consequences of poor sleep, (3) unrealistic sleep expectations, (4) diminished perceptions of control and predictability of sleep, and (5) faulty beliefs about sleep-promotion practices (Morin, 1993). Treatment involves providing accurate information and having the insomniac identify and rehearse alternative belief statements.

Paradoxical intention. A cognitive intervention that has been frequently evaluated is paradoxical intention (PI). Many insomniacs exacerbate their problem by worrying about whether they will be able to fall asleep and by 'trying' to fall asleep. In a study on the ironic effects of trying to fall asleep, Ansfield, Wegner, and Bowser (1996) found that individuals under high mental load took longer to fall asleep when trying to do so than individuals under low mental load. High mental load is analogous to being under stress. Insomniacs, who are worried about sleep and who are often trying hard to fall asleep, may be making their insomnia worse.

To reduce the anticipatory anxiety associated with 'trying' to fall asleep, insomniacs who are given paradoxical intention are instructed to get into bed and stay awake rather than to try to fall asleep. Since this would presumably reduce the anxiety associated with trying to fall asleep, the insomniac should become more relaxed and fall asleep faster than they would otherwise.

Paradoxical instructions tend to be most effective with patients who are resistant and reactant to therapeutic suggestions (Shoham, Bootzin, Rohrbaugh & Urry, 1995). The rationale provided by the therapist for the paradoxical instruction may be a crucial component of its effectiveness. In a meta-analysis of the application of PI to a number of different problems, Shoham-Salomon and Rosenthal (1987) found that rationales that emphasize a positive benefit or the positive qualities of the person having the problem are more effective than rationales that are neutral or that emphasize negative aspects of the problem.

Thought-stopping and articulatory suppression. Most insomniacs complain of cognitive intrusions when trying to sleep. Two techniques that have been used to help insomniacs suppress cognitive intrusions are thought-stopping and articulatory suppression. In thought-stopping the insomniac says, 'Stop!' forcefully every time obsessive rumination occurs (Wolpe, 1973). This briefly disrupts the chain of thought, and repetitions decrease the frequency of subsequent cognitive intrusions. A related procedure is articulatory suppression (Levey, Aldaz, Watts & Coyle, 1991). In this procedure, insomniacs are instructed to repeat a word such as 'the' subvocally three to four times a second until sleep occurs. This is based on cognitive research that indicates that articulatory suppression interferes with short-term memory. It has been effectively used in insomnia treatments to reduce cognitive intrusions that interfere with sleep.

A combination of cognitive interventions (cognitive restructuring, PI, and thought-stopping) has been found to be effective. In fact, it has been shown to produce as much improvement in sleep as EMG biofeedback or the combination of stimulus control and progressive muscle relaxation training (Sanavio, et al., 1990).

Multicomponent Treatments

A commonly employed multicomponent package has been to combine stimulus control instructions, relaxation training, and sleep education. In one evaluation, this combination of stimulus control instructions and relaxation training produced more overall improvement than stimulus control instructions alone, although the difference was not statistically significant (Jacobs et al., 1993). This combination has also been evaluated as a self-help treatment delivered by audio-tape (Morawetz, 1989). The audio tape treatment produced as much improvement in sleep as did the same treatments with a live therapist for insomniacs who were not on hypnotics. For those on hypnotics, the live therapist produced more improvement than the tapes.

A multicomponent treatment consisting of stimulus control instructions, sleep restriction, cognitive restructuring and sleep education has been found to be effective for adult (Chambers & Alexander, 1992; Morin, Stone, McDonald, & Jones 1994) and elderly insomniacs (Edinger et al., 1990; Morin, Kowatch, Berry & Walton, 1993). Epstein (1994) used this combination of interventions with 22 older insomniacs in a six week treatment program following a small group format. After treatment, there was significant improvement in wake after sleep onset, sleep efficiency, and total sleep time. These gains were maintained at a three month follow-up.

Because of the multifaceted etiology of insomnia, the tailoring of treatments to patient needs would seem to be appealing. Each causal mechanism, however, must be tested and evaluated. For example, one might assume that relaxation techniques should be recommended for an insomniac who is in a stressful situation and, therefore, experiences tension. Nevertheless, relaxation treatments have not been found to be significantly more effective than other behavioral treatments, even for those who are tense and under stress (Espie, Brooks & Lindsay, 1989). There is no advantage for tailoring treatments if more effective treatments are omitted and less effective ones are included.

Combining Behavioral and Pharmacological Treatments

Many insomniacs who request treatment at sleep disorder centers are reluctant to withdraw from hypnotics for fear that their sleep will become substantially worse. This fear is not entirely unfounded since benzodiazepine withdrawal symptoms have been well documented and may last as long as 4 or 5 weeks following abrupt discontinuation (Espie, Lindsay & Brooks, 1988; Rickels, Schweizer, Case & Greenblatt, 1990).

Behavioral treatment has been shown to be effective when patients either withdraw from hypnotics or maintain a consistent dose of the hypnotic throughout the behavioral treatment (Espie, Lindsay, et al., 1989). There is also an accumulating literature to indicate that behavioral treatments can be used to both help patients withdraw from hypnotics and improve their sleep (Gilbert, Innes, Owen & Sansom, 1993; Lichstein & Johnson, 1993).

There have been few controlled studies that compare a hypnotic with a nonpharmacological treatment. In a comparison of triazolam with a combination of stimulus control instructions and relaxation training, triazolam had an immediate effect whereas the nonpharmacological treatment took three weeks to have an equivalent effect (McClusky et al., 1991). At a one-month follow-up, however, the nonpharmacological treatment was more effective than triazolam at maintaining improvement.

The differential course and effects of pharmacological and behavioral treatments for insomnia suggested that it might be possible to use them together. To examine this hypothesis, the investigators assigned 15 insomniacs to either triazolam with behavioral therapy or triazolam with sleep-related information (Milby et al., 1993). At follow-up, triazolam plus behavioral therapy produced greater improvement in total sleep and restedness in the morning than did triazolam plus sleep-related information. These results suggest that hypnotics and behavior therapy might be effectively combined.

The possibility of using hypnotics and cognitive-behavioral treatment together was also evaluated in a large, controlled study by Morin et al.

(1995). Seventy-eight community-resident older adults (average age of 64.5 years) with chronic insomnia were randomly assigned to temazepam pharmacotherapy, cognitive-behavioral therapy, combined pharmacotherapy and cognitive-behavioral therapy, and a medication placebo group. All treatments lasted eight weeks. Cognitive-behavioral therapy consisted of 'cognitive restructuring aimed at altering dysfunctional beliefs and attitudes about sleep and, combined stimulus control and sleep restriction aimed at regulating sleep schedules, curtailing sleep-incompatible behaviors, and consolidating sleep over shorter periods of time spent in bed' (p. 303).

The results at posttest were that patients in all three active treatment groups had improved sleep compared to those receiving the placebo treatment. The combined treatment showed a nonsignificant trend to produce more improvement than the cognitive-behavioral treatment which was itself nonsignificantly superior to pharmacotherapy. The pattern of results was similar for both sleep diary and polysomnography measures.

Even though cognitive-behavioral and pharmacological therapies, either alone or in combination, were about equally effective in the short-term treatment of insomnia, patients reported greater subjective improvement and more satisfaction with the cognitive-behavioral and combined treatment than with the pharmacotherapy and placebo condition. Further, preliminary results at the 12 month and 24 month follow-ups suggested that only patients who received cognitive-behavioral treatment alone maintained their gains over time. Patients who received either pharmacotherapy or the combined treatment showed more relapse. Thus, it is possible that pharmacotherapy, while working in the short-run, may undermine the capacity of cognitive-behavioral treatment to maintain improvement over the long term.

It is too early to conclude whether or not pharmacotherapy and behavioral therapies can be effectively combined in the treatment of insomnia. More studies of the quality of Morin et al. (1995) are needed. However, caution in the prescription of hypnotics and other substances for sleep would be prudent. Cognitive-behavioral treatments have typically been found to be most effective with patients who are not currently taking hypnotics (Murtagh & Greenwood, 1995). Similarly, not using anxiolytic or barbiturate medications has been found to predict a higher likelihood of the resolution of insomnia in the elderly (Monjan & Foley, 1997). It would appear that in the absence of physical sleep disorders, educational and cognitive-behavioral treatments should be the first set of interventions in the clinician's algorithm for the treatment of persistent insomnia.

CONCLUSION

In recent years there have been enormous advances in our understanding of the etiology and treatment of sleep disorders, including advances in the neurophysiology and pharmacology of sleep, the processes and mechanisms of biological rhythms, and documentation of the effectiveness of cognitive-behavioral treatments on the sleep of insomniacs through comparative outcome studies. The field of sleep disorders is diverse and there is still much to be learned.

An important focus for the future will be whether treatments investigated in controlled experiments can be effective when applied in the field. This is often called effectiveness, as opposed to efficacy, research. It is not sufficient that a treatment be shown to have efficacy with highly selected patients, under tightly controlled conditions, with narrowly defined outcome measures, and over short follow-up periods. It is important to know whether treatments can be delivered and complied with as part of usual clinical practice and whether treatment effects persist for years, not just for months. It is equally important to know whether treatments that improve sleep also reduce the problems associated with persistent sleep loss. Does treatment for insomnia improve mood and emotional well-being, reduce absences from work due to illness, increase memory, concentration, and performance, reduce work-related accidents and injuries, and generally improve quality of life? These questions have yet to be investigated and provide an exciting research agenda.

References

American Psychiatric Association (1994) *Diagnostic and Statistical Manual of Mental Disorders: DMS IV*. Washington, D.C.: American Psychiatric Association.

American Sleep Disorders Association (1997) *The International Classification of Sleep Disorders: Diagnostic and Coding Manual, Revised*. Rochester, MN: ASDA.

Ansfield, M. E., Wegner, D. M. & Bowser, R. (1996) Ironic effects of sleep urgency. *Behaviour Research and Therapy*, **34**, 523–531.

Armitage, R., Trivedi, M., Rush, A. J. & Hoffmann, R. (1995) The effects of fluoxetine on period-analyzed sleep EEG in depression. *Sleep Research*, **24**, 381.

Balter, M. B. & Uhlenhuth, E. H. (1992) New epidemiologic findings about insomnia and its treatment. *Journal of Clinical Psychiatry*, **53**(Suppl.), 34–42.

Beck, A. T., Ward, C. H., Mendelson, M., Mock, J. E. & Erbaugh, J. K. (1961) An inventory for measuring depression. *Archives of General Psychiatry*, **4**, 561–571.

Benca, R. M., Obermeyer, W. H., Thisted, R. A. & Gillin, J. C. (1992) Sleep and psychiatric disorders: A meta-analysis. *Archives of General Psychiatry*, **49**, 651–668.

Bliwise, D. L. (1993) Sleep in normal aging and dementia. *Sleep*, **16**, 40–81.

Bonnet, M. H. & Arand, D. C. (1995) 24-hour metabolic rate in insomniacs and matched normal sleepers. *Sleep*, **18**, 581–588.

Bootzin, R. R., Engle-Friedman, M. & Hazlewood, L. (1983) Insomnia. In *Clinical Geropsychology: New Directions in Assessment and Treatment*, pp. 81–115, edited by P. M. Lewinsohn & L. Teri. New York: Pergamon Press.

Bootzin, R. R., Epstein, D., Engle-Friedman, M. & Salvio, M. (1996) Sleep disturbances. In *The Practical Handbook of Clinical Gerontology*, edited by L. Carstensen, B. Edelstein & L. Dornband, pp. 398–420. Thousand Oaks, CA: Sage Publications.

Bootzin, R. R., Epstein, D. & Wood, J. M. (1991) Stimulus control instructions. In *Case Studies in Insomnia*, pp. 19–28, edited by P. J. Hauri. New York: Plenum Press.

Bootzin, R. R., Manber, R., Perlis, M. L., Salvio, M. & Wyatt, J. K. (1993) Sleep disorders. In *Comprehensive Handbook of Psychopathology*, edited by P. B. Sutker & H. E. Adams, 2nd edn. (pp. 531–561). New York: Plenum Press.

Bootzin, R. R. & Nicassio, P. (1978) Behavioral treatments for insomnia. In *Progress in Behavior Modification*, pp. 1–45, edited by M. Hersen, R. M. Eisler & P. M. Miller, vol. 6. New York: Academic Press.

Bootzin, R. R., Quan, S. F., Bamford, C. R. & Wyatt, J. K. (1995) Sleep disorders. *Comprehensive Therapy*, **21**, 401–406.

Bootzin, R. R. & Rider, S. P. (1997) Behavioral techniques and biofeedback for insomnia. In *Understanding Sleep: The Evaluation and Treatment of Sleep Disorders*, edited by M. R. Pressman & W. C. Orr, (pp. 315–338). Washington, D.C.: American Psychological Association

Bootzin, R. R., Shoham, V. & Kuo, T. F. (1994) Sleep Anticipatory Anxiety Questionnaire: A measure of anxiety about sleep. *Sleep Research*, **23**, 188.

Borkovec, T. D., Grayson, J. B., O'Brien, G. T. & Weerts, T. C. (1979) Relaxation treatment of pseudoinsomnia and idiopathic insomnia: An electroencephalographic evaluation. *Journal of Applied Behavior Analysis*, **12**, 37–54.

Brown, S. L., Salive, M. E., Pahor, M., Foley, D. J., Corti, C., Langlois, J. A., Wallace, R. B. & Harris, T. B. (1995) Occult caffeine as a source of sleep problems in an older population. *Journal of the American Geriatric Society*, **43**, 860–864.

Campbell, S. S., Dawson, D. & Anderson, M. W. (1993) Alleviation of sleep maintenance insomnia with time exposure to bright light. *Journal of the American Geriatrics Society*, **41**, 829–836.

Chambers, M. J. & Alexander, S. D. (1992) Assessment and prediction of outcome for a brief behavioral insomnia treatment program. *Journal of Behavior Therapy and Experimental Psychiatry*, **23**, 289–297.

Derogatis, L. R. & Melisaratos, N. (1983) The Brief Symptom Inventory: An introductory report. *Psychological Medicine*, **13**, 595–605.

Edinger, J. D., Hoelscher, T. J., Marsh, G. R., Lipper, S. & Ionescou-Pioggia, M. (1990) A cognitive-behavioral therapy for sleep-maintenance insomnia. *Psychology and Aging*, **7**, 282–289.

Edinger, J. D., Morey, M. C., Sullivan, R. J., Higginbotham, M. B., Marsh, G. R., Dailey, D. S. & McCall, W. V. (1993) Aerobic fitness, acute exercise and sleep in older men. *Sleep*, **16**, 351–359.

Epstein, D. R. (1994) *A Behavioral Intervention to Enhance the Sleep-wake Patterns of Older Adults with Insomnia*. Unpublished dissertation, Tucson, AZ: University of Arizona.

Espie, C. A., Brooks, D. N. & Lindsay, W. R. (1989) An evaluation of tailored psychological treatment of insomnia. *Journal of Behavior Therapy and Experimental Psychiatry*, **20**, 143–154.

Espie, C. A., Lindsay, W. R. & Brooks, D. N. (1988) Substituting behavioural treatment for drugs in the treatment of insomnia: An exploratory study. *Journal of Behavior Therapy and Experimental Psychiatry*, **19**, 51–56.

Espie, C. A., Lindsay, W. R., Brooks, D. N., Hood. E. M. & Turvey, T. (1989) A controlled comparative investigation of psychological treatments for chronic sleep-onset insomnia. *Behavour Research and Therapy*, **27**, 79–88.

Ford, D. E. & Kamerow, D. W. (1989) Epidemiological study of sleep disturbances and psychiatric disorders. *Journal of the American Medical Association*, **262**, 1479–1484.

Freedman, R. R. & Sattler, H. L. (1982) Physiological and psychological factors in sleep-onset insomnia. *Journal of Abnormal Psychology*, **91**, 380–389.

Friedman, L., Bliwise, D. L., Yesavage, J. A. & Salom, S. R. (1991) A preliminary study comparing sleep restriction and relaxation treatments for insomnia in older adults. *Journal of Gerontology: Psychological Sciences*, **46**, 1–8.

Gilbert, A., Innes, J. M., Owen, N. & Sansom, L. (1993) Trial of an intervention to reduce chronic benzodiazepine use among residents of aged-care accommodation. *Australia New Zealand Journal of Medicine*, **23**, 343–347.

Good, R. (1975) Frontalis muscle tension and sleep latency. *Psychophysiology*, **12**, 465–467.

Guilleminault, C., Clerk, A., Black, J., Labanowski, M., Pelayo, R. & Claman, D. (1995) Nondrug treatment trials in psychophysiologic insomnia. *Archives of Internal Medicine*, **155**, 838–844.

Haimov, I., Lavie, P., Laudon, M., Herer, P., Vigder, C. & Zisapel (1995) Melatonin replacement therapy of elderly insomnaics. *Sleep*, **18**, 589–598.

Hauri, P. (1981) Treating psychophysiologic insomnia with biofeedback. *Archives of General Psychiatry*, **38**, 752–758.

Hauri, P., Percy, L., Hellekson, C., Hartmann, E. & Russ, D. (1982) The treatment of psychophysiologic insomnia: A replication study. *Biofeedback and Self-Regulation*, **7**, 223–235.

Haynes, S. N., Follingstad, D. R. & McGowan, W. T. (1974) Insomnia: Sleep patterns and anxiety level. *Journal of Psychosomatic Research*, **18**, 69–74.

Jacobs, G. D., Rosenberg, P. A., Friedman, R., Matheson, J., Peavy, G. M., Domar, A. D. & Benson, H. (1993) Multifactor behavioral treatment of chronic sleep-onset insomnia using stimulus control and the relaxation response. A preliminary study. *Behavior Modification*, **17**(4), 498–509.

Jacobson, E. (1938) *Progressive Relaxation*. Chicago: University of Chicago Press.

Kopta, S. M., Howard, K. I., Lowry, J. L. & Beutler, L. E. (1994) Patterns of symptomatic recovery in psychotherapy. *Journal of Consulting and Clinical Psychology*, **62**, 1009–1016.

Kupfer, D. J. & Reynolds III, C. F. (1997) Management of insomnia. *New England Journal of Medicine*, **336**, 341–346.

Lack, L. & Wright, H. (1993) The effect of evening bright light in delaying the circadian rhythms and lengthening the sleep of early morning awakening insomniacs. *Sleep*, **16**, 436–443.

Lack, L., Wright, H. & Paynter, D. (1995) The treatment of sleep onset insomnia with morning bright light. *Sleep Research*, **24A**, 338.

Lacks, P. & Morin, C. M. (1992) Recent advances in the assessment and treatment of insomnia. *Journal of Consulting and Clinical Psychology*, **60**, 586–594.

Leger, D., Le Pen, C., Thebault, C., Loos, F., Levy, E. & Paillard, M. (1997) Economical consequences of insomnia. *Sleep Research*, **26**, 412.

Levey, A. B., Aldaz, J. A., Watts, F. N. & Coyle, K. (1991) Articulatory suppression and the treatment of insomnia. *Behaviour Research and Therapy*, **29**, 85–89.

Lichstein, K. L. & Johnson, R. S. (1993) Relaxation for insomnia and hypnotic medication use in older women. *Psychology and Aging*, **8**, 103–111.

Lichstein, K. L. & Riedel, B. W. (1994) Behavioral assessment and treatment of insomnia: A review with an emphasis on clinical application. *Behavior Therapy*, **25**, 659–688.

Manber, R. & Bootzin, R. R. (1997) Sleep and the menstrual cycle. *Health Psychology*, **16**, 209–214.

Manber, R., Bootzin, R. R., Acebo, C. & Carskadon, M. A. (1996) Reducing daytime sleepiness by regularizing sleep-wake schedules of college students. *Sleep*, **19**, 432–441.

Matalon, A., Yinnon, A. M. & Hurwitz, A. (1990) Chronic use of hypnotics in a family practice: Patients' reluctance to stop treatment. *Family Practice*, **7**, 258–260.

McClusky, H. Y., Milby, J. B., Switzer, P. K., Williams, V. & Wooten, V. (1991) Efficacy of behavioral versus triazolam treatment inpersistent sleep-onset insomnia. *American Journal of Psychiatry*, **48**, 121–126.

Mellinger, G. D., Balter, M. B. & Uhlenhuth, E. H. (1985) Insomnia and its treatment: Prevalence and correlates. *Archives of General Psychiatry*, **42**, 225–232.

Mendelson, W. B. (1993) Pharmacologic alteration of the perception of being awake or asleep. *Sleep*, **16**, 641–646.

Mendelson, W. B. (1995) Effects of flurazepam and zolpidem on the perception of sleep in insomniacs. *Sleep*, **18**, 92–96.

Milby, J. B., Williams, V., Hall, W. V., Khuder, S., McGill, T. & Wooten, V. (1993) Effectiveness of combined triazolam-behavioral therapy for primary insomnia. *American Journal of Psychiatry*, **105**, 1259–1260.

Monjan, A. A. & Foley, D. J. (1997) Resolution of chronic complaints of insomnia: An epidemiologic study among older adults. Paper presented at the annual meeting of the Association of Professional Sleep Societies, San Francisco.

Monti, J. M, Attali, P., Monti, D., Zipfel, A., de la Giclais, B. & Morselli, P. L. (1994) Zolpidem and rebound insomnia—a double-blind, controlled polysomnographic study in chronic insomniac patients. *Pharmacopsychiatry*, **27**, 166–175.

Morawetz, D. (1989) Behavioral self-help treatment for insomnia: A controlled evaluation. *Behavior Therapy*, **20**, 365–379.

Morin, C. M. (1993) *Insomnia: Psychological Assessment and Management*. New York: Guilford Press.

Morin, C. M., Colecchi, C. A., Stone, J., Sood, R. & Brink, D. (1995) Cognitive-behavior therapy and pharmacotherapy for insomnia: Update of a placebo-controlled clinical trial. *Sleep Research*, **24**, 303.

Morin, C. M., Culbert, J. P. & Schwartz, S. M. (1994) Nonpharmacological interventions for insomnia: A meta-analysis of treatment efficacy. *American Journal of Psychiatry*, **151**, 1172–1180.

Morin, C. M., Kowatch, R., Berry, T. & Walton, E. (1993) Cognitive-behavior therapy for late-life insomnia. *Journal of Consulting and Clinical Psychology*, **61**, 137–146.

Morin, C.M., Stone, J., McDonald, K., & Jones, S. (1994). Psychological management of insomnia: A clinical replication series with 100 patients. Behavior Therapy, 25, 291-309.

Morris, M., Lack, L. & Dawson, D. (1990) Sleep-onset insomniacs have delayed temperature rhythms. *Sleep*, **13**, 1–14.

Murtagh, D. R. R. & Greenwood, K. M. (1995) Identifying effective psychological treatments for insomnia: A meta-analysis. *Journal of Consulting and Clinical Psychology*, **63**, 79–89.

Nicassio, P. M. & Bootzin, R. R. (1974) A comparison of progressive relaxation and autogenic training as treatments for insomnia. *Journal of Abnormal Psychology*, **83**, 253–260.

Nicholson, A. N. (1994) Hypnotics: Clinical pharmacology and therapeutics. In *Principles and Practice of Sleep Medicine*, 2nd edn, edited by M. H. Kryger, T. Roth & W. C. Dement, pp. 355–363. Philadelphia: W. B. Saunders.

Penn, P. E. & Bootzin, R. R. (1990) Behavioural techniques for enhancing alertness and performance in shift work. *Work & Stress*, **4**, 213–226.

Perlis, M. L., Giles, D. E., Buysse, D. J., Tu, X. & Kupfer, D. J. (1997) Self-reported sleep disturbance as a prodromal symptom in recurrent depression. *Journal of Affective Disorders*, **42**, 209–212.

Quera-Salva, M. A., Orluc, A., Goldenberg, F. & Guilleminault, C. (1991) Insomnia and use of hypnotics: Study of a French population. *Sleep*, **14**, 386–391.

Reynolds III, C. F. (1989) Sleep in Affective Disorders. In *Principles and Practice of Sleep Medicine*, edited by M. H. Kryger, T. Roth & W. C. Dement, pp. 413–415. Philadelphia: W. B. Saunders Company.

Reynolds III, C. F., Buysse, D. J., Nofzinger, E. A. & Kupfer, D. J. (1995) Treatment of persistent insomnia in psychiatric patients: Effect of antidepressant therapies on sleep in mood disorders. In *Textbook on Psychopharmacology*, edited by A. Schatzberg. Washington, D.C.: American Psychiatric Press, Inc.

Reynolds III, C. F. & Kupfer, D. (1987) Sleep research in affective illness: State of the art circa 1987. *Sleep*, **10**, 199–215.

Rickles, K., Schweizer, E., Case, W. G. & Greenblatt, D. J. (1990) Long-term therapeutic use of benzodiazepines, I: Effects of abrupt discontinuation. *Archives of General Psychiatry*, **47**, 899–907.

Sanavio, E., Vidotto, G., Bettinardi, O., Rolletto, T. & Zorzi, M. (1990) Behaviour therapy for DIMS: Comparison of three treatment procedures with follow-up. *Behavioural Psychotherapy*, **18**, 151–167.

Sanchez, R. & Bootzin, R. R. (1985) A comparison of white noise and music: Effects of predictable and unpredictable sounds on sleep. *Sleep Research*, **14**, 121.

Schweizer, E., Rickels, K., Case, W. G. & Greenblatt, D. J. (1990) Long-term use of benzodiazepines, II: Effects of gradual taper. *Archives of General Psychiatry*, **47**, 908–915.

Shader, R. I. & Greenblatt, D. J. (1993) Use of benzodiazepines in anxiety disorders. *New England Journal of Medicine*, **328**, 1398–1405.

Shoham, V., Bootzin, R. R., Rohrbaugh, M. & Urry, H. (1995) Paradoxical versus relaxation treatment for insomnia: The moderating role of reactance. *Sleep Research*, **24a**, 365.

Shoham-Salomon, V. & Rosenthal, R. (1987) Paradoxical interventions: A meta-analysis. *Journal of Consulting and Clinical Psychology*, **55**, 22–28.

Silva, J. A. C. E., Chase, M., Sartorius, N. & Roth, T. (1996) Special report from a symposium held by the World Health Organization and the World Federation of Sleep Research Societies: An overview of insomnias and related disorders—recognition, edpidemiology, and rational management. *Sleep*, **19**, 412–416.

Spielman, A. J., Saskin, P & Thorpy, M. J. (1987) Treatment of chronic insomnia by restriction of time in bed. *Sleep*, **10**, 45–56.

Terman, M. (1994) Light therapy. In *Principles and Practice of Sleep Medicine*, (2nd edn) edited by M. H. Kryger, T. Roth & W C. Dement, pp. 1012–1029. Philadelphia: W. B. Saunders Company.

Vitiello, M. V., Schwartz, R. S., Davis, M. W., Ward, R. R., Ralph, D. D. & Prinz, P. N. (1992) Sleep quality and increased aerobic fitness in healthy aged men: preliminary findings. *Journal of Sleep Research*, **1**(Suppl.), 245.

Wetter, D. W., Fiore, M. C., Baker, T. B. & Young, T. B. (1995) Tobacco withdrawal and nicotine replacement influence objective measures of sleep. *Journal of Consulting and Clinical Psychology*, **63**, 58–67.

Wolpe, J. (1973) *The Practice of Behavior Therapy*, 2nd edn. New York: Pergamon Press.

Youngstedt, S. D., O'Connor, P. J. & Dishman, R. K. (1997) The effects of acute exercise on sleep: A quantitative synthesis. *Sleep*, **20**, 203–214.

Chapter 15

COGNITIVE-BEHAVIORAL THEORY, RESEARCH AND TREATMENT OF TRAUMA DISORDERS

John G. Carlson, PhD and Claude M. Chemtob

THEORETICAL BACKGROUND

This chapter is a review of a cognitive-behavioral theoretical perspective on symptoms related to exposure to trauma, in particular the features of posttraumatic stress disorder (PTSD), and a comprehensive review of related research conducted mainly in our laboratory. These studies were aimed at investigating implications of our model in both an experimental context and in controlled outcome clinical studies. The populations from which our samples have been drawn include primarily war veterans with histories of traumatic combat experiences and a unique group of young survivors of an extremely intense hurricane.

Definition

Posttraumatic stress disorder (PTSD) is an anxiety disorder owing to exposure to events that threaten life or injury and evoke intense fear or helplessness. PTSD characterized by a pattern of responses including: (a) reexperiencing of events of trauma in the form of memories or flashbacks, along with psychological and physiological distress (arousal) when exposed to stimuli that are related; (b) avoidance of stimuli that are trauma-relevant and/or periods of emotional detachment; and (c) physiological arousal characterized by such problems as hypervigilance, sleep disorders, or inappropriate anger (American Psychiatric Association, 1994, pp. 427–429). The disorder is a serious one both symptomatically and in terms of chronic prevalence among some groups of veterans, in particular those of the Vietnam era. A conservative estimate of prevalence of PTSD based on epidemiological data is that 15% of the 3.5 million Vietnam veterans in the U.S. are afflicted (Kulka, Schlenger, Fairbank, Hough, Jordan, Marmar, & Weiss, 1988), resulting in high demand for related medical and mental health services within the Veterans Administration and the health field generally.

Cognitive/Behavioral Perspectives

The theoretical orientation for this research is a cognitive-behavioral perspective, grounded in an appreciation of the evolutionary perspective of sociobiology, first proposed by Chemtob, Roitblat, Hamada, Carlson & Twentyman (1988) and later elaborated (Chemtob, 1997; Chemtob & Carlson, 1994). We maintain that PTSD arises in consequence of an incompletely resolved challenge to a person's survival. Specifically, when a person perceives or expects an event to be threatening to survival a number of psychobiological subsystems are activated, taken together defining what we term the *survival system*. When the survival system is activated, we describe the person as functioning in 'survival mode'. The components of the survival system include behavioral, physiological, and cognitive (though not necessarily conscious) responses to trauma, and they have a primary and dominant quality over other reactions in traumatic situations because they serve to support primitive biological functions. The system is relatively nonvolitional owing to its origins in the history of the species, its onset is rapid and general in effect (reflecting the underlying biology of the stress response, e.g. Carlson & Hatfield, 1992), and its offset is slow in action and response-specific. Moreover, as arousal increases, the survival system gains access to the control of information processing resources that might be functional in more normal psychological environments (Chemtob et al., 1988). In PTSD, the activation of survival mode remains facilitated and the PTSD sufferer reacts to normative environments as if they were life-threatening. Consequently, the PTSD patient frequently processes the world through a cognitive organization which provides built in confirmation of vigilance for the presence of threat.

We maintain further that within the survival system are five subsystems: (1) Early warning; (2) threat perception/evaluation; (3) social attachment; (4) defense (aggression or withdrawal); and (5) arousal. A problem for the survival system is that it must be both inhibitory as well as activating in effect. People with PTSD have difficulties with the regulation of activation and inhibition, for example, shifting into 'survival mode' at slight provocations and becoming highly activated. They also have difficulty with overattention to certain details, inhibiting irrelevant information, a form of 'dissociation' from ongoing events. Thus, when a memory of a traumatic event attempts to resurface into consciousness, it is as if the events are played out in "real-time"; both the events themselves as well as the emotions attached to them are inhibited in the service of maximizing adaptive motor responses and cognitive efficiency. As a result, they are split off during the trauma and stored separately. Another manifestation of the impact of trauma, which is often neglected, is a deficit in the synthetic capacity to create a unified and consistent sense of self. Traumatic experiences overwhelm the self both during the trauma because of the intensity of the experience and after the trauma because of the dyscontrol experience induced by intrusive experiences and dysregulated affect and arousal. The self must go about the normal business of daily life but nevertheless remain in a perpetual state of readiness for survival. The shifts in experience are both intense and unpredictable. Again, it is the dysregulation of inhibition/activation that is at the heart of the conflict.

Thus PTSD is not a simple unitary disorder—it is a complex compound disorder that involves the disordering of a number of systems within the person that are linked together through activation of the superordinate survival system. The individual with PTSD must be treated through attempts to (1) redevelop a cohesive sense of self; (2) alter conceptions of the nature of threat and its evaluation; (3) receive attention for disordered attachment and bonding behaviors; (4) have the defense system altered to lower the likelihood of aggression and withdrawal; (5) be treated for arousal (activation) reduction. In our experience, treatment of each these subsystems may not impact on other subsystems but require individual attention. Moreover, secondary effects of PTSD symptoms, such as social difficulties owing to hyperactivation or substance abuse, must also be attended to, not as aspects of the disorder itself but as consequences of the fundamental dysregulation of activating and inhibitory processes.

Therefore, this model predicts the potential effectiveness of several types of related treatment, specifically generalized and trauma-specific arousal reduction through direct and indirect effects on the sympathetic and adrenocortical arousal mechanisms (Carlson & Hatfield, 1992) achieved through clinical exposure to traumatic material, clinical rehearsal of traumatic material to facilitate reprocessing of related memories and other trauma reactions, cognitive restructuring, and specific training with respect to associated trauma symptoms, such as, anger. It also predicts that the subsystems activated in the survival mode of cognitive organization each require system specific treatment protocols to address the particular form of dysregulation induced in each. Conversely, treatment primarily directed at one system will typically only partially carry over to the other subsystems.

In earlier behavioral formulations, consistent with our model but with little emphasis on cognitive processing, the conditions responsible for the development of arousal and avoidance symptoms of trauma exposure were seen to be Pavlovian conditioning and two-process learning theory (e.g. Keane, Zimering & Caddell, 1985). In our view, this more limited approach provides a basis for certain of the learned components of the 'survival system' and suggests mechanisms for the effectiveness of some specific aspects of exposure therapy, discussed below. In a Pavlovian view of events that determine the development of trauma reactions, incidents in trauma may function as biologically significant 'unconditional stimuli' that serve to classically condition fear and its attendant autonomic arousal responses to visual, auditory, and olfactory 'conditional stimuli' present at the time of the trauma. Through stimulus generalization, related events may trigger conditioned anxiety at later times and in other places, including responses mediated through stored memories. Some aspects of behavioral and psychological 'avoidance' of trauma-associated stimuli (including drug and alcohol abuse), as well as emotional numbing, may also be accounted for in learning terms. In an application of the two-factor learning view, instrumental avoidance and escape behavior may be negatively reinforced through successful attenuation or elimination of aversive events, in this case, those associated with trauma. In this way, a number of the defining criteria for the disorder may be understood as acts that temporarily reduce the discomfort of the conditioned reactions in trauma but that may, themselves, be counterproductive for the PTSD victim.

VARIABLES RELATED TO PTSD: EXPERIMENTAL STUDIES

A number of research studies on aspects of PTSD that have relevance for theoretical mechanisms and for treatment have been conducted in our laboratory. In this section we mainly describe several empirical studies aimed at delineating dimensions of stress-related stimuli in PTSD, examining physiological aspects of the disorder, and showing attentional distortions due to this disorder that follow from our model.

The Honolulu Posttraumatic Stress Disorder Stimulus Set

In accordance with the DSM-IV criteria for PTSD, a patient may experience psychological distress upon exposure to external cues that resemble or symbolize the original trauma. A number of stimuli have been investigated for their effects on the PTSD sufferer including sounds of combat (e.g. Blanchard, Kolb, Pallmeyer & Gerardi, 1982) and imaginal material (Pitman, Orr, Forgue, de Jong & Claiborn, 1987). However, no validated lists of picture or word cues have been available for the study of PTSD reactions in the laboratory or clinic. For this reason, with our coworkers, we initiated two related studies that investigated reactions to an assortment of such stimuli (Chemtob, Roitblat, Hamada, Carlson, Muraoka & Bauer, 1997). In the first, a large number of pictures and words, including Vietnam-related photos, threat-related words, and neutral stimuli of both types were first presented to Vietnam combat veterans recruited from the community. Their task was to rate the stimuli on a 7-point scale of Vietnam relatedness. Stimuli with ratings of 5.5 or greater (highly related) and 2.0 and less (highly nonrelated, 'neutral') were selected for the second study. Next, new groups of combat veterans with PTSD, with other psychiatric disorders, with no disorders, or veterans without combat experience were recruited. Stimuli consisting of 91 threat-related pictures, 59 threat-related words, 83 neutral pictures and a like number of neutral words were presented via prepared slides. The stimuli were rated by the veterans along four dimensions—unpleasantness, relevance, stressfulness, and memorability.

Comparing the threat-related and neutral stimuli, for the words, the veterans with PTSD rated the former stimuli higher on all dimensions of stimulus rating; for the pictures, there were significant differences between the PTSD participants and the other groups on all except the unpleasantness dimension. In addition, using a signal detection statistic it was shown that the pictures somewhat more effectively differentiated the veterans with PTSD from the other veterans than did the word stimuli. With these materials, it is now possible to present stimuli with known memorability, unpleasantness, Vietnam relevance, and stressfulness in research on PTSD-based reactions in Vietnam veterans. The Stimulus Set also has the potential for use as a diagnostic instrument in this arena.

Physiological Dimensions of PTSD

Facial Expression and PTSD
Among the diagnostic criteria for PTSD listed in DSM-IV and predicted from our survival system model are possible symptoms of heightened arousal and physiological reactivity upon exposure to stimuli related to the event. Relatedly, in a number of previous studies in this area, general autonomic nervous system sensitivity to trauma related cues has been the main focus (Orr, 1994), and autonomic measures were also incorporated into our some of our controlled treatment outcome studies, outlined in a later section. We reasoned that an additional direction for the application of psychophysiological methods to the study of PTSD is in the arena of muscle patterning, specifically in the facial musculature, a method that has had numerous applications in other studies of emotional behavior (Cacioppo, Bush & Tassinary, 1992). Therefore, we set out to incorporate measures of a number of facial muscles during exposure of veterans with PTSD to a known set of combat-related stimuli, specifically, picture stimuli from the Honolulu PTSD Stimulus Set (Carlson, Singelis & Chemtob, 1997). It was hypothesized that distinctive facial muscle patterns may provide more sensitive physiological indices than autonomic indicators of PTSD and enable documentation of more specific underlying emotional reactions in the combat veteran than available through autonomic assessment. Moreover, based on earlier failures to show autonomic effects of purely visual trauma stimuli in this clinic (unpublished data), it was hypothesized that measures of general autonomic reactivity to the visual stimuli would actually show no effects in this application.

The 15 most threatening and 15 least threatening (neutral) slides from the Honolulu Stimulus Set provided the combat- and noncombat-related stimuli, respectively. Ten veterans with previously diagnosed PTSD and ten veterans without PTSD were administered additional tests for PTSD reactions to confirm the diagnoses as well as to reveal certain associated symptoms, namely depression and anxiety. The participants were then tested individually with electrodes for muscle potential (electromyographic, EMG, responses) on the forehead, above the eyebrows, on the cheek, and on the jaw, along with measures of skin conductance and heart rate during presentation of the slides. The participants were also queried on their levels of distress on a five-point scale following slide presentation.

The primary results of this study were that relative to the non-PTSD control group, veterans with PTSD showed greater reactivity to the combat related pictures in muscles of the cheek (zygomaticus major), forehead (lateral frontalis) and jaw (masseter). At the same time, skin conductance and heart rate failed to show differential effects due to the stimuli. Moreover, the PTSD-afflicted veterans reported significantly greater distress owing to the combat slide presentation than did the control group. The sensitivity of some parts of the facial musculature to the visually traumatic material in this study, along with the verbally reported distress, is consistent with the negative emotionality presumed to characterize the survival system in PTSD. In particular, the obtained activity in the forehead and cheek regions possibly reflects the effects of viewing very unpleasant imagery, such as reported by others working in the area of facial muscle reactivity (e.g. Cacioppo et al., 1992). Similarly, increased activity in the masseter (clenching of the jaw) may have some bearing on the results of other studies in this laboratory showing exaggerated anger symptoms associated with PTSD (Chemtob, Hamada, Roitblat & Muraoka, 1994). The fact that several facial muscles differentiated the combat stimuli in this study, despite the general absence of autonomic effects, suggests the sensitivity of the facial musculature to subtle emotional effects in this application.

Ambulatory Cardiovascular Assessment and PTSD
Further evidence of physiological involvement of the survival system in PTSD has been obtained in studies examining cardiovascular variables. Averaging across eight earlier studies of PTSD patients assessed at baseline in the laboratory, Blanchard (1990) found elevated heart rates in the range of 10 beats per minute, and elevated systolic and diastolic blood pressures in the approximate range of 7 mmHg. In an effort to extend these observations to natural settings outside the clinic, such as home, work, or other contexts, our colleague, M. Muraoka, initiated a study of cardiovascular responses in a total of 18 veterans with and without PTSD using the first reported ambulatory physiological monitoring in this area (Muraoka, Carlson & Chemtob, 1998). Following initial psychometric assessment, the veterans were asked to wear an ambulatory blood pressure/heart rate monitor for a period of 24 hours outside of the laboratory/clinic during all activities except strenuous exercise and bathing. When the subjects returned to the clinic, the data were downloaded directly into a computer—no clinic measures were included.

Upon analysis of the ambulatory observations, as shown in Table 15.1, it was found that the PTSD-afflicted veterans exhibited significantly higher heart rate and diastolic blood pressure during awake periods and higher heart rate during sleep periods than the nonPTSD group. Systolic blood pressure, while elevated during the awake period for the PTSD subjects, was not statistically significantly increased for these subjects during either awake or asleep periods. This study validated the use of physiological measures in the assessment of PTSD, in particular aimed at aspects of the physiological arousal component of this disorder. This study also demonstrates the persistence of chronic arousal outside of the clinic, complementing previous research demonstrating physiological reactivity confined to the laboratory or clinic setting, and further showing the broad impact of PTSD on the life of the sufferer.

An interesting uncontrolled variable in this and all studies to date in the PTSD area is the possibility that veterans with combat PTSD are less fit in cardiovascular terms owing to lower levels of regular active exercise or overall daily physical activity. Relatedly, the PTSD participants in the Muraoka et al. study were significantly more likely to report being unemployed than those in the nonPTSD condition—see also the demographic study of a large group of Vietnam veterans below—perhaps implying that the former individuals were somewhat less active overall. This is an important topic for further research since it has implications for the assessment of arousal variables in PTSD more generally, whether physiologically or psychometrically.

Attentional Effects Related to PTSD

Earlier research has indicated the possibility that patients with PTSD and

Table 15.1   Mean blood pressure and heart rate obtained from combat veterans with and without PTSD by way of ambulatory monitoring methods outside of the laboratory[1].

	Overall	Awake	Asleep
Heart rate			
PTSD	80.8	83.9	71.0
NonPTSD	71.9	74.3	62.8
Systolic blood pressure			
PTSD	123.0	126.1	107.9
NonPTSD	119.3	122.4	109.0
Diastolic blood pressure			
PTSD	80.1	83.0	67.8
NonPTSD	71.5	73.7	64.0

[1]After Muraoka, Carlson & Chemtob (1998), Table 15.2.

other anxiety disorders may tend to process information about threat at the expense of information processing relative to other, nonthreat material. In the area of PTSD, most of the research has been done using a Stroop color naming task in which a word in a given color spells out, say, a combat related event (e.g. FIREFIGHT, AMBUSH). The task is to identify the color irrespective of the word. Relative to noncombat related words (e.g. INPUT, DETENTION), the general trend of this research suggests that responding with the color name to threat-related words is slower in veterans with PTSD than various control populations, suggesting the impact of the disorder on cognitive processing (e.g. McNally, Kaspi, Riemann & Zeitlin, 1990; Litz, Weathers et al., 1996). Given some technical difficulties in interpreting data from the Stroop task that are beyond the scope of this review, the present authors and colleagues conducted a study further aimed at determining cognitive deficits, specifically attentional difficulties, that may be attributable to features of PTSD (Chemtob et al., in press).

Again using the Honolulu PTSD Stimulus Set, both word and picture stimuli (most and least Vietnam-related) were displayed by a tachistoscope to 79 Vietnam era veterans, including a group with PTSD and three control groups (combat experience without PTSD, nonPTSD with other diagnoses, and veterans without combat experience or diagnoses). Additionally displayed in one of the four quandrants (randomly) of the pictures or words were sets of five digits. The principal task for the participants was to identify the digit '4' in a set of digits by pressing a button for YES (present) or NO (not present). It was found that the veterans with PTSD took longer than the control groups to identify the primary digit when Vietnam-related pictures—but not Vietnam-related words—were presented as distracters. The effect was restricted to Vietnam-related stimulus slides and did not carry over to non-related slides. Moreover, in a separate task the PTSD group tended to recall more Vietnam-related stimuli in a free recall test suggesting they were, in fact, attentionally biased towards these cues.

This study demonstrates the importance of cognitive factors in PTSD, in particular, the impelling, distractive effect of trauma-laden material on the ability of PTSD sufferers to focus on other material, in this case digits. (As with other studies in our laboratory cited in this review, it also appeared that the pictorial threat information was more salient than the verbal threat information for reasons that remain to be researched.) These data are consistent with those obtained using other avenues to study attention bias, such as the Stroop color task. It is notable that these results are also consistent with our survival system model for PTSD outlined earlier. Specifically, it appears that individuals with PTSD have a level of threat-seeking activation that is more sensitive than those without PTSD such that, at least in early stages of stimulation, there is an attention-compelling aspect of threat cues that may be cognitively disruptive (Chemtob et al., 1988; Chemtob & Carlson, 1994). Interestingly, it is possible that, after some time has elapsed, an opposite 'inhibitory' tendency may become dominant that corresponds to the tendency for individuals with anxiety disorders to regain equilibrium through avoidance of threat cues, one of the defining criteria for PTSD in DSM-IV.

Other Predictors of PTSD

Additional research in this laboratory has focused on relationships between a number of variables and the likelihood of PTSD in combat veterans. In the earliest of these studies, Chemtob, Bauer et al. (1990) examined a group of highly selected, highly motivated, intensively trained and 'fit' Vietnam Veterans in order to determine the role of selection factors and personality variables in likelihood of PTSD. A group of 57 veterans of the Special Forces (Green Berets) were rigorously diagnosed for PTSD and then completed a comprehensive battery of questionnaires covering such areas as childhood history, health characteristics of service, employment history, and others. Approximately 25% of the veterans were diagnosed with PTSD. The data were subjected to correlational and regression analysis that yielded a number of highly significant predictors of PTSD (dichotomous scores) including less family closeness, poor relationships with others, having friends missing in action, and guilt over the death of a friend. Additionally, using continuous scores for PTSD, additional variables that emerged as highly significant included number of times wounded, being wounded shortly after returning to combat after a leave, and being emotionally unprepared to leave service. Failure to discuss feelings about the war upon returning home was also a significant variable. These results show a complex picture of relevant variables in the development of PTSD, including prior family and social adjustment, intense combat exposure with wounding, and opportunities to resolve combat-related emotionality (such as, guilt) or issues regarding separation from service through expression of feelings with others. The authors conclude that 'even the rigorous selection and training required to be an elite professional soldier do not provide absolute immunity from the long-term effects of traumatic stress' (p. 20). In short, the cognitive, behavioral, and physiological variables underlying PTSD undoubtedly include aspects of prior history and post-trauma experiences as well as the trauma itself. (For further efforts in this laboratory to refine knowledge of predictor variables for PTSD, see studies on the determination of relationships between cultural variables and PTSD, Chemtob, 1996; the role of head injury in this disorder, Chemtob et al., (1998); and the examination of PTSD as a sequelae of Guillain-Barre syndrome, Chemtob & Herriott, 1994.)

PTSD TREATMENT: CONTROLLED OUTCOME RESEARCH

Several lines of controlled outcome clinical research also have been conducted in this laboratory in relation to our cognitive-behavioral model for treating symptoms of PTSD. These studies have been aimed at examining a therapeutic approach to PTSD that emphasizes traumatic memory exposure and cognitive restructuring in combat veterans and children, and at a cognitive-behavioral method for the management of anger reactions in veterans. As discussed at the outset of this chapter, our model emphasizes a multidimensional approach to both the symptoms and the modes of therapeutic treatment for PTSD, on the assumption that survival subsystems may coexist and, while linked together, may require multiple forms of treatment that may or may not generalize across subsystems. Accordingly, across these studies multimodal assessment strategies and multiple treatment modalities were investigated.

A Demographic Study of the Veteran PTSD Patient Population

Among war veterans, the seriousness of PTSD has been made most evident by survivors of combat in Vietnam. About 500,000 Vietnam veterans overall in the United States meet the diagnostic criteria for PTSD. Of those with high exposure to combat, estimates of prevalence of PTSD range as high as 38% (Kulka et al., 1988). Moreover, it has been estimated that about one-fourth of all mental health outpatient visits and 20% of inpatient discharges in the Veterans Administration health system are attributable to PTSD.

In order to document the characteristics of our patient samples and to relate them to national samples, we conducted the first systematic study of both demographic and psychological characteristics of the Vietnam veteran population in Hawaii. In this effort we compared a large sample of veterans with PTSD to a sample of those without PTSD, both of whom were seeking services at the Veterans Administration Medical Center (Carlson, Chemtob, Hedlund, Denny & Rusnak, 1994). A total of 118 combat veterans were assessed with several measures of trauma disorder, including the Mississippi Scale for Combat-Related PTSD (Keane, Caddell & Taylor, 1988), and an instrument for general personality assessment, the Minnesota Multiphasic Personality Inventory, MMPI-2 (Butcher, Dahlstrom et al., 1989). In addition, a number of demographic measures were taken. The purpose was to determine the extent and severity of diagnostic indicators of PTSD in our clinical population of veterans and to ascertain if our treatment should focus on particular parameters of the disorder.

In summary of some of the main demographic results of this study, the typical Hawaii combat veteran with PTSD we assessed was: 1) about 45 years of age at the time of the study (significantly younger, by about 4 years, than a combat veteran without PTSD); 2) more likely to be unemployed than employed, and unmarried (divorced or separated) than married; 3) more likely to have been in the Vietnam theatre than another theatre of war; 4) more likely to have been recently hospitalized for a psychiatric problem than a veteran without PTSD; and 5) as likely as not to report a substance abuse problem. In addition, most of these veterans were

Caucasian or Hawaiian (in lesser numbers, Asian-American) in ethnic extraction and all were male.

On the Mississippi instrument for assessment of PTSD, the mean for the veterans in the PTSD group in this study was 130.6. For those in the non-PTSD group the mean was 90.8. The recommended cutoff for PTSD on this instrument is 107 (Malloy, Fairbank & Keane, 1983). On the MMPI-2, the veterans with PTSD were significantly elevated relative to the veterans without PTSD on all except the masculinity-femininity and hypomania scales. They were also significantly elevated on the MMPI on measures of symptom reporting (the F scale), anxiety, and the Keane scale for PTSD. No ethnic differences in symptom presentation were found, although sample sizes were small in the comparisons.

In short, this study amply demonstrates that the population of combat veterans with PTSD from which our clinical samples are drawn is a seriously disordered group of veterans with well-documented symptoms of PTSD in accordance with all DSM-IV criteria as well as a number of areas of psychological distress and social maladjustment. In measured respects, these men resemble comparable populations in other demographic studies on a national level (Kulka et al., 1988).

Treatment Methods: Flooding, Desensitization, and EMDR therapy.

Three therapies emphasizing exposure to imagined traumatic material—imaginal flooding, systematic desensitization, and eye movement desensitization and reprocessing (EMDR)—have origins in the cognitive/behavioral perspectives outlined earlier. One rationale for such approaches is that repeated exposure to stimuli that have traumatic effects will lead to extinction, counterconditioning, and adaptation, ameliorating especially the emotional impact of early memories. We have argued that cognitive reprocessing of traumatic material is assisted within desensitization versions of these therapies in which both negative and positive aspects of related cognitions also are emphasized (Carlson, Chemtob, Rusnak & Hedlund, 1996).

The effectiveness of the flooding method—essentially repeated imaginal rehearsal of vivid traumatic memories along with related and sometimes intense anxiety—in terms of various client self-reports, behavioral changes, and (in some instances) psychophysiological indices of modest improvement in this context has been demonstrated in a few case reports (e.g. Black & Keane, 1982; Fairbank, Gross & Keane, 1983; and Keane & Kaloupek,1982) and in several controlled treatment outcome studies (Boudewyns &Hyer, 1990; Cooper & Clum, 1989; Keane, Fairbank, Caddell & Zimering, 1989). By contrast with the flooding method, systematic desensitization for anxiety disturbance involves, first, relaxation training followed by a more gradual introduction of trauma-related stimuli, and a deliberate effort to minimize anxiety. Peniston (1986) used a systematic desensitization technique with veterans with PTSD and found that even two years following treatment there was a significant advantage of the treatment for the desensitized subjects in terms of reduced reports of nightmares and intrusive images.

A third exposure method, recently applied to traumatized populations is eye movement desensitization and reprocessing (EMDR), first described by Shapiro (1989). The technique essentially involves having a subject identify a traumatic memory and then assessing its related level of distress (e.g. anxiety) on a 0–10 point Subjective Units of Distress (SUD) scale where 10 indicates maximum distress. Current memory-related negative cognitions are identified (e.g. 'I am helpless'), as well as corresponding desired positive cognitions (e.g. 'I can handle it'), the latter given a 1–7 rating of believability or 'validity' (a VOC rating) prior to therapy. Next, periods of eye movements are administered in which the client is asked to visually track the back and forth movements of the therapist's hand for short periods of time while concentrating on an image of the memory, the negative belief and related bodily sensations. In later stages of treatment, following reduction of SUD ratings to very low levels (0–2), during 'reprocessing' the client is asked to focus on the positive belief during further periods of induced eye movements and attention to the original memory until the validity of the positive belief is established (say, a rating of 5–7).

As pointed out by Puk (1991), the procedure does not *require* (nor does it preclude) many of the features of the other exposure techniques, including extended exposure to fear stimuli and attendant anxiety (as in flooding), or hierarchy construction and relaxation training (as in systematic desensitization). For these reasons, EMDR may be a lower risk procedure with potentially a reduced rate of attrition relative to other exposure therapies for PTSD. On the other hand, the data with respect to the application of EMDR to combat PTSD is mixed. Favorable results have been reported in a number of case studies (see Shapiro, 1995), but in controlled outcome studies EMDR has yielded effects ranging from positive (Shapiro, 1989), to mixed (Boudewyns et al., 1993; Pitman, Orr, Altman, Longpre, Poire & Lasko, 1993), to negative (Jensen, 1994).

Our treatment program with veterans with PTSD has focused on several types of related interventions suggested by cognitive-behavioral theory, namely, EMDR exposure treatment, relaxation training, and anger management. As discussed later, with children manifesting symptoms of PTSD, we have employed EMDR treatment exclusively. These studies are outlined in the following sections.

EMDR with Combat Veterans

Given the potential for treatment of PTSD offered by certain cognitive-behavioral procedures, especially exposure therapy in the form of flooding and EMDR, we initiated a comparison of two treatment methods designed to focus on different aspects of the disorder (Carlson, Chemtob, Rusnak, Hedlund & Muraoka, 1998). As noted, EMDR is especially directed at the cognitive, reexperiencing features of PTSD, that is, the traumatic memories themselves. By contrast, systematic desensitization (and the flooding method of Keane et al., 1989) incorporates training in relaxation, whose effects focus on the physiological arousal aspects of PTSD during exposure treatment. In the first case, the recent mixed effects of EMDR in application to PTSD in combat veterans suggested to us that, while the method overall was potentially effective, perhaps some particular aspect of this form of treatment in this context may be problematic. In a review of the relevant studies, we observed that just one or two sessions of treatment had typically been administered, an amount of therapy that we judged to be potentially inadequate considering the chronic and severe nature of combat PTSD in many patients. Therefore we opted for a 12-session protocol that brought our procedures more in line with studies using other exposure conditions, such as flooding interventions, and also with usual clinical standards for short-term psychotherapy.

Additionally, we compared EMDR with a relatively straightforward relaxation procedure, biofeedback-assisted progressive relaxation, which had several potential advantages in this context. One, this was an active procedure that provided a control for certain attentional effects due to treatment. Two, and more importantly, this condition was designed to impact primarily on the autonomic arousal associated with PTSD, free from other procedures that may be more cognitive in impact (such as, desensitization). Three, other studies have shown the potential value of biofeedback-assisted relaxation by itself in chronic anxiety (Townsend, House & Addario, 1975), suggesting its possible value with PTSD. (See also Carlson, Chemtob & Hedlund, 1994.) An additional treatment comparison in this study was with a group that was wait-listed and that received routine clinical care in the Veterans Administration or other health facilities.

Thirty-five combat veterans diagnosed with combat-related PTSD were treated with either (a) 12 sessions of eye movement desensitization and reprocessing, EMDR, (b) 12 sessions of biofeedback-assisted muscle relaxation, or (c) routine clinical care (the control condition). The EMDR treatment focused on the veterans' worst and second-worst combat memories. (For specific examples, see Carlson et al., 1996.) A comprehensive multimodal battery of assessment procedures was administered before and after treatment, including standardized questionnaires, self-reports, a structured clinical interview based on DSM-IV criteria, and physiological assessment. The subjects were assessed at pretreatment, posttreatment, 3-month follow-up, and 9-month follow-up.

Figure 15.1 depicts a few results for the three groups through the 3-month follow-up on (a) one of the PTSD questionnaires (the Mississippi scale, cited earlier), (b) the interview for symptoms of PTSD (Clinician

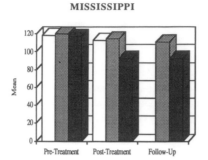

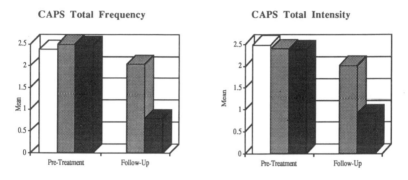

Figure 15.1 Means of groups treated with EMDR (EMD), biofeedback-assisted relaxation (RXT), or maintained on routine clinical care (CON) at pretreatment, posttreatment, and follow-up on questionnaire and structured interview measures of PTSD and associated features (depression).

Administered PTSD Survey, CAPS, Blake, Weathers, Nagy, Kaloupek, Klauminzer, Charney & Keane, 1990), and (c) a measure of depression, the Beck Depression Inventory (Beck, Ward, Mendelson, Mock & Erbaugh, 1961). The pattern of outcomes seen in Figure 15.1 was replicated as well in virtually every other psychometric measure of symptoms used in this study. Compared with the relaxation and control conditions, it can be seen in the figure that substantial positive treatment effects in the EMDR condition were obtained at posttreatment and follow-up on a number of the measures of PTSD. Further, at posttreatment, it was found that 70% of the veterans in the EMDR group no longer met the criteria for PTSD on the Mississippi scale. Effects due to EMDR relative to relaxation treatment were generally maintained at the 9-month follow-up conducted by a blind clinical assessor. In addition, it was found at that time that patient treatment satisfaction and amount of clinician-assessed improvement also significantly favored the EMDR procedure. The failure in this study to obtain substantial treatment effects owing to relaxation alone, a procedure aimed strictly at physiological arousal symptoms, also suggests the importance of a mode of exposure treatment for PTSD, such as EMDR, that includes cognitive aspects of this disorder, in particular some form of exposure technique.

Interestingly, an additional feature of this study provided for a large number of psychophysiological measures—including muscle potentials, skin conductance levels, heart rate, and others—to be taken during exposure of the patients to their combat-related memories. While some of these measures reflected apparent habituation from pretreatment to posttreatment, the physiological decreases appeared in all of the groups and did not favor the treatment conditions. Again, as discussed earlier, the survival systems model predicts that treatment along one modality may not transfer to another modality and that special attention to several of the dimensions of PTSD may be required to impact on the disorder in a clinically meaningful way.

Individual effects of EMDR treatment for PTSD in four cases were also reported by Carlson et al. (1996), demonstrating complete symptom reduction in some instances and an overall success rate of the treatment method that was substantially greater than normally reported in the area of combat PTSD using other treatment procedures. These results may owe to the extended 12 sessions of treatment by comparison with more mixed effects obtained in veteran populations with substantially less EMDR treatment, but this possibility is open to further controlled investigation.

The results obtained in our laboratory parallel those obtained in one other recent large group EMDR study conducted with a somewhat broader population of traumatized individuals, including abused women (Wilson, Becker & Tinker, 1995). In that study, 4–5 hours of EMDR treatment were found to be effective in ameliorating trauma (reexperiencing and other symptoms) on a number of standardized measures, effects that persisted at an 15-month follow-up (Wilson, Becker & Tinker, 1997).

Anger Management in Combat Veterans

Anger is considered one of the aspects of arousal disorder in the DSM-IV classification of PTSD and it constitutes a significant concern of Vietnam veterans seeking clinical assistance (Blum, Kelly, Meyer, Carlson & Hodson, 1984). In one effort to document the significance of anger reactions among veterans, Kulka et al., (1988) determined that veterans with PTSD scored higher on a measure of hostility and evidenced more violent acts than veterans without PTSD. Following up on some of these earlier and less systematic efforts, in our laboratory an empirical investigation was initiated (Chemtob, Hamada, Roitblat & Muraoka, 1994) comparing 24 Vietnam veterans with PTSD to 23 combat veterans without this disorder and 12 veterans with other psychiatric diagnoses (and no history of combat). Five measures of anger were used including the State-Trait Anger Scale (Spielberger, Jacobs, Russell & Crane, 1983) and a scale developed by Novaco (1975). It was found that the veterans with PTSD exhibited significantly higher scores than the other groups on an anger factor consisting of a number of measures of anger from the individual scales. The effects were found not to owe to simple impulsivity and also to be independent of amount of exposure to combat itself.

In a later, related study in this laboratory, an attempt was made to develop a typology of regulatory deficits associated with anger (Chemtob, Novaco, Hamada, Gross & Smith, 1997). Specifically, cognitive, behavioral, and arousal deficits in anger regulation plus a severe 'ball of rage' pattern were observed in 77 PTSD patients who manifested high anger on the Novaco Anger Scale (Novaco, 1994). Our survival model for PTSD served as a conceptual focus for this study, linking anger to the 'survival mode' of functioning for these veterans. In this view, spreading activation due to threat schemas strongly potentiates anger and has implications for coping urgency, strong arousal, and a biasing of cognitive processes towards confirmation of expectation of threat, among other effects. Several case studies are reviewed in this paper in an effort to demonstrate specific anger regulation deficit subsystems as they operate at the individual patient level.

Accordingly, with our coworkers, a first controlled outcome treatment effort in the combat PTSD area also was initiated that was aimed at systematically targeting anger symptoms as an arousal component of PTSD (Chemtob, Novaco, Hamada & Gross, 1997). Fifteen veterans were measured for anger levels along a number of dimensions including anger control, anger reaction and anger disposition, as well as for anxiety and depression. The patients were then randomly assigned to a multimodal anger treatment protocol—including self-monitoring, relaxation, cognitive restructuring, skills training, and other methods of self-regulation of anger—or maintained in a group that received routine clinical care.

As shown in Table 15.2, which depicts a few of the results of this study, veterans who received multimodal anger management therapy showed reduced anger scores on several scales (total anger, anger-in, and anger-out) and increased anger control on the Speilberger State-Trait Anger Scale, as

Table 15.2 Group means for anger (AX) and anxiety (STAI) measures[1]

Measure	Anger treatment group		Routine clinical care group	
	Pretreatment	Posttreatment	Pretreatment	Posttreatment
AX-Total	45.00	33.12	42.57	41.71
AX-Control	14.88	21.38	16.71	16.00
AX-Out	20.88	17.50	20.14	19.57
AX-In	23.00	21.00	23.14	22.14
STAI-State	51.50	38.14	51.50	56.57

[1]After Chemtob, Novaco, Hamada & Gross (1997), Table 15.2.

well as reduced state anxiety scores. Controlling for pretreatment levels, significant effects between groups were found on the anger reaction and anger control measures (but not for anger-out or -in), as well as on state anxiety. These results were maintained at an 18-month follow-up. Hence, again a cognitive-behavioral intervention strategy was found effective in ameliorating symptoms of PTSD, in this case, associated anger reactions which are not normally targeted for treatment but often are a source of considerable distress for the Vietnam veteran.

Treating Hurricane Trauma

Based on positive outcomes of our multimodal assessment and treatment strategies grounded in the survival model of PTSD, still more recent proposals for research in this laboratory have begun an attempt to generalize the model to new patient populations. In one direction of treatment research, schoolchildren on the island of Kauai, Hawaii ($N =$ 10,460), were first screened for symptoms of exposure to trauma in the wake of a devastating level 5 hurricane that struck the island and their homes approximately two years previously (Chemtob, Nakashima & Hamada, 1996; Chemtob, Tomas, Law & Cremnniter, 1997). Those identified as needing services were treated by way of a brief, manual-guided, counseling protocol and were followed up one year later. Despite positive gains overall at posttreatment for the group of children who received trauma counseling, the follow-up also revealed a subgroup of children who were still showing significant post-trauma distress on a measure of PTSD (the Kauai Recovery Inventory, KRI, Hamada, Kameoka & Yanagida, 1966). Consequently, it was determined that these children would receive an additional psychological intervention, specifically EMDR—based on the previous powerful effects with this form of treatment obtained in our laboratory with veterans (Carlson et al., 1998) and with other civilian populations (e.g. Wilson et al., 1995).

At the start of the study, approximately 3½ years post-hurricane, identified children were assessed via a measure of PTSD for children (the

Children's Reaction Inventory, CRI, Pynoos, Frederick, Nader et al., 1987), a measure of depression (the Children's Depression Inventory, CDI, Kovas, 1992), and a measure of anxiety (the Revised Children's Manifest Anxiety Scale, RCMAS, Reynolds & Richmond, 1985). A subset of the children met our criteria for trauma based on scores on the KRI and the CRI, and parental consent for treatment was obtained for 32 of these children. The study was conducted using an ABAA design (Preassessment, Treatment, Postassessment, Follow-up). Two groups of the children of approximately equal size were formed through random assignment. In one group, wait-list control, children were placed on a waiting list for treatment until the first treatment phase for the other group was completed. In the other group, the first treatment condition, the children were administered three 50-min. sessions of EMDR treatment in accordance with a manualized protocol. The therapists were all trained in the general EMDR protocol independently and then were trained together in a subsequent specially designed protocol for children. With all the children, following identification of the 'worst' hurricane-related memory, an attempt was made to begin a standardized eye movement procedure similar to that described above (Carlson et al., 1998). If the child was unable to track the therapist's fingers, usually for reasons of incomplete motor development in the case of younger children, a 'hand tapping' procedure was used as an alternative. In this method, the child touches one and then the other hand of the therapist's hands, alternating left-right, twenty times or more, *in lieu* of back- and-forth eye movements. Following reduction of SUD ratings to 0 and increase in VOC ratings to 5–7, the protocol called next for a focus on other current reminders of the hurricane (such as, heavy windstorms) and then on future concerns a child may have (such as, severe rain storms that might happen) in subsequent treatment sessions. In these cases, also, the criterion levels of SUD and VOC ratings were in effect. All treatment sessions were conducted in an assigned room in the child's school building during the school day and were videotaped for purposes of maintaining treatment integrity (Chemtob, Nakashima, Hamada & Carlson, 1996).

Figure 15.2 shows results from the Pynoos measure of PTSD, the measure of anxiety, and the measure of depression prior to treatment, at posttreatment, and at a three-month follow-up for the group treated first (group 1) and the wait-listed group treated one month later (group 2). The two groups did not differ at pretreatment (with assessments approximately 1-month apart), showing the similar levels obtained with the measure of PTSD and therefore the reliability of the preassessment. However, both groups showed dramatic (and statistically significant) reductions in symptoms of PTSD at posttreatment, effects that were essentially maintained at follow-up. The Pynoos measure of PTSD showed that at follow-up 18 of the children (56%) overall were in the nonsymptomatic range (scores less than 12) versus none at pretreatment. It was also found that the children whose symptoms of PTSD had remitted had significantly

PYNOOS CHILDHOOD REACTION INVENTORY

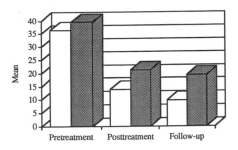

REVISED CHILD MANIFEST ANXIETY SCALE

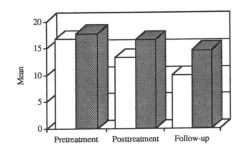

CHILDHOOD DEPRESSION INVENTORY

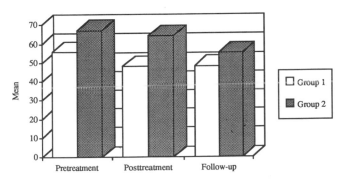

Figure 15.2 Means of a group of children of children diagnosed with PTSD and treated with EMDR (Group 1) and a group wait-listed then treated with EMDR (Group 2) at pretreatment, posttreatment, and follow-up. Measures of PTSD and associated features (anxiety and depression) are shown. (After Chemtob et al., 1996)

fewer health visits to the school nurse in the following year than the children who still met criteria for PTSD.

This controlled study is the first of its kind to attempt to provide treatment to a group of children who were hurricane survivors and who had proved resistant to prior treatment. The very persistence of the trauma disorder up until this treatment in these children, as well as the reliability of the preassessment measure within the study, helped demonstrate the effectiveness of the EMDR procedure in application to the manifestations of PTSD shown in the figure. Moreover, the multimodal assessment and several other rigorous details of the experimental design provide additional sources of strength to the conclusion that this cognitive-behaviorally based exposure intervention was effective in this context.

CONCLUSIONS

Posttraumatic stress disorder is a potentially debilitating, chronic emotional disorder with implications for disturbances in multiple aspects of the victim's life. A cognitive-behavioral perspective on PTSD offers a means to integrate a wide assortment of experimental and treatment observations that mirror the range of the disturbance. In particular, the 'survival model' emphasizes the functional value of behaviors, physiological reactions, and cognitions in the etiology and maintenance of the disorder. Thus the model encourages multimodal assessment and multi-faceted treatment procedures including arousal reduction, exposure to and rehearsal of traumatic material, cognitive restructuring, and special attention to specific aspects of PTSD, among other interventions.

Our research shows the importance of specifying the stimuli that evoke trauma along dimensions that have potential uses in studying reactions in controlled settings. Using the Honolulu PTSD Stimulus Set, the model also has fostered research on physiological manifestations of PTSD in the form of distinct facial expressions and cardiovascular disturbances in daily life situations. Additional research in this laboratory has shown the attention-compelling aspects of traumatic stimuli, demonstrating a dysregulation of activation/inhibition said to characterize PTSD from the survival model.

Treatment efforts in relation to the survival model have similarly emphasized the multiple dimensions of PTSD. One recent controlled study has shown the relative ineffectiveness of treatment directed strictly at arousal processes in the absence of attention to cognitive disturbances in one treatment group. By contrast, both in this study of combat veterans and in another of young survivors of a natural disaster, a cognitive-behavioral technique (EMDR) emphasizing memory processes, exposure treatment, and cognitive restructuring proved dramatically effective in addressing multiple cognitive aspects of PTSD. Interestingly, the failure of this method to show generalized effects of treatment across modalities—specifically on physiological reactions—further supports the notion of the survival model that attention to one survival subsystem may not produce effects in another. An alternative cognitive-behavioral treatment method used in an effort to address anger symptoms in PTSD patients combined arousal reduction and cognitive procedures and demonstrated broad treatment effects as measured multi-modally.

Developing a cognitive-behavioral approach to PTSD through research designed to clarify experimental and clinical implications has enormous potential for understanding and ameliorating this potentially severe and disabling emotional disorder. Fruitful future directions of research and theory will focus on the underlying psychological, social, and biological origins and dynamics of PTSD, more diverse patient populations, and systematic refinement of successful treatment protocols.

References

American Psychiatric Association, Committee on Nomenclature and Statistics. (1994) *Diagnostic and Statistical Manual of Mental Disorders*, Ed. 4. Washington, D. C.: Author.

Beck, A. T., Ward, C. H., Mendelson, M., Mock, J. & Erbaugh, J. (1961) An inventory for measuring depression. *Archives of General Psychiatry*, **4**, 561–571.

Black, J. L. & Keane, T. M. (1982) Implosive therapy in the treatment of combat-related fears in a World War II veteran. *Journal of Behavior Therapy and Experimental Psychiatry*, **13**, 163.

Blake, D., Weathers, F., Nagy, L., Kaloupek, D., Klauminzer, G., Charney, D. & Keane, T. (1990) A clinician rating scale for assessing current and lifetime PTSD: The CAPS-1. *Behavioral Assessment Review*, **September**, 187–188.

Blanchard, E. B. (1990) Elevated basal levels of cardiovascular responses in Vietnam veterans with PTSD: A health problem in the making? *Journal of Anxiety Disorders*, **4**, 223–237.

Blanchard, E. B., Kolb, L. C., Pallmeyer, T. P. & Gerardi, R. J. (1982) A psychophysiology study of post traumatic stress disorder in Vietnam veterans. *Psychiatric Quarterly*, **54**, 220–229.

Blum, M. D., Kelly, E. M., Meyer, K., Carlson, C. R. & Hodson, L. (1984) An assessment of the treatment needs of Vietnam-era veterans. *Hospital and Community Psychiatry*, **35**, 691–696.

Boudewyns, P. A. & Hyer, L. (1990) Physiological response to combat memories and preliminary treatment outcome in Vietnam veteran PTSD patients treated with direct therapeutic exposure. *Behavior Therapy*, **21**, 63–87.

Boudewyns, P. A., Stwertka, S. A., Hyer, L. A., Albrecht, J. W. & Sperr, E. V. (1993) Eye movement desensitization for PTSD of combat: A treatment outcome pilot study. *The Behavior Therapist*, **16**, 29–33.

Butcher, J. N., Dahlstrom, W. G. et al. (1989) *Manual for the Restandardized Minnesota Multiphasic Personality Inventory: MMPI-2*. Minneapolis, Minn.: University of Minnesota Press,.

Cacioppo, J. T., Bush, L. K. & Tassinary, L. G. (1992) Microexpressive facial actions as a function of affective stimuli: Replication and extension. *Personality and Social Psychology Bulletin*, **18**, 515–526.

Carlson, J. G., Chemtob, C. M. & Hedlund, N. L. (1994) A multisite EMG feedback protocol in the treatment of posttraumatic stress disorder in Vietnam combat veterans. *Biofeedback and Self-Regulation*, **19**, 288, abstract.

Carlson, J. G., Chemtob, C. M., Hedlund, N. L., Denny, D. R. & Rusnak, K. (1994) Characteristics of veterans in Hawaii with and without diagnoses of post-traumatic stress disorder. *Hawaii Medical Journal*, **83**, 314–318.

Carlson, J. G., Chemtob, C. M., Rusnak, K. & Hedlund, N. L. (1996) Eye movement desensitization and reprocessing treatment for combat-related PTSD. *Psychotherapy*, **33**, 104–113.

Carlson, J. G., Chemtob, C. M., Rusnak, K., Hedlund, N. L. & Muraoka, M. (1998) Eye movement desensitization/reprocessing (EMDR) for combat-related posttraumatic stress disorder. *Journal of Traumatic Stress*, **11**, 3–24.

Carlson, J. G. & Hatfield, E. (1992) *Psychology of Emotion*. New York: Harcourt Brace Jovanovich (formerly Holt Rinehart & Winston).

Carlson, J. G., Singelis, T. & Chemtob, C. M. (1997) Facial EMG responses to combat- and noncombat-related stimuli in veterans with PTSD. *Journal of Applied Psychophysiology and Biofeedback*, **22**, 247–259.

Chemtob, C. M. (1997) *Joining Heart and Mind: A Clinical and Research Agenda for Psychological Debriefing*. Paper presented at the April meeting of the International Society for Critical Incident Debriefing.

Chemtob, C. M. (1996) Posttraumatic stress disorder, trauma, and culture. In *International Review of Psychiatry*, edited by F. LehMac & C. Nadelson, vol. 2. pp. XX–XX. Washington, DC: American Psychiatric Press.

Chemtob, C. M., Bauer, G. B., Neller, G., Hamada, R., Glisson, C. & Stevens, V. (1990) Posttraumatic stress disorder among Special Forces Vietnam veterans. *Military Medicine*, **155**, 16–20.

Chemtob, C. M. & Carlson, J. G. (1994) *A Theoretical Model for the Systematic Treatment of PTSD*. Annual Meeting of the Western Psychological Association, Kona, HI.

Chemtob, C. M., Hamada, R. Roitblat, H. & Muraoka, M. (1994) Anger, impulsivity, and anger control in combat-related Posttraumatic stress disorder. *Journal of Consulting and Clinical Psychology*, **62**, 827–832.

Chemtob, C. M. & Herriott, M. (1994) PTSD as a sequelae of Guillain-Barre Syndrome. *Journal of Traumatic Stress*, **7**, 705–712.

Chemtob, C. M., Nakashima, J. & Hamada, R. (1996) *The Maile Project: A Community-wide Psychosocial Intervention for Elementary School Children with Disaster-related Psychological Distress*. Paper presented at the August meeting of the American Psychological Association, Toronto.

Chemtob, C. M., Novaco, R. W., Hamada, R. S. & Gross, D. M. (1997) Cognitive-behavioral treatment of severe anger in posttraumatic stress disorder. *Journal of Consulting and Clinical Psychology*, **65**, 184–189.

Chemtob, C. M., Novaco, R. W., Hamada, R. S., Gross, D. M. & Smith, G. (1997) Anger regulation deficits in combat-related Posttraumatic stress disorder. *Journal of Traumatic Stress*, **10**, 17–36.

Chemtob, C. M., Roitblat, H. L., Hamada, R. B., Carlson, J. G., Muraoka, M. Y. Bauer, G. (In press). Compelled attention: The effects of viewing trauma-related stimuli on concurrent task performance. *Journal of Trauma Stress*.

Chemtob, C. M., Roitblat, H. L., Hamada, R. M., Carlson, J. G., Muraoka, M. Y. & Bauer, G. B. (1997) The Honolulu Post-Traumatic Stress Disorder Stimul. *Validation: Journal of Traumatic Stress*, **10**, 337–343.

Chemtob, C., Roitblat, H., Hamada, R., Carlson, J. & Twentyman, C. (1988) A cognitive action theory of post-traumatic stress disorder. *Journal of Anxiety Disorders*, **2**, 253–275.

Chemtob, C., Nakashima, J., Hamada, R. & Carlson, J. G. (1996) Calming the storm: Eye movement desensitization treatment for treatment-resistant children with posttraumatic stress disorder, paper presented at the annual meeting of the International Society for the Study of Traumatic Stress, San Francisco, CA.

Chemtob, C. M., Muraoka, M. Y., Holt, P. W., Hamada, R. S., Keane, T. M. & Fairbank, J. A. (1998) Head injury and combat-related PTSD. *Nervous and Mental Disease*, **186**, 701–708.

Chemtob, C. M., Tomas, S., Law, W. & Cremeniter, D. (1997) A field study of the impact of psychological debriefing on post-hurricane psychological distress. *American Journal of Psychiatry*, **154**, 415–417.

Cooper, N. A. & Clum, G. A. (1989) Imaginal flooding as a supplementary treatment for PTSD in combat veterans: A controlled study. *Behavior Therapy*, **20**, 381–391.

Fairbank, J. A., Gross, R. T. & Keane, T. M. (1983) Treatment of posttraumatic stress disorder. Evaluating outcome with a behavioral code. *Behavior Modification*, **7**, 557–568.

Hamada, R. S., Kameoka, V. & Yanagida, E. (1996, November). The Kauai Recovery Index (KRI): Screening for post-disaster adjustment problems in elementary-aged populaations. Paper presented at the 12th annual meeting of the International Society for the Study of Traumatic Stress, San Francisco, CA.

Jensen, J. A. (1994) An investigation of eye movement desensitization and reprocessing (EMD/R) as a treatment for posttraumatic stress disorder (PTSD) symptoms of Vietnam combat veterans. *Behavior Therapy*, **24**, 311–325.

Keane, T. M. & Kaloupek, D. G. (1982) Imaginal flooding in the treatment of a postraumatic stress disorder. *Journal of Consulting and Clinical Psychology*, **50**, 138–140.

Keane, T. M., Caddell, J.M. & Taylor, K.L. (1988) The Missisippi scale for combat-related PTSD: Three studies in reliability and validity. *Journal of Consulting and Clinical Psychology*, **56**, 85–90.

Keane, T. M., Fairbank, J. A., Caddell, J. M. & Zimering, R. T. (1989) Implosive (flooding) therapy reduces symptoms of PTSD in Vietnam combat veterans. *Behavior Therapy*, **20**, 245–260.

Keane, T. M., Zimering, R. T. & Caddell, J. M. (1985) A behavioral formulation of posttraumatic stress disorder in Vietnam veterans. *Behavior Therapist*, **8**, 9 12.

Kovas, M. (1992) *Chidren's Depression Inventory*. North Tonawanda, NY: Multi-Health Systems.

Kulka, R., Schlenger, W., Fairbank, J. A., Hough, R. L., Jordan, B. K., Marmar, C. R. & Weiss, D. S. (1988) *National Vietnam Veterans Readjustment Study Advance Data Report: Preliminary Findings from the National Survey of the Vietnam Generation*. Executive Summary. Washington, D. C.: Veterans Administration.

Litz, B. T., Weathers, F. W., Monaco, V., Herman, D. A., Wulfson, M., Marx, B. & Keane, T. M. (1996) Attention, arousal, and memory in posttraumatic stress disorder. *Journal of Traumatic Stress*, **9**, 497–519.

Malloy, P. F., Fairbank, J. A. & Keane, T. M. (1983) Validation of a multimethod assessment of posttraumatic stress disorders in Vietnam veterans. *Journal of Consulting and Clinical Psychology*, **51**, 488–494.

McNally, R. J., Kaspi, S. P., Rieman, B. C. & Zeitlin, S. B. (1990) Selective processing of threat cues in posttraumatic stress disorder. *Journal of Abnormal Psychology*, **99**, 398–402.

Muraoka, M. Y., Carlson, J. G. & Chemtob, C. M. (1998). Twenty-four hour ambulatory blood pressure and heart rate monitoring in combat-related posttraumatic stress disorder: An exploratory study. *Journal of Traumatic Stress*, **11**, 473–484.

Novaco, R. W. (1975) *Anger Control: The Development and Evaluation of an Experimental Treatment*. Lexington, MA: Heath.

Novaco, R. W. (1994) Clinical problems of anger and its assessment and regulation through a stress coping skills approach. In *Handbook of Psychological Skills Training: Clinical Techniques and Applications*, edited by W. O'Donohue & L. Krasner, (pp. 320–338). Boston: Allyn & Bacon.

Orr, S. P. (1994) An overview of psychophysiological studies of PTSD. *PTSD Research Quarterly*, **5**, 1–7.

Peniston, E. G. (1986) EMG biofeedback-assisted desensitization treatment for Vietnam combat veterans post-traumatic stress disorder. *Clinical Biofeedback and Health*, **9**, 35–41.

Pitman, R. K., Orr, S. P., Altman, B., Longpre, R. E., Poire, R. E. & Lasko, N. B. (1993) *A Controlled Study of Eye Movement Desensitization/Reprocessing (EDMR) Treatment for Post-traumatic Stress Disorder*. Paper presented at the annual meeting of the American Psychiatric Association, Washington, D. C.

Pitman, R. K., Orr, S. P., Forgue, D. F., de Jong, J. B. & Claiborn, J. M. (1987) Psychophysiological assessment of postraumatic stress disorder imagery in Vietnam combat veterans. *Archives of General Psychiatry*, **44**, 970–975.

Puk, G. (1991) Treating traumatic memories: A case report on the eye movement desensitization procedure. *Journal of Behavior Therapy and Experimental Psychiatry*, **22**, 149–151.

Pynoos, R. S., Frederick, C., Nader, K. et al. (1987) Life threat and posttraumatic stress in school-age children. *Archives of General Psychiatry*, **44**, 1057–1063.

Reynolds, C. R. & Richmond, B. O. (1985) *Revised Children's Manifest Anxiety Scale (RCMAS)* (3rd ed. rev.). Washington, D.C.: Author.

Shapiro, F. (1989) Eye movement desensitization: A new treatment for post-traumatic stress disorder. *Journal of Behavior Therapy and Experimental Psychiatry*, **20**, 211–217.

Shapiro, F. (1995) *Eye Movement Desensitization and Reprocessing*. New York: Guilford Press.

Spielberger, C. D., Jacobs, G. A., Russell, S. & Crane, R. (1983) Assessment of anger: The State-Trait Anger Scale. In *Advances in Personality Assessment*, edited by J. D. Butcher & C. D. Spielberger, vol. 2. Hillsdale, NJ: Lawrence Erlbaum.

Townsend, R. E., House, J. F. & Addario, D. (1975) A comparison of biofeedback-mediated relaxation and group therapy in the treatment of chronic anxiety. *American Journal of Psychiatry*, **132**, 598–601.

Wilson, S. A., Becker, L. A. & Tinker, R. H. (1995) Eye movement desensitization and reprocessing (EMDR) treatment for psychologically traumatized individuals. *Journal of Consulting and Clinical Psychology*, **63**, 928–937.

Wilson, S. A., Becker, L. A. & Tinker, R. H. (1997) Fifteen-month follow-up of eye movement desensitization and reprocessing (EMDR) treatment for posttraumatic stress disorder and psychological trauma. *Journal of Consulting and Clinical Psychology*, **65**, 1047–1056.

Chapter 16

PERSONALITY AS A RISK FACTOR IN CANCER AND CORONARY HEART DISEASE

H. J. Eysenck, PhD, DSc

INTRODUCTION

Over hundreds of years, medical orthodoxy believed firmly in the existence of a strong relation between personality and specific diseases, like cancer; the cancer-prone personality was described as repressing emotions and finding it difficult to cope with stress, giving up easily and developing feelings of hopelessness and helplessness (Eysenck, 1991; Temoshok & Dreher, 1992). As Sir William Osler, often called the father of English Medicine, said in 1906: 'It is very often much more important what person has the disease, than what disease the person has'. During the first 50 years of this century this belief has come under fierce criticism by the new medical orthodoxy, partly because it was based largely on purely observational data without benefit of clinical trials or statistical elaboration, but partly because of the success of methods of diagnosis and treatment introduced by Pasteur involving specificity of illness.

In the 1950s, serious scientific study began to show that the anecdotal evidence of past centuries had a hard backing of truth. The work of pioneers like Bahnsen (1969, 1976, 1980), Le Shan (1959, 1977; Le Shan & Le Shan, 1971; Le Shan & Reznikoff, 1960), Kissen (1963a, 1963b, 1964; Kissen & Eysenck, 1962) verified many of the old theories in relation to cancer, and the Type A concept of Friedman and Rosenman (1959, 1974) and Rosenman and Chesney (1980) did the same for coronary heart disease, although only parts of their concept (aggressiveness, hostility, anger) appear to have survived replication (Eysenck, 1990). Grossarth-Maticek (1976, 1979, 1986, 1989; Grossarth-Maticek, Eysenck & Vetter, 1988) is another such pioneer, spanning in his work both cancer and cardiovascular disease and pointing out specific similarities and differences between them. He has also provided much the largest body of material on follow-up studies of healthy probands in existence (Eysenck, 1991, 1993), demonstrated the possibility of using behaviour therapy for the prevention of illness in cancer-prone and coronary heart disease-prone probands (Eysenck & Grossarth-Maticek, 1991), and demonstrated the synergistic interaction of psychosocial and physical risk factors in the causation of cancer and CHD (Eysenck, 1994a; Eysenck, Grossarth-Maticek & Everitt, 1991; Grossarth-Maticek, 1980b). Most important, he has created instruments for measuring objectively the personality characteristics relevant to disease.

I have given a detailed survey of the available evidence elsewhere (Eysenck, 1994b) and do not propose to do so again. I will instead concentrate on recent studies, and on considering methodological problems that are of fundamental importance in trying to understand the apparent contradictions that have arisen in the field (Fox, 1981, 1983, 1988; Fox & Temoshok, 1988). Without such an understanding it would be impossible to arrive at a meaningful and comprehensive picture of the position as it obtains at present. There exist certain theories regarding the psychosocial factors that predict or accompany cancer and coronary heart disease (CHD) and it will be useful to consider the nature of the theories before considering the methodologies used to test the theories, and the results obtained using these methodologies. Temoshok & Dreher (1992), Eysenck (1991) and Baltrush, Stangel & Waltz (1988) have listed some of the personality traits that characterize the cancer-prone type, or C type; such a person is likely to be over-cooperative, appeasing, unassertive, over-patient, seeking for harmony, avoiding conflict, unable to express his emotions, compliant and conforming, and having difficulties in coping with (mainly interpersonal) stress, leading to feelings of helplessness, hopelessness and finally depression. The CHD-prone person, on the other hand, is characaterized by easily-aroused feelings of anger, hostility and aggression; not repressed as Freud and his followers mistakenly assumed, but openly expressed and consciously felt (Johnston, 1993; Williams & Williams, 1993; Siegman & Smith, 1994). This is the Friedman & Rosenman Type A, with irrelevant traits omitted. Both Type A and Type C can be contrasted with Type B, a healthy personality type not given to the neurotic excesses of Types A and C. How can we test these theories?

The most obvious method, of course, is a comparison of cases and controls (Eysenck, 1985). Case studies can support the theories in question, but are subject to the argument that perhaps the disease process has influenced personality, rather than the other way about. This seems unlikely; there is no theory that would predict that CHD patients should develop strong feelings of anger, hostility and aggression, while cancer patients would develop strongly altruistic, peaceful, conformist feelings. The relationship would make just as much sense if reversed - cancer making you angry, and CHD making you more peaceful! In addition, there is good evidence to show that even serious, life-threatening operations do not alter scores on personality scales (e.g. Weinryb, Gustafsson, Asburg &

Rissel, 1992). But the criticism has to be met more directly, and this can only be done by prospective studies, in which healthy people are studied, and then followed up to see who dies of what. Prospective studies are of course vastly more complex and expensive than case studies, but they constitute the gold standard of epidemiology.

A somewhat intermediary method starts with patients, thus resembling the case-control method of study, but after obtaining relevant information follows up the patients' progress to see if progress is related to personality. The expectation would be that a C-type patient would die earlier of cancer than a non-C type, while an A-type CHD patient would die earlier than a non-A type. There are problems here of identifying the stage of illness at diagnosis, and matching medical treatments received, but in principle this is an acceptable method of study (Eysenck, 1994b).

All three methods are essentially correlational; they associate illness with personality; but even if such an association could be established quite firmly, causation could not necessarily be inferred. A fourth method involving intervention can make a causal interpretation much more likely. This method has two variants. In the first we ascertain groups of healthy A-type or C-type probands, match individuals on age, sex and score on A or C inventory, and assign one member of each pair to a control, the other to an intervention group, using a random method of assignment. The method of treatment would of course be intended to alter the A or C personality in the direction of B; if successful, this would strengthen the causal hypothesis. There are problems here, but they are not insuperable.

As regards differentiation, we must consider 3 stages of inclusiveness. The theories mentioned would suggest a differentiation along psychosocial lines between cancer and CHD. A more inclusive differentiation would be mortality from all causes, assuming that these were important aspects of personality (e.g. high neuroticism, poor coping behaviour) common to cancer and CHD, and other causes of death as well. A more analytic theory might suggest that different types of cancer might be related to different aspects of personality—stress, coping. All three types of theory will be considered.

Case-control Studies

Following a number of studies using anecdotal and subjective methods of investigation, the first double-blind investigation to be reported was designed to look at the theory that lung cancer patients have difficulties in expressing their emotions, and repress or deny them (Kissen & Eysenck, 1962). Prior to diagnosing patients coming to Kissen's clinic complaining of chest pains, they were tested with the Maudsley Personality Inventory, which contains a neuroticism scale; it was predicted that, if the theory was true, those later diagnosed as suffering from lung cancer would have lower scores than those later diagnosed as suffering from a benign disease.

Results bore out prediction at an acceptable level of statistical significance, and several repetitions of the study by Kissen replicated the finding. Roughly a 6 to 1 difference appeared between low scorers on the scale and high scorers, a difference not due to smoking. Smoking and personality interacted in a synergistic manner, in that cancer-prone persons needed fewer cigarettes to develop lung cancer. Thus the theory is quite strongly supported by these results. Many other studies have since added support (Eysenck, 1985).

The major contributions to be discussed derive from the work of Grossarth-Maticek (1979; Grossarth-Maticek et al., 1988; Eysenck, 1991). Essentially he devised questionnaires for testing the theoretical notions outlined above along two lines. In the first place he constructed short inventories to measure specific traits assumed to be connected with cancer or CHD, such as 'Need for Harmony' and 'Rational/Antiemotional', where cancer-prone persons, or persons suffering from cancer, are predicted to have high scores on both 'Need for Harmony' and 'Rational/ Antiemotional' behaviour, i.e. suppression or denial of emotion. As an alternative approach, he designed 'Type' questionnaires, responses to which would assign people to one of 4 (later 6) types. Type 1 is cancer-prone, Type 2 CHD-prone. Type 3 has a hysterical personality, but is otherwise healthy, Type 4 is psychologically healthy, Type 5 is rational/antiemotional, and Type 6 is psychopathic-antisocial (Grossarth-Maticek & Eysenck, 1990). Scales are reliable (Schmitz, 1992, 1993; Spielberger, 1988). Types 1 + 2 + 5 together define an unhealthy personality type, Types 3 + 4 + 6 a healthy personality type, i.e. 1 + 2 + 5 predict illness and mortality, 3 + 4 + 6 predict health. Such 'type' approaches, like the Friedman and Rosenbaum Types A and B, are obviously subject to psychological statistical criticisms, but appeal to medical practitioners in that they resemble the 'medical model'.

Vitally important for a proper understanding of the published work of Grossarth-Maticek is the fact that his studies were carried out by specially-trained students who first established trust by talking with prospective subjects about the project, and then stayed to explain any items that were not completely clear to the subjects. This combination of trust and explanation contrasts vividly with the usual habit of just dishing out questionnaires with little preparation, and no chance to explain sometimes very complex concepts. It must also be remembered that the subjects in Grossarth-Maticek's studies are health, randomly selected people between certain age categories (usually with a cut-off at 40), so that roughly half would have an IQ of below 100, and correspondingly little education. Thus the need for explanation, especially because the items in Grossarth-Maticek's scales tend to be highly complex, and difficult to understand.

Two studies were carried out to test the hypothesis that this method of administration would give better prediction in prospective studies than simple handing out of questionnaires (Grossarth-Maticek, Eysenck &

Barrett, 1993; Grossarth-Maticek, Eysenck & Boyle, 1995). Actually, four methods were used in all. In addition to the two methods mentioned above, one method used establishment of trust, but no explanation, and the other explanation, but no establishment of trust. As expected, it was found that simply handing out questionnaires gave very poor results; interviewer administration with establishment of trust and explanation gave very good results in the prediction of cancer and CHD. Explanation was more important than establishment of trust, but both were intermediate between the other two methods. It is clear that a proper replication of Grossarth-Maticek's work must employ the method of interviewer-assisted administration; simply handing out questionnaires will give relatively poor or non-significant results. This should be borne in mind in assessing results of replication studies. It may be interesting to present two such replications to illustrate good and bad methodology. The bad study was carried out by Amelang and Schmidt-Rathgens (1992). There were 204 subjects who responded to a questionnaire, one-third students, the others acquaintances and relatives of these. Ages ranged from 19 to 72 years for the 74 men and from 17 to 71 for the 130 women, with mean ages of 36.8 and 36.1 respectively. Two additional samples consisted of 10 men who suffered from various types of cancer, and 20 men showing various signs of coronary disease. The questionnaire consisted of 291 items extracted from various Grossarth-Maticek inventories, using a rather complex selection procedure that is difficult to follow or justify. The end results showed a high discrimination between ill and healthy (p < .001), but no differentiation between cancer and CHD patients.

There are many weaknesses in this study regarded as a 'replication'. The choice of measuring instruments is very unusual; no such combination had ever been used by Grossarth-Maticek. The number of questions is excessive; few people are willing to answer nearly 300 complex and lengthy questions without getting restive and losing patience, and possibly answering pretty randomly at the end. The choice of subjects is very far removed from that used by Grossarth-Maticek; the mean age is below the lowest age used by Grossarth-Maticek, and very few would be in the interesting age groups where cancer and CHD are common. The fact that there were many more women than men make the choice of only male cancer and CHD patients as cases incomprehensible; there were only 30 men over 40 in the healthy group. This drastically reduces the statistical power of any tests of significance. The method of administration was badly chosen, giving the least chance for positive results to emerge. Finally, a case study was being used to replicate a prospective study. Under these circumstances it seems remarkable that there was such a successful discrimination of cases from controls; it is not surprising that different types of disease were not successfully resolved.

An interesting contrast with this poorly conceived and even more poorly executed study is the work of Fernandez-Ballesteros (Fernandez-Ballesteros,

Zamarron, Ruiz, Sebastian & Spielberger, 1997; Fernandez-Ballesteros, Ruiz & Garde, in press). In the first of these two studies, the population consisted of 96 healthy women, 90 women with benign disease, and 122 women with breast cancer, as well as another group of 210 female students. The questionnaires were an adaptation of the Grossarth-Maticek's 'Need for Harmony' and 'Rationality/Antiemotionality' scales undertaken originally by Spielberger (1988), and used by Swan, Carmelli, Dame, Rosenman & Spielberger (1991, 1992). The main changes were improvement in wording (making it simpler to understand), but the old and new versions were found to correlate so highly that clearly there was no essential change in meaning. Factor analysis by Spielberger and Fernandez-Ballesteros of the Rationality/antiemotionality scale revealed that the scale broke down into two correlated sub-scales (Rationality and Emotional Defensiveness); hence the new scale was called R/ED; it consisted of 15 items in the Fernandez-Ballesteros version, 12 items in the Spielberger version. Reliabilities for the sub-scales and the total scale were high (above .80), as was retest reliability. (Information on these and other important psychometric points was missing from the original Grossarth-Maticek studies.)

The group differences between healthy, benign, cancer and student samples, for the R/ED scale suggest the following: (1) cancer patients are over two standard deviations higher on R/ED and NH than the other groups, which do not differ among themselves. (2) All items by themselves show a similar difference. (3) Looking only at the highest scores on the R/ED scale, there are 88.3% of the breast cancer cases in this category, but only 12.0% of healthy women, 11.9% of 'benign' women, and 11.4% of female students. These are truly remarkable results, and fully supportive of the Grossarth-Maticek theory.

Fernandez-Ballesteros took care to rule out social desirability and dissimulation as important contributing factors, both were tested and failed to correlate with the R/ED scale. This is important in ruling out willful deceit in filling in questionnaires.

It will be obvious why the Fernandez-Ballesteros study is objectively better than the Amelang one. (1) The selection of participants is aimed directly at the problem of discrimination, rather than involving quite irrelevant groups; in the Amelang study the majority of participation was female, but the cases were all men. (2) The numbers involved guaranteed proper statistical power, involving several hundred cases and controls in the Fernandez-Ballesteros study, while in the Amelang study numbers were miniscule, there being only 10 cancer patients! (3) The choice of test instrument was rational in the Fernandez-Ballesteros study, each inventory being very short, and easily understandable, while the Amelang study used far too many questions, arbitrarily thrown together from several different inventories and not at all easy to comprehend. (4) The whole study would have made sense to the participants in the Fernandez-Ballesteros group, because they were members of a mammography group, while the motivation of the Amelang group is questionable. These are some of the criteria by which I propose to judge other studies.

In her second replication, Fernandez-Ballesteros, Ruitt & Garez (in press) obtained even better results, again contrasting women suffering from cancer of the breast with women having less serious growths, or being healthy. The sample included 319 women diagnosed as suffering from breast cancer, and 103 healthy women, similar in professional status and education. All participants were initially screened by mammograph for breast tumours, and were 40 years or older at the time. On the Rationality/Antiemotionality scale, women with low scores had a 2.1% cancer rate; women with high scores a 69.5% cancer rate! On a short Need for Harmony scale, the figures were 17.5% vs. 84.5%. These are remarkable differences to find in a case-control study, and they fully support the Kissen and Grossarth-Maticek theory.

An interesting feature of the Swann et al. (1991) study is the failure of the R/ED scale to discriminate between cancer patients and controls, in spite of the large numbers involved (over 300 cancer cases, over 2,000 controls). This is instructive in view of the many 'failure to replicate' studies in this field. Usually it is easy to discover a good reason for this failure. In this case, the reason is likely to be found in the age of the probands, averaging over 70. It is a well-known prediction, often suggested in research studies, that differences between cases and controls on psychosocial measures are largest in the youngest group, falling away, and occasionally reversed, with the oldest groups. The theoretical reason is of course the simple fact that psychosocial factors are added to all the genetic, environmental and behavioural risk factors involved in cancer and CHD, making the appearance of the disease more probable at an earlier age than would otherwise occur. Those lacking these psychosocial risk factors would succumb to the other risk factors at a later date. In the seventies, when most if not all of the probands under threat from psychosocial risk factors had already died, a null or even inverse correlation might appear between mortality and psychosocial risk factors. (It should be remembered that the cancer patients involved in this study were still alive, and able to answer questionnaires; mortality might be as late as 80 or over!) Thus this negative outcome of the study was not unexpected; all analyses of outcome studies should indicate age of probands as a most important consideration.

To illustrate this effect, consider figures for smoking-related mortality. British doctors (Doll & Peto, 1976) found that for those who died at <45 years of age, the risk ratio for smoking was 8.71, for those 45–54, it was 3.62; for those 55–64, it was 1.54; for those 65–74, it was 1.27; and for those 75+ it was 1.01. Thus risk ratios for any factor affecting survival decrease linearly with increasing age, and the Swann et al. figures are exactly what might have been expected.

Other independent replication studies giving support to the validity of the Grossarth-Maticek questionnaire are Van der Ploeg et al. (1989),

Wirsching et al. (1982), Schmitz (1992, 1993), Bleiker (1995) and many more. There is little doubt that even studies less well designed and carried out than those of Grossarth-Maticek give results very similar to his own, leaving little doubt that personality-stress-coping variables play a paramount part in cancer and heart disease.

Prospective Studies

So far I have commented on replication of the Grossarth-Maticek studies, because they have so often been criticized; a special issue of Psychological Inquiry, 1991, 2,3, was devoted to an explication of Grossarth-Maticek's theories and findings, criticisms of both and replies. Such arguments seldom settle the question, but independent replications surely do; hence their importance. I will now go on to a brief discussion of prospective studies, which originated in the famous Baltimore investigation of Caroline Thomas (1976; Thomas & Greenstreet, 1973; Shaffer et al., 1987). Thomas in 1946 evaluated some thirteen hundred healthy medical students by using tests, interviews, etc. and then followed them up for over three decades, looking for psychological traits that would predispose them to disease. Cancer was predicted in terms of prone-students being 'loners', having lacked closeness to their parents in childhood, reporting little demonstrative activity in their families, having the poorest capacity to accept negative and positive emotions in oneself and others in close relationships, and who suppressed their emotions 'beneath a bland exterior'. The loners were sixteen times more likely to develop cancer than those who 'gave vent to their emotions'. These findings of a risk ratio of 16 gives powerful support to the Kissen and Eysenck, and the Grossarth-Maticek theories and studies, and indeed pre-dated them, and continued follow-up for a much longer period. The risk-ratio factors for personality factors is seven times as high as that for smoking and cancer (2.4) or CHD (2.0), a result very much in agreement with a similar one concerned with a ten-year follow-up study using the Grossarth-Maticek inventories (Grossarth-Maticek et al., 1988), where personality factors were 6 times as important as smoking.

Thomas also found that all causes of death could be reliably predicted from her questionnaires, suggesting that an underlying neurotic personality might be responsible for early mortality. Such a conclusion agrees well with the results of a study by Hinckle & Woolf (1959), who analyzed the medical histories of some three thousand probands. They concluded that there was an 'unhealthy person', i.e. one subject to all sorts of minor and major diseases; this conclusion was based on the negative binomial distribution of episodes of illness per year. Here the most interesting finding of the study was that those people who had the greater number of bodily illnesses'... were the ones who experienced the greater number of disturbances of mood, thought and behaviour .... There was a parallel in between the occurrence of psychoneuroses and psychoses and the occurrence of bodily diseases' (p. 446). This observation clearly suggests the existence of a healthy personality, mens sana in corpore sano, and there has been much interest recently in measuring this healthy personality. Ryff & Keyes (1995) suggested six major categories of well-being: self-acceptance, environmental mastery, positive relations, purpose in life, personal growth, and autonomy; all were found positively correlated and defining a common factor.

Grossarth-Maticek & Eysenck (1995) constructed a 105-item questionnaire in 1980 labelled 'Self-regulation' which contained items related to all six categories; and this was administered to randomly chosen healthy men and women in Heidelberg, who were then followed up for fifteen years when mortality and cause of death were established. Figures 16.1 and 16.2 show the results. There is a linear relationship between self-

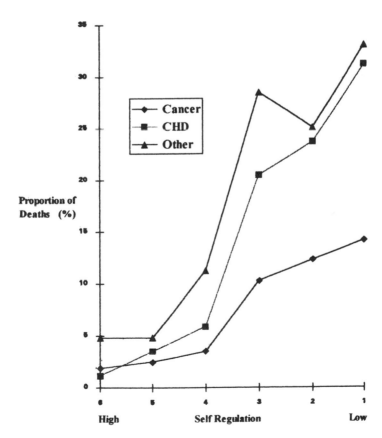

Prospective 1973-1988 Study: Males (N=3,108)

Figure 16.1 Effects of self-regulation in mortality in fifteen-year follow-up: males (Grossarth-Maticek & Eysenck, 1995)

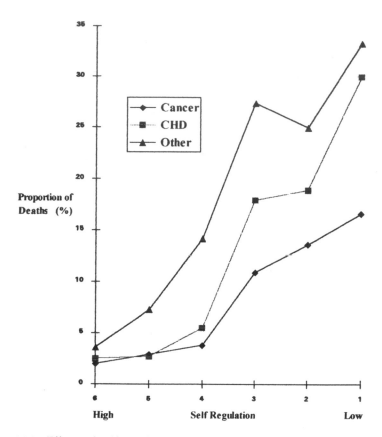

Figure 16.2   Effects of self-regulation in mortality in fifteen-year follow-up: females (Grossarth-Maticek & Eysenck, 1995)

regulation and mortality, with high self-regulation, predicting good health. Clearly there is a general factor of psychological health that correlates well with physical health in general. This correlation is not due to cigarette smoking!

Concerning the next step, namely the differentiation of cancer and CHD-proneness, the essential studies are those carried out by Grossarth-Maticek, Kanazin, Schmidt and Vetter (1982), Grossarth-Maticek, Frentzel-Beyme & Becker (1984), Grossarth-Maticek, Bastiaans and Kanazir (1985), and Grossarth-Maticek, Schmidt, Vetter and Arndt (1984); see also Eysenck (1988, 1991) and Grossarth-Maticek et al. (1988). We are dealing with three prospective studies on healthy randomly selected populations followed for many years. The first sample was selected from a small Yugoslav town, and followed up for 30 years; the second from Heidelberg, the third also from

Heidelberg, but instead of being randomly selected chosen for their degree of stress. Both individual scales and 'type' scales (types 1 to 4) were administered by interviewers. The Heidelberg studies were followed up for 23 years (Grossarth-Maticek, in press).

Results for the Yugoslav study are shown in Table 16.1. Shown are the types (1 = cancer-prone; 2 = CHD-prone; 3 and 4 = healthy), the numbers falling into each type, and their fate after 30 years—alive and healthy, alive but chronically ill; died of cancer; died of stroke or infarct; died of other causes. Some probands could not be located, in spite of the fact that in this small Yugoslav village hardly anyone moved elsewhere. It is clear that of those who died of cancer, the great majority were of type one, while of those who died of stroke or infarct, the great majority were of type two. Of those still alive and healthy, most were of type four and (somewhat less) of type three. These data support Grossarth-Maticek's theory very conspicuously.

Table 16.2 gives the same information for the Heidelberg study in which probands were chosen randomly by reference to registry tables. Mortality is much lower because the mean age was around 50, as compared with 60 in the Yugoslav group. Otherwise the data are very similar to those in Table 16.1. Table 16.3 shows data for the second Heidelberg group, differing from the first one on the basis that they were nominated by members of the first

Table 16.1   Thirty year follow-up of healthy probands diagnosed as cancer-prone (Type 1), coronary heart disease-prone (Type 2), neither (Type 3) and healthy (Type 4). Yugoslav sample.

| Type | N | Still living | | Deceased | | |
		Alive & well	Alive but ill	Cancer	Cause of death Stroke/infarct	Other
I	303	1 (3%)	2 (7%)	174 (57.4%)	41 (13.5%)	85 (28%)
II	339	2 (5%)	1 (3%)	34 (10%)	161 (47.4%)	141 (41.5%)
III	217	48 (22.1%)	36 (16.6%)	8 (3.7%)	27 (12.4%)	98 (45.1%)
IV	482	181 (37.5%)	69 (14.3%)	7 (1.4%)	29 (6%)	196 (40.6%)
Not scored	12	1	2	5	3	
Total:	1353	233 (17.2%)	109 (8.1%)	225 (16.6%)	263 (19.4%)	523 (38.6%)

Source: Grossarth-Maticek, in press.

Table 16.2 Twenty-three year follow-up of healthy probands diagnosed as cancer-prone (Type 1), coronary heart disease-prone (Type 2), neither (Type 3) and healthy (Type 4). Heidelberg normal sample.

Type	N	Still living		Deceased		
		Alive & well	Alive but ill	Cancer	Cause of death Stroke/infarct	Other
I	109	12 (11%)	11 (10%)	41 (37.6%)	18 (16.5%)	21 (19.3%)
II	170	13 (7.6%)	12 (7.1%)	20 (11.8%)	51 (30%)	66 (38.6%)
III	188	80 (42.8%)	65 (34.6%)	4 (2.1%)	8 (4.3%)	25 (13.3%)
IV	391	191 (48.8%)	107 (27.4%)	19 (4.9%)	13 (3.3%)	51 (13%)
Not scored	14	9	—	1	—	4
Total:	872 8	305 (35%)	195 (22.4%)	85 (9.7%)	90 (10.3%)	167 (19.1%)

Note: 30 persons could not be traced 1995/96.
Source: (Grossarth-Maticek, in press).

Table 16.3 Twenty-three year follow-up of healthy probands diagnosed as cancer-prone (Type 1), coronary heart disease-prone (Type 2), neither (Type 3) and healthy (Type 4). Heidelberg stressed sample.

Type	N	Still living		Deceased		
		Alive & well	Alive but ill	Cancer	Cause of death Stroke/infarct	Other
I	489	11 (2.2%)	14 (2.9%)	266 (54.4%)	62 (12.7%)	131 (26.8%)
II	309	12 (3.9%)	15 (4.8%)	36 (11.6%)	129 (41.7%)	106 (34.3%)
III	165	30 (18.2%)	21 (12.7%)	16 (9.8%)	31 (18.8%)	59 (35.7%)
IV	73	32 (43.8%)	9 (12.3%)	2 (2.7%)	7 (9.6%)	20 (27.4%)
Not scored	4	—	—	3	—	1
Total:	1042	85 (8.2%)	59 (5.7%)	323 (31%)	229 (22%)	317 (30.5%)

Note: 27 persons could not be traced 1995/96.
Source: Grossarth-Maticek, in press.

Heidelberg group as being severely stressed. Age being similar to the normal Heidelberg sample, the greater mortality of this sample is likely due to the much greater stress under which they lived. Otherwise the data are again similar to those in Tables 16.1 and 16.2.

There are several similar studies in the literature, and a more detailed description is given elsewhere (Eysenck, 1991). They all support to a varying degree the theory in question, and leave little doubt that cancer and CHD are linked with certain personality types, and can be predicted with remarkable accuracy, even though our data do not quite reach the impressive size of the Caroline Thomas data mentioned earlier.

One further study may be worth mentioning as it used two additional 'types', namely Type 5 (rational-antiemotional) and Type 6 (psychopathic). I am not sure that these additions are very useful in this connection, but Grossarth-Maticek has used the 6-type inventory quite widely, and hence it is of interest to include follow-up data here. We are dealing with another randomized sample of Heidelberg inhabitants, 3,231 in all, who were tested when healthy and followed-up for 15 years (i.e. less than the Heidelberg group discussed earlier). Table 16.4 gives the results, which again show that Type 1 probands tend to die of cancer, Type 2 probands of CHD. Survivors tend to be Type 4 and, somewhat less, Type 3.

Table 16.4 Fifteen year follow-up of probands diagnosed as cancer-prone (Type 1), coronary heart disease-prone (Type 2), neither (Type 3) and healthy (Type 4), rational/antiemotional (Type 5), or psychopathic (Type 6). Heidelberg normal study.

	Type I	Type II	Type III	Type IV	Type V	Type VI	Total
N	652	607	453	529	856	134	3240
Cancer	121	54	20	12	84	123	304
%	(18.5)	(8.9)	(4.4)	(2.2)	(9.7)	(9.7)	(9.4)
Infarct	55	204	26	12	71	11	379
%	(8.4)	(33.6)	(5.7)	(2.3)	(8.2)	(8.2)	(11.7)
Cause of death:							
Other:	122	126	53	47	143	32	523
%	(18.7)	(20.8)	(11.7)	(8.9)	(16.5)	(23.9)	(16.1)
Total mortality	298	384	99	71	298	56	1206
%	(45.7)	(63.2)	(21.8)	(13.4)	(34.4)	(41.7)	(37.2)
Living & healthy	67	72	210	302	193	37	910
%	(10.2)	(11.8)	(46.3)	(57.0)	(21.9)	(27.6)	(28.0)
Living but ill	287	151	144	156	365	41	1124
%	(44.0)	(24.8)	(31.7)	(29.4)	(42.1)	(30.5)	(34.6)
Average age in year	53	53	53	54	52	52	

Source: Grossarth-Maticek, in press.

Can we sub-divide personality factors even further, so as to predict specific types of cancer? In a recent study Grossarth-Maticek, Schmidt, Keppel & Eysenck (1997) posited certain personality aspects that would predict specifically cancer of the cervix, cancer of the breast, and cancer of the uterus. Figures 16.3, 16.4, 16.5 show the results of a follow-up study. The

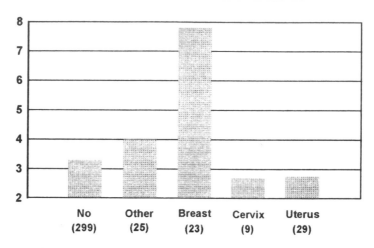

Figure 16.3 Cancer of the breast, as related to blocking by father; females (Grossarth-Maticek et al. 1997).

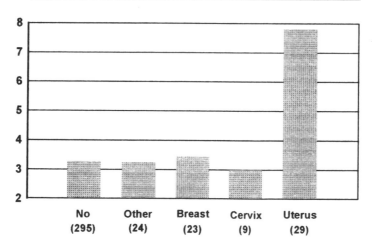

Figure 16.4 Cancer of the uterus, as related to ambivalence of mother role (Grossarth-Maticek et al. 1997).

Type of Cancer And Sado-Masochistic Tendency

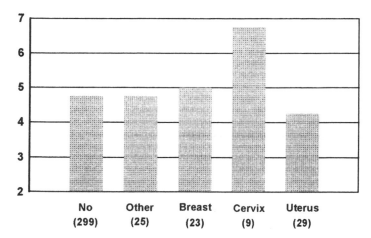

Figure 16.5   Cancer of cervix and sado-masochistic tendency (Grossarth-Maticek et al. 1997).

total number of the women, in the Yugoslav study already mentioned, was small (385 in all), so that the number of specific cancers is very small indeed, ranging from 9 (cervical) to 29 (uterus). The nature of the hypothesis tested was that ambivalence of mother role would be prediction of cancer of the uterus, blocking by father of cancer of the breast, and sado-masochistic tendencies of cancer of the cervix. Results are significant (except for cervical cancer, where there are only 9 women), and all in the predicted direction. Obviously these results require replication, in view of the small sample resulting in insufficient statistical power, but they certainly support the possibility of substantiating cancer-prone subjects according to specific types of cancer.

On the basis of personality inventories, prediction of duration of illness has also been possible for both cancer and CHD (Eysenck, 1991; Temoshok & Dreher, 1992). There is also evidence for the synergistic interaction between stress and smoking, already referred to in connection with the work of Kissen (Kissen & Eysenck, 1962; Grossarth-Maticek, 1980b). I have dealt with this topic in some detail elsewhere (Eysenck, 1994a), but two Figures (16.6, 16.7) may indicate the importance of the interaction. One deals with lung cancer, the other with coronary heart disease. In each case the total group is split-up into smokers and non-smokers, and into stress and non-stress. Stress is measured by using the Grossarth-Maticek scales appropriate for cancer and CHD, respectively. Proportion of sample dying of lung cancer and CHD respectively is indicated on the ordinate, and it will be seen that while smoking and stress have a small contribution to

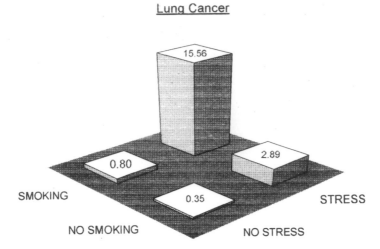

Figure 16.6 Synergistic interaction of smoking and stress on Lung Cancer (Eysenck, 1994a).

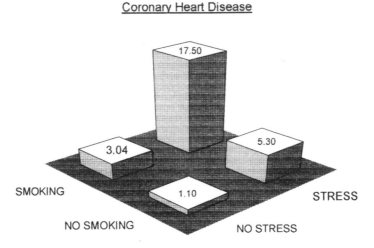

Figure 16.7 Synergistic interaction of smoking and stress on Coronary Heart Disease (Eysenck, 1994a).

make towards mortality, when compared with the no stress/no smoking group, it is the synergistic interaction that produces much of the most horrifying rise in mortality. This simple fact indicates the inadequacy of univariate analysis in blaming so many deaths on a single cause, such as smoking.

Autonomy Training and the Prevention of Cancer and CHD

The fact that personality-stress-coping are clearly relevant to cancer and CHD is of scientific interest, but of comparatively little social importance. On the scientific side too, it merely reports a correlation, and cannot be interpreted necessarily in terms of causation. Both scientifically and socially, intervention studies are necessary to establish a causal link and to demonstrate that cancer and CHD can be prevented in many cases by psychological therapy. The method used in the studies to be summarized here has been called autonomy training, a term that seemed more appropriate than the earlier appelation, 'creative novation behaviour therapy' (Eysenck & Grossarth-Maticek, 1991; Grossarth-Maticek & Eysenck, 1991). These earlier descriptions and summaries of published work were extended in Grossarth-Maticek's (in press) recent book. In all the studies mentioned, healthy probands were selected on the basis of very high Type 1 (cancer-prone) or Type 2 (CHD-prone) scores. They were then allocated to a therapy or control group on a random basis, and treatment was administered to the members of the therapy group. Follow-up investigations after varying periods ranging from 13 years to 23 years were then instituted to establish the status of probands (living healthily; living but chronically ill, dead of cancer, CHD, or other causes).

The therapy was designed to alter the behaviour of the proband, away from typical Type 1 or Type 2 behaviour, and closer to Type 4 behaviour. Details are given in Grossarth-Maticek and Eysenck (1991) and Grossarth-Maticek (in press). Grossarth-Maticek was nearly always the acting therapist; leaving open the question of whether it was the method or the charismatic therapist that was responsible for the observed effects, or perhaps both. This is of course an eternal problem in all forms of psychotherapy.

Table 16.5 shows the effects of autonomy training in a 23-year follow-up of 100 Type 1 probands. Of the therapy group, 8 died of cancer, of the control group 19. Clearly, and significantly the therapy group has much less mortality than the control group. Therapy consisted of roughly 30 hours of individual treatment (Grossarth-Maticek, in press).

In a similar experiment, using 92 probands of Type 2 and followed up over 13 years, results were similar (Table 16.6). Clearly autonomy training is as successful in preventing CHD as it was in preventing cancer (Eysenck & Grossarth-Maticek, 1991).

In a rather smaller experiment, using a mixed Type 1-Type 2 group, Grossarth-Maticek obtained similar results after a 20 year follow-up (Grossarth-Maticek, in press); results are shown in Table 16.7.

A rather different approach was used in another prophylactic experiment, in which probands were selected on the basis of a new questionnaire attempting to measure psychological well-being. Probands were selected on the basis of very low scores in this inventory, and followed

Table 16.5 Survival rates of 50 controls and 50 therapy subjects after twenty-three years.

	N	Living healthy	Living ill	Died of: Cancer	Other causes
Control	50	3 (6%)	7 (14%)	19 (38%)	21 (42%)
Therapy	50	19 (38%)	8 (16%)	8 (16%)	15 (30%)
Total	100	21	15	27	36

Source: Grossarth-Maticek, in press.

Table 16.6 Survival rates of 46 controls and 46 therapy subjects after thirteen years.

	N	Death from CHD.	Diseased	Other causes of death	Living
Control	46	16 (34.8%)	20 (43.5%)	13 (28.3%)	17 (36.9%)
Therapy	46	3 (6.5%)	11 (23.9%)	6 (13.0%)	37 (80.4%)
Total	92	19 (20.6%)	31 (33.7%)	19 (20.7%)	54 (58.7%)

Source: Eysenck & Grossarth-Maticek, in press.

Table 16.7 Effect of autonomy training of probands with exceptionally high scores on Type 1 or Type 2, after twenty-year follow-up.

	N	Death from: Cancer	CHD	Other causes	Living: Ill	Well
Control	29	5 (17.2%)	4 (13.7%)	7 (24.1%)	10 (34.4%)	3 (10.3%)
Therapy	29	1 (3.4%)	1 (3.4%)	4 (13.7%)	8 (27.5%)	15 (51.7%)

Source: Grossarth-Maticek, in press.

up for 19 years. Results are shown in Table 16.8, with results very similar to those of the other prophylactic experiments (Grossarth-Maticek, in press). What is of interest in this and the preceding experiments is that the questionnaire was administered twice—once before training, and once after training. In both the control and the therapy groups there was no change in those who died later on, but a marked shift towards higher psychological well-being in those who survived. The difference between therapy and

Table 16.8   Effect of autonomy training of probands with very low scores on psychological well-being and pleasure-taking, after nineteen years.

	N	Death from:			Living:
		Cancer	CHD	Other causes	Healthy
Control	49	14	8	10	5
		(28.5%)	(16.3%)	(20.4%)	(10.2%)
Therapy	49	4	3	4	30
		(8.1%)	(6.1%)	(8.1%)	(61.7%)

Source: Grossarth-Maticek, in press.

control groups was simply that many more survived in the therapy group. This demonstrates the causal connection between personality and survival; apparently events in a person's life other than therapy can produce this effect.

Yet another choice of probands is shown in Table 16.9, where probands were chosen on the basis of a combination of prognosticators, namely low scores on self-regulation, cigarette smoking, uses of CNS depressant drugs, genetic predisposition (as shown by mortality from cancer of close family members), poor nutrition, contact with traffic pollution. Again, we find strong therapy effects, and a marked change in score on the self-regulation inventory in those who are still alive. Like all the therapy experiments, statistical evaluation shows a p < 0.0000 value.

Table 16.10 shows the results of a rather different type of experiment, using carcinoma of the stomach as the terminal point in groups predisposed to the disorder on the basis of genetic predisposition, chronic gastritis and/or ulcus ventriculi, physical risk factor in nutrition, and very low scores on self-regulation. There are four different therapy groups, of which that using nutritional advice clearly had no effect by itself. Autonomy training almost halved the mortality rate, and did even better when combined with nutritional advice. Best of all was a combination with

Table 16.9   Follow-up study of probands with several risk-factors for cancer, including stress, smoking, wrong nutrition, etc. Plotted is the outcome comparison of thirty controls and thirty therapy probands.

	N	Death from:		Still living:
		Cancer	Other causes	
Control	30	19 (63.3%)	10 (33.3%)	1 (3.3%)
Therapy	30	8 (26.6%)	5 (16.6%)	17 (56.6%)

Source: Grossarth-Maticek, in press.

Table 16.10 Fifteen-year follow-up of eighty probands with strong risk factors for stomach cancer, divided into five groups, one control and four groups subjected to different types of therapy.

	Control group	Autonomy training (1)	Advice (2)	Nutritional intervention (1 + 2)	Intervention 1 + 2 & multi- vitamins administered (3)
N	16	16	16	16	16
Died from Cancer of Stomach	8 (50%)	5 (31.2%)	8 (50%)	3 (18.7%)	1 (6.2%)

Source: Grossarth-Maticek, in press.

added multi-vitamin administration. The overall effect is significant (p < 0.02), with control vs. treatment 3 (combining all 3 treatment methods) giving p < 0.006.

A similar experiment on lung cancer, again using highly predisposed probands (genetic predisposition, bronchitis, low self-regulation, heavy cigarette consumption), gave results shown in Table 16.11. Simply testing the giving up of cigarettes fell just short of significance; all other treatments were significantly better than control. Overall p < 0.001 indicates the effectiveness of the various treatments.

In his book, Grossarth-Maticek gives several tables suggesting autonomy training leading to prophylactic success in probands prone to cancer of the liver and other cancers, but the samples studied are too small to give statistically significant results, although they go in the expected direction. We will now discuss the effects of group administration of autonomy training, i.e. using groups of some 20 or more probands in a series of 2 to 3 hour-long group meetings (Grossarth-Maticek & Eysenck, 1991). Results are shown in Table 16.12 (Eysenck & Grossarth-Maticek, 1991). The probands

Table 16.11 Fifteen-year follow-up of 105 probands with strong risk factors for lung cancer, divided into five groups, one control and four therapy groups.

	Training to cease smoking (1)	Autonomy train (2)	Intervention 1 + 2 (1 + 2)	Intervention 1 + 2 + M/Vit. administered (3) 1 + 2	M/Vit.
N	21	21	21	21	21
Bronchial carcinoma mortality	14 (66.6%)	8 (38%)	6 (28.5%)	4 (19%)	2 (9.5%)

Source: Grossarth-Maticek, in press.

Table 16.12 Comparison of death and incidence in control and therapy group subjected to group autonomy training.

	Therapy		Control	
n	245		245	
Not Contacted	6		11	
	Mortality	Incidence	Mortality	Incidence
	239	235	234	231
Cancer	18	75	111	129
	7.5%	31.9%	47.4%	55.8%
CHD	10	29	36	45
	4.2%	12.3%	15.4%	19.5%
Other causes of death	20	—	33	—
	8.4%		14.1%	
Living	191		56	
	79.9%	23.9%		

Source: Eysenck & Grossarth-Maticek, 1991.

were selected on the basis of high Type 1 and/or Type 2 scores. Statistical significance is high, and clearly group therapy is not inferior to individual therapy.

Surprisingly, bibliotherapy is also very successful in preventing cancer and CHD. A specially prepared short account on the implication of personality and behaviour in disease was prepared, going on to methods of avoiding these dangers. This was administered by trained interviewers who spent one hour going over the material with probands answering questions, and tendering advice. They returned twice, again for one hour, to answer questions, tender advice, and discuss behaviour changes inaugurated by the probands. In thus involving interviewer-therapists, this is much more than a simple example of bibliotherapy, but the success rate is reassuring (see Table 16.13). Randomly selected probands, high on Type 1 and/or Type 2 scores, made up the control group and the therapy group. There were 600 probands in the therapy group, and 500 in the control group. Another 100 probands made up a special control group who were administered a different script, using 'dynamic' terminology and given 'dynamic advice'. It was anticipated, and found, that this placebo treatment would have no effect (Eysenck & Grossarth-Maticek, 1990, 1991).

In a more recent set of experiments, Grossarth-Maticek used three different methods to demonstrate the uses of bibliotherapy. In the first of these, using 125 therapy—125 control subjects, the text used related to improving self-regulatory behaviour. In the second experiment, using 343 therapy and 343 control subjects, the self-regulation questionnaire was administered several times. In the third experiment, both text and inventory

Table 16.13 Comparison of controls and therapy group using autonomy training by means of interviewer-assisted bibliotherapy.

	Cancer		Causes of death: CHD		Other	
	D*	I*	D*	I*	D*	I*
Control = 500	156	162	145	203	164	–
	(21.5%)	(33.4%)	(29.4%)	(41.8%)	(33.3%)	–
Control with use of psychoanalytic text N = 100	22 (22%)	37 (37.7%)	31 (31.%)	40 (40.8%)	28 (28.%)	–
Therapy group w. behaviour therapy text N = 600	27 (4.5%)	99 (16.9%)	47 (7.9%)	132 (22.5%)	115 (19.2%)	–

D* = died of   I* = incidence

	Total	Living		Not investigated
		M*	D*	
Control N = 500	415 (84.2%)	78 (15.8%)	7 (1.4%)	15 (3%)
Control w. use of psychoanalytic text N = 100 (placebo gp.)	81 (81%)	19 (19%)	– –	2 (2%)
Therapy group w. behaviour therapy text. N = 600	189 (31.6%)	409 (68.4%)	2 (3%)	14 (2.3%)

M = mortality   D = diseased

Source: (Eysenck & Grossarth-Maticek, 1991)

were presented several times. The group differed in many details, and these as well as specific results from the various studies, are given in Grossarth-Maticek's (in press) book. Here I will only cite his table putting all these data together (Table 16.14); there are no great differences in the specific results of the three separate experiments.

These results are not only of interest because of the fact that a very cheap method of bibliotherapy is capable of having a very definite prophylactic effect, but also because interaction with probands was exclusively by students specially trained by Grossarth-Maticek. This suggests that while in individual and group therapy, his charismatic personality might have had a marked influence on the success of the treatment, the method itself and the underlying theory must also have played an important role, as otherwise the administration by students would not have been successful.

Autonomy training can also be used to ensure longer life in patients suffering from incurable cancer. Grossarth-Maticek (1980a) published

Table 16.14   Comparison of control and therapy group after twenty-two years follow-up. Therapy used multiple presentation of self-regulation inventory and of special brochure (bibliotherapy).

	N	Cancer		Other causes of death	Still living
		Mortaloity	Incidence		
Therapy	596	58 (9.7%)	62 (10.4%)	204 (34.2%)	334 (56%)
Control	596	137 (22.5%)	130 (21.8%)	292 (49%)	167 (28%)

Source: Grossarth-Maticek, in press.

details of an experiment in which 24 pairs of cancer sufferers were established, suffering from similar types of cancer. On a chance basis, one of each pair was included in a control, the other in a therapy group. Survival in years was 5.07 in the therapy group, and 3.09 in the control group. Table 16.15 shows the details.

In a later experiment (Grossarth-Maticek, in press), 66 women suffering from mammary carcinomas with metasteses, were randomly divided into therapy and control groups. Duration of survival is shown in Table 16.16. Changes in self-regulation in the direction of higher scores were noted to correlate with better prognosis; the greater the improvement in score, the greater the probability of survival. Other studies are cited in Eysenck & Grossarth-Maticek (1991). It may be noted that other types of intervention in independent studies have also been at least as successful as those mentioned (e.g. Spiegel et al., 1989); clearly we can prolong life of terminal cancer patients by something between 50% and 100%.

In this field, too, bibliotherapy was found useful. As Table 16.17 shows, in a group of patients suffering from cancer without metasteses, the three-times administration of the self-regulation inventory and script had an important influence on survival, and again upward change in score on the self-regulation inventory was correlated with survival.

In summary, it may be useful to state that there cannot be any doubt that psychosocial factors (personality, stress, coping) are closely related to physical health and physical disease, with more specific types of personality being related to specific diseases, such as cancer and CHD. Possibly even more specific relations exist between different types of cancer and different types of personality; there is too little evidence to decide. These relations are particularly important because of their synergistic interaction between physical and psychosocial factors, and the demonstrated possibility of intervention through psychological treatment reducing the psychosocial risk factors, and thus preserving life through prevention (Eysenck & Grossarth-Maticek, 1991; Grossarth-Maticek & Eysenck, 1991). Clearly, only the beginnings have been made in this quest,

Table 16.15 Survival (in years) of twenty-four pairs of matched cancer patients, allocated at random to control and therapy group.

Type of cancer	Number of pair of patients	Survival time, years		Sex	Age	
		Therapy group	Control group		Therapy group	Control group
Scrotal cancer	1	5.8	3.2+	M	34	35
Stomach cancer	1	4.8	1.8+	M	64	63
	2	2.4	2.3+	M	59	59
Bronchiolar	1	1.7	2.4−	M	42	42
	2	5.6	1.5+	M	59	60
	3	4.2	1.6+	M	60	60
	4	3.2	1.1+	M	47	46
	5	1.7	1.7−	M	39	39
	6	4.5	1.2+	M	58	98
	7	5.2	1.0+	M	63	64
Corpus uteri	1	6.8	4.2+	F	64	65
	2	4.5	4.8−	F	66	66
	3	7.2	3.5+	F	49	48
	4	8.2	3.1+	F	50	51
Cervical	1	5.5	4.2+	F	41	41
	2	6.1	4.0+	F	46	46
	3	3.2	3.3−	F	38	37
	4	4.5	4.1+	F	50	49
	5	2.8	3.6−	F	39	40
Colon and rectum carcinoma	1	9.5	4.2+	M	64	64
	2	7.5	2.1+	F	56	56
	3	6.3	4.9+	M	55	56
	4	4.8	4.3+	F	61	60
	5	5.7	4.1+	F	52	52
Total	24	5.07	3.09			

Source: (Grossarth-Maticek, in press).

Table 16.16 Duration of survival (in years) for women suffering from cancer of the breast, divided into control and therapy groups.

Duration of survival in years	Therapy N = 33	Control N = 33
1–5	6	16
6–10	6	14
11–15	14	2
16+	7	1

Source: Grossarth-Maticek, in press.

Table 16.17 Duration of survival (in years) for patients divided into control and bibliotherapy group.

Duration of survival in years	Therapy group N = 68	Control group N = 68
1–5	9	18
6–10	26	17
11–15	23	10
16+	10	3

Source: Grossarth-Maticek, in press.

but its social and scientific importance will hardly be questioned any longer.

I have in this chapter concentrated on the contribution of Grossarth-Maticek, not because it is the only support for my thesis regarding the importance of psychosocial factors in cancer and CHD (there is a large volume of support for this view, as shown by Eysenck, 1991, Temoshok & Dreher, 1992, Siegman & Smith, 1994 and many others), but because his work, having been published largely in Germany, has not become sufficiently known in English-speaking countries to exert the influence it should. His work has been criticized—no pioneering studies fail to be subjected to criticism, both just and unjust—but there are now sufficient successful replications of his work to make it clear that here we are dealing with an outstanding set of studies that well deserve to be taken seriously. Furthermore, the results fit extremely well into the framework constructed by a large body of American, British, Australian, Canadian, German, Spanish and Scandinavian psychologists, epidemiologists, oncologists, and psychiatrists—amazingly well, as when Grossarth-Maticek began his work in the late 1950s, this structure did not yet exist, and he had to construct his own framework. It is to be hoped that his work will give rise to many more replications, and in due course improvements on the necessarily primitive theories he and we are perforce working with.

References

Amelang, M. & Schmidt-Rathgens, C. (1992) Personality, stress and disease: Some results on the psychometric properties of the Grossarth-Maticek and Eysenck inventories. *Psychological Reports*, **71**, 1251–1263.

Bahnsen, C. B. (1969) Psychophysiological complementary malignancies: past work and future vistas. *Annals of the New York Academy of Sciences*, **164**, 319–337.

Bahnsen, C. B. (1976) Emotional and personality characteristics of cancer patients. In *Oncological Medicine*, edited by A. I. Southick & P. Engstrom, pp. 357–378. Baltimore: University Park Press.

Bahnsen, C. B. (1980) Stress and cancer: The state of the art. *Psychosomatics*, **21**, 975–981; **22**, 207–220.

Baltrush, H., Stangel, W. & Waltz, M. (1988) Cancer from the behavioural perspective: The type C pattern. *Activitas Nervosa Superior*, **30**, 18–20.

Bleiker, E. (1995) *Personality Factors and Breast Cancer*. Amsterdam: Vrije Universiteit.

Doll, R. & Peto, R. (1976) Mortality in relation to smoking: 20 years' observation on male British doctors. *British Medical Journal*, 25 December, 1525–1536.

Eysenck, H. J. (1985) Personality, cancer and cardiovascular disease: A causal analysis. *Personality and Individual Differences*, **5**, 535–557.

Eysenck, H. J. (1988) The respective importance of personality, cigarette smoking and interaction effects for the genesis of cancer and coronary heart disease. *Personality and Individual Differences*, **9**, 453–464.

Eysenck, H. J. (1990) Type A behaviour and coronary heart disease. The third stage. *Journal of Social Behaviour and Personality*, **5**, 25–44.

Eysenck, H. J. (1991) *Smoking, Personality and Stress: Psychosocial Factors in the Prevention of Cancer and Coronary Heart Disease*. New York: Springer Verlag.

Eysenck, H. J. (1993) Prediction of cancer and coronary heart disease mortality by means of a personality inventory. Results of a 15-year follow-up study. *Psychological Reports*, **72**, 499–516.

Eysenck, H. J. (1994a) Synergistic interaction between psychosocial and physical factors in the causation of lung cancer. In *The Psychoimmunology of Cancer*, edited by C. Lewis, C. O'Sullivan & J. Barraclough, pp. 163–178. Oxford: Oxford University Press.

Eysenck, H. J. (1994b) Cancer, personality and stress: Prediction and prevention. *Advances in Behaviour Research and Therapy*, **16**, 167–215.

Eysenck, H. J. & Grossarth-Maticek, R. (1990) Personality, stress and disease: description and validation of a new inventory. *Psychological Reports*, **66**, 355–373.

Eysenck, H. J. & Grossarth-Maticek, R. (1991) Creative novation behaviour therapy as a prophylactic treatment for cancer and coronary heart disease: II. Effects of treatment. *Behaviour Research and Therapy*, **29**, 17–31.

Eysenck, H. J., Grossarth-Maticek, R. & Everitt, B. (1991) Personality, stress, smoking and genetic predisposition as synergistic risk factors for cancer and coronary heart disease. *Integrative Physiological and Behavioural Sciences*, **26**, 309–322.

Fernandez-Ballesteros, R., Ruiz, M. & Garde, M. (in press) Emotional expression in breast cancer and healthy women.

Fernandez-Ballesteros, R., Zamarron, M. D., Ruiz, M. A., Sebastian, J. & Spielberger, C. D. (1997) Assessing emotional expression: Spanish adaptation of the Rationality/Emotional Defensiveness Scale. *Personality and Individual Differences*, **22**(5), 719–729.

Fox, B. H. (1981) Psychosocial factors and the immune system in human cancer. In *Psychoneuroimmunology*, edited by R. Ader, pp. 103–158. Orlando, Fl.: Academic Press.

Fox, B. H. (1983) Current theory of psychogenic effects on cancer incidence and prognosis. *Journal of Psychosocial Oncology*, **1**, 17–31.

Fox, B. H. (1988) Psychogenic factors in cancer, especially its incidence., In *Topics in Health Psychology*, edited by S. Maes, C. D. Spielberger, T. B. Defares & I. G. Sarason, pp. 37–55. London: Wiley.

Fox, B. H. & Temoshok, L. (1988) Mind-body and behaviour in cancer incidence. *Advances, Institute for the Advancement of Health*, **5**, 41–56.

Friedman, M. & Rosenman, R. H. (1959) Association of specific overt behaviour patterns with blood and cardiovascular findings. *Journal of the American Medical Association*, **169**, 1286–1296.

Friedman, M. & Rosenman, R. H. (1974) *Type A Behaviour and Your Heart*. London: Wildwood.

Grossarth-Maticek, R. (1976) *Das Verhalten als Krebsrisikofactor*. Heidelberg: Reihe Sozialwissenschaftliche Onkologie.

Grossarth-Maticek, R. (1979) *Sozialen Verhalten und die Krebserkrankung*. Weinheim: Beltz.

Grossarth-Maticek, R. (1980a) Social psychopathology and course of the disease. *Psychotherapy and Psychosomatics*, **33**, 129–138.

Grossarth-Maticek, R. (1980b) Synergistic effects of cigarette smoking, systolic blood pressure, and psychosocial risk factors for lung cancer, cardiac infarct, and apoplexy cerebri. *Psychotherapy and Psychosomatics*, **34**, 267–272.

Grossarth-Maticek, R. (1986) Psychosoziale Verhaltenstypen und Chronische Erkrankungen. *Der Kassenarzt*, **39**, 26–35.

Grossarth-Maticek, R. (1989) Disposition, Exposition, Verhaltensmuster, Organschadigung und Stimulierung des Zentralen Nervensystems in der Atiologie des Antiologie des Bronchial-, Magen-und Leberkarzinoma. *Deutsche Zeitschrift fur Onkologie*, **2**, 62–78.

Grossarth-Maticek, R. (in press) Die Psychosomatische Dimension im Krebproblem.

Grossarth-Maticek, R., Bastiaans, J. & Kanazir, D. T. (1985) Psychosocial factors as strong predictors of mortality from cancer, ischaemic heart disease and stroke: The Yugoslav Prospective Study. *Journal of Psychosomatic Research*, **29**, 167–176.

Grossarth-Maticek, R. & Eysenck, H. J. (1990) Personality, stress and disease description and validation of a new inventory. *Psychological Reports*, **66**, 355–373.

Grossarth-Maticek, R. & Eysenck, H. J. (1991) Creative novation behaviour therapy as a prophylactic treatment for cancer and coronary heart disease: I. Description of treatment. *Behaviour Research and Therapy*, **29**, 1–16.

Grossarth-Maticek, R. & Eysenck, H. J. (1995) Self-regulation and mortality from cancer, coronary heart disease and other causes: A prospective study. *Personality and Individual Differences*, **19**, 781–795.

Grossarth-Maticek, R., Eysenck, H. J. & Barrett, P. (1993) Prediction of cancer and coronary heart disease as a function of method of questionnaire administration. *Psychological Reports*, **73**, 943–959.

Grossarth-Maticek, R., Eysenck, H. J. & Boyle, G. J. (1995) Method of test administration as a factor in test validity: The use of a personality questionnaire in the prediction of cancer and coronary heart disease. *Behaviour Research and Therapy*, **33**, 705–710.

Grossarth-Maticek, R., Eysenck, H. J. & Vetter, H. (1988) Personality type, smoking habit and their interaction as predictors of cancer and coronary heart disease. *Personality and Individual Differences*, **9**, 479–495.

Grossarth-Maticek, R., Eysenck, H. J., Ppfeifer, A., Schmidt, P. & Kappel, C. (1997) The specific action of different personality risk factors on cancer of the breast, cervix, corpus uteri, and other types of cancer: A prospective investigation. *Personality and Individual Differences*, **23**(6), 949–960.

Grossarth-Maticek, R., Frentzel-Beyme, R. & Becker, N. (1984) Cancer risks associated with life events and conflict solutions. *Cancer Detection and Prevention*, **7**, 201–209.

Grossarth-Maticek, R., Kanazir, D. T., Schmidt, P. & Vetter, H. (1982) Psychosomatic factors in the process of cancerogenesis. *Psychotherapy and Psychosomatics*, **38**, 284–302.

Grossarth-Maticek, R., Pfeifer, A., Schmidt, P. & Koppel, G. (1983) Psychosomatic predictors for breast, cervix, corpus uteri and other types of cancer. Paper presented at the 7th International Congress on Psychosomatic Obstetrics and Gynaecology, 11–15 September 1983, Dublin.

Grossarth-Maticek, R., Schmidt, P., Vetter, H. & Arndt (1984) Psychotherapy research in oncology. In *Health Care and Human Behaviour*, edited by A. Steptoe & A. Mathews, pp. 325–341. London: Academic Press.

Hinckle, L. & Woolf, H. (1959) The nature of man's adaptation to his total environment and the relation of this to illness. *Archives of Internal Medicine*, **99**, 442–460.

Johnston, D. W. (1993) The current status of the coronary-prone behaviour pattern. *Journal of the Royal Society of Medicine*, **86**(7), 406–409.

Kissen, D. M. (1963a) Personality characteristics in males conducive to lung cancer. *British Journal of Medical Psychology*, **36**, 27–36.

Kissen, D. M. (1963b) Aspects of personality of men with lung cancer. *Actas Psychotherapeutica, Psychosomatics et Orthopaedagogica*, **11**, 200–210.

Kissen, D. M. (1964) Relationship between lung cancer, cigarette smoking, inhalation and personality. *British Journal of Medical Psychology*, **37**, 203–216.

Kissen, D. M. & Eysenck, H. J. (1962) Personality in male lung cancer patients. *Journal of Psychosomatic Research*, **6**, 123–137.

Le Shan, L. (1959) Psychological states as factors in the development of malignant disease: A critical review. *Journal of the National Cancer Institute*, **22**, 1–18.

Le Shan, L. (1977) *You can fight for your life: Emotional factors in the causation of cancer.* New York: M. Evans.

Le Shan, L. & Le Shan, E. (1971) Psychotherapy and the patient with a limited life span. *Psychiatry*, **24**, 318–326.

Le Shan, L. & Reznikoff, M. (1960) A psychological factor apparently associated with neoplastic disease. *Journal of Abnormal and Social Psychology*, **60**, 439–440.

Osler, W. (1906) *Aequanimitas*, p. 258. New York: McGraw-Hill.

Rosenman, R. H. & Chesney, M. A. (1980) The relationship of type of behaviour to coronary heart disease. *Activitas Nervosa Superior*, **22**, 1–45.

Ryff, C. & Keyes, C. (1995) The structure of psychological well-being revisited. *Journal of Personality and Social Psychology*, **6a**, 719–727.

Schmitz, P. (1992) Personality, stress reaction and disease. *Personality and Individual Differences*, **213**, 683–691.

Schmitz, P. (1993) Personality, stress-reaction, and psychosomatic complaints. In A. van Heck, P. Bonainto, I. Deary & W. Novack (eds). *Personality Psychology in Europe*, **4**, 321–242. Tilburg: Tilburg University Press.

Shaffer, J., Graves, P., Swanck, R. & Pearson, T. (1987) Clustering of personality traits in youth and the subsequent developmental cancer among physicians. *Journal of Behavioural Medicine*, **10**, 441–447.

Siegman, A. W. & Smith, T. W. (eds.) (1994) *Anger, Hostility, and The Heart.* Hillsdale, N.J.: Lawrence Erlbaum Associates.

Spiegel, D., Bloom, J., Kraemer, H. J. & Gottleib, E. (1989) Effects of psychosocial treatment on survival of patients with metastatic breast cancer. *Lancet*, **Oct. 14**, 888–891.

Spielberger, C. (1988) Rationality/Emotional Defensiveness Scale and Need for Harmony Preliminary Manual. Tampa: Institute for Research on Behavioral Medicine and Health Psychology, South Florida University.

Swan, G., Carmelli, D., Dame, A., Rosenman, R. & Spielberger, C. (1991) The rationality/emotional defensiveness scale—I. Internal structure and stability. *Journal of Psychosomatic Research*, **35**, 545–557.

Swan, G., Carmelli, D., Dame, A., Rosenman, R. & Spielberger, C. (1992) The rationality/defensiveness scale—II. Convergent and division of correlational analysis in males and females with or without cancer. *Journal of Psychosomatic Research*, **36**, 349–359.

Temoshok, L. L. & Dreher, H. (1992) *The Type C Connection.* New York: Random Houe.

Thomas. C. B. (1976) Precursors of premature disease and death. *Annals of Internal Medicine*, **85**, 653–658.

Thomas, C. B. & Greenstreet, R. L. (1973) Psychological characteristics in youth as predictors of five disease states: Suicide, mental illness, hypertension, coronary heart disease and tumor. *The Johns Hopkins Medical Journal*, **132**, 16–43.

Van der Ploeg, H., Kleign, W., Mook, J., Dauge, M., Pieters, A. & Leer, W. (1989) Positivity of antiemotionality as a risk factor for cancer: Concept and differentiation. *Journal of Psychosomatic Research*, **33**, 217–225.

Weinryb, R., Gustafsson, J., Asberg, M. & Rissel, R. (1992) Stability over time of character assessment using a psychodynamic and personality inventory. *Acta Psychiatrica Scandinavica*, **86**, 179–184.

Williams, R. & Williams, V. (1993) *Cancer Kills.* New York: Random House.

Wirsching, M., Sterlin, M., Hoffmann, E., Weber, G. & Wirsching, B. (1982) Psychological identifications of breast cancer patients before biopsy. *Journal of Psychosomatic Research*, **26**, 1–10.

Chapter 17

PSYCHOSOCIAL ASPECTS OF CANCER CONTROL

R. W. Sanson-Fisher, PhD and Billie Bonevski BA (Hons)

INTRODUCTION

Cancer is a major cause of death throughout the world, although the mortality rates attributable to cancer vary from country to country (Sanson-Fisher, 1993). Similarly, there is considerable variation across countries with regard to the types of cancer causing most deaths. For example, although female breast cancer is a major cause of death in many developed countries, it is rare in much of Asia and Africa (Muir et al., 1987). Despite these variations, there is agreement that the burden of illness imposed by cancer across the world is likely to increase. Projections estimate that worldwide, cancer will cause another 200 million deaths and affect another 300 million people in the next 25 years. There are three main strategies in cancer control: primary prevention, or the reduction of the incidence of the disease; secondary prevention, the early detection and treatment of the disease; and tertiary care which relates to minimisation of the impact of the established disease (Sanson-Fisher, 1993).

To date, when resources and energy are directed towards the tertiary aspects of cancer control, they have been dominated by the biomedical approach to cure (Sanson-Fisher, 1993). However, with little promise in sight for a cure to all cancer in the near future, it is important that efforts in tertiary care are orientated towards patient care. The main focus of this broad domain should be minimisation of the psychosocial impact of cancer and its treatments to the patient. Certainly, there has been a steady increase in the research efforts in this aspect of tertiary care. A count of the number of articles listed in MEDLINE, the computerised medical database of published articles, using the keywords of *Psychosoc*, Quality of Life, Psycholog* and Cancer, Oncolog*, Neoplas** revealed an increasing trend in publishing related research. Figure 17.1 shows that the number of articles extracted by the search rose from 38 to 1,068 in two decades (1970–1990).

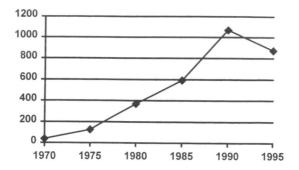

Figure 17.1 Number of articles listed in MEDLINE in the area of psychosocial cancer care, by year.

Note though, that this search is a comment merely on the amount of research conducted in the area and not the quality of the articles.

To explore the type of research being published in this area across time, the articles were categorised into several groups; commentaries and reviews, measures, descriptive, case studies, and program evaluation. This process revealed that most of the research published in 1975, 1985 and 1995 was commentary and review (see Figure 17.2). Although 10% of the 1985 research and 22% of the 1995 research was descriptive, no research reporting the development and evaluation of measures had been published in any year. Less than 20% of the research was based on evaluation studies.

With a large bulk of research on the psychosocial care of patients with cancer, one would expect a concomitant improvement in related patient outcomes. Afterall, is not the purpose of this research to decrease the burden experienced by patients with cancer? This paper will argue that the expected improvements in care and outcomes are not yet evident. To do this, research needs to encompass a number of areas: development and use

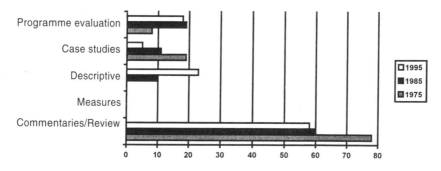

Figure 17.2 Proportion of published research on psychosocial therapies categorised by type of research study.

of credible measurement tools; establishment of baseline levels of burden of illness; quality assurance for providers; development of cost-effective interventions for patients; implementation of systems of routine feedback; and provision of effective provider training. By researching these areas, we provide the health care system and its workers with tools by which to decrease the burden experienced by patients with cancer.

DECREASING THE BURDEN FOR PATIENTS WITH CANCER

1. Credible Measures

There are a number of reasons why credible measures of patient psychosocial outcomes are necessary (Foot, 1996; Lindley, 1992). With adequate measurement tools, patient progress is able to be monitored across time. For example, using a reliable measurement instrument, changes in patient needs may be compared before and after treatment. Similarly the natural history of psychosocial aspects of the disease and its treatment effects may be measured. For example, there is now sufficient evidence which suggests that anxiety changes across time and is different for various diseases (Johnston, 1980). By obtaining this type of information, hospitals and clinicians are able to execute their own quality assurance activities, reacting to the experiences of patients. Using measures which are valid and reliable provide clinics with outcome indicators with meaning. Furthermore, uniform application of the measure across treatment facilities and clinics allows reliable comparisons across settings to be made. Such comparisons provide information which aid resource allocation to those areas most in need.

There are various domains of psychosocial patient outcomes which may be measured (Foot, 1996). Measures of anxiety and depression give an indication of the psychological impact of cancer to the person and his or her coping abilities. Other important domains which should be included in the armament of measures are quality of life, patient satisfaction with care and patient perceived needs. Quality of life is a multidimensional construct that is generally accepted to include several important areas or domains of a person's life: physical functioning, psychological functioning, social functioning, spiritual or existential concerns, sexual functioning and body image (World Health Organisation, 1958). Quality of life measures allow clinicians and patients to base treatment decisions not only on the prolongation of life, but also on the impact these treatments would have on the patients' overall well-being. Patient satisfaction has been defined as patient reactions to salient aspects of care involving measurement of the patients' cognitive evaluations of and emotional reactions to the structure, process and/or outcomes of care (Linder-Pelz, 1982). There are problems associated with patient's desires not to provide critical feedback on the care provided. Numerous studies have shown patient perceptions of quality of care are positively skewed when satisfaction measures are used (Ware & Davies, 1983; Wigger et al., 1990). Patient needs refer to what the patient perceives he or she must have or be able to do in order to resolve or improve the mental health and physical outcomes associated with having cancer (Foot, 1996). Needs information collected directly from the patient allows the development of a comprehensive picture of the existing and potential problems experienced by individuals or groups thereby providing information on the sorts of interventions that might be developed and implemented.

Regardless of the domain under investigation, it is imperative that the measure possess a number of traits (Aaronson et al., 1991; Anastasi, 1976; Foot, 1996; Lindley, 1992; Moinpour et al., 1989). First, it is important that the measure takes into account the patients' perspective of the psychosocial outcome of interest. Due to the subjective nature of some psychosocial indicators such as quality of life and perceived needs, a true assessment can only be obtained through instruments completed by the patient concerned. Recent research has revealed significant discrepancies between patients' and others' perceptions of aspects related to quality of life. In order to avoid observer biases, it is essential that measures used are based on patients' self-reports whenever possible.

Second, the measures given to patients should be user-friendly in order to increase the likelihood that they are understood, completed and that accurate responses are given. Ease of completion refers to the issues of delivery and presentation of the measurement instrument. As some patients have limited physical resources, the survey should not take a long time to complete. It should be easy to complete and score. The survey should also be written in a manner which is comprehensible to the majority of the target population and assessed in terms of its reading age.

Third, the measure should contain a well defined temporal frame. There are two main reasons why it is important to apply a specific timeframe to responses. First, by doing so, patient recall is aided as patients need only think back to how they felt or what they needed in the amount of time requested rather than an indefinite amount of time. Second, psychosocial outcomes are likely to change with time and by asking patients to refer to one specific timeslot, it allows a snapshot of needs or distress which may be compared with a snapshot taken at another time.

Fourth, a number of psychosocial domains should be included in the measurement process. Inclusion of only one outcome such as depression or satisfaction with care will fail to show the spectrum of outcomes the patient is experiencing. In addition, inclusion of only one or two measures may miss the indicator which is of concern to that patient.

Fifth, it is important that the measures have demonstrated validity and reliability. Validity refers to the extent to which a measurement instrument actually measures the concept that it claims to measure. Many instruments have purported to be measures of quality of life, but a close inspection of the items used often reveals that the scale is only measuring one aspect of quality of life, such as physical discomfort, and should only be considered valid in that area. Reliability is the extent to which an instrument produces results that are free of random error. For example, a patient's quality of life scores should not be influenced by other factors (such as the weather) and should remain relatively stable unless there has been an actual change in quality of life.

Other traits which are equally important include the ability to detect small changes in outcomes, that the measure be easily adopted into routine practice and that the measure be 'systems-friendly' in order to promote its regular use.

2. Establish Burden of Suffering

Why do providers need to know about the level of psychosocial distress their patients are experiencing? Because before we may attempt to change a system, we must know its current level of functioning. For example, it has been estimated that up to one third of patients will abandon chemotherapy prematurely as a result of side-effects, despite the potentially life-threatening consequences of such action (Shapiro, 1987). Equipped with the knowledge to identify 'at risk' patients, providers are able to act to prevent detrimental patient behaviours by treating side-effect.

There are now considerable data which provide a clear picture of the psychosocial morbidity experienced by patients with cancer (Derogatis et al., 1983; Fallowfield, 1995; Foot & Sanson-Fisher, 1995; Wiggers et al., 1990). Past reports have indicated that patients with cancer have to confront many problems associated with having a potentially life-threatening diagnosis and coping with treatments which can be mutilating and/or highly toxic. All of these problems are exacerbated by a variety of other factors which include witnessing the distress of family and friends, confusing media reports, a lack of information or even too much information presented inappropriately (Fallowfield, 1995). Some reports have suggested that between 20–30% of patients with cancer experience anxiety and/or depression during the course of their treatment of significant severity to warrant psychological intervention such as counselling or drug therapy with anxiolytics or antidepressants (Derogatis et al., 1983; Fallowfield, 1988).

More recent research using standardised measures and innovative data collection techniques has revealed similarly high rates of psychological distress. Perkins et al. (unpublished) surveyed 374 patients about to undergo their radiotherapy treatment about a number of psychosocial and symptom related outcomes. Patients completed the survey on a touchscreen computer program located in the clinic waiting area. The group found that 54% of patients experienced fatigue in the week prior to the survey and

18% reported that the fatigue was debilitating. Also, 27% of patients reported experiencing nausea in the last week, with 10% of patients reporting that the nausea was debilitating. Using the Hospital Anxiety and Depression Scale (Zigmund & Snaith, 1983), the survey found that 52% of patients reported borderline or clinical levels of anxiety and 88% of patients reported borderline or clinical levels of depression.

High levels of perceived needs have also been reported by patients with cancer (Foot & Sanson-Fisher, 1995). One Australian study with a heterogeneous sample of 358 ambulatory cancer patients using a reliable and valid needs assessment instrument found that of the ten items most commonly reported as being high unmet needs, eight were needs for more information (Foot & Sanson-Fisher, 1995). For example, 49% of patients reported moderate to high need for more information about cancer remission, 49% reported need for test results as soon as possible, 48% reported needs for information about things to help themselves get well, and 47% reported needs for more information about the possible effects of the cancer on the length of your life. Patients also reported high levels of need for more services and resources: 47% needed easy car parking at the hospital or clinic; 44% needed brochures; 40% books and videos; and 39% needed a 24-hour telephone support and cancer advisory service.

3. Quality Assurance

Quality assurance is a process whereby systems can determine whether the care they are providing is adequate (Donabedian, 1980). If care is adequate, they may continue as they have done so. If care is less than adequate, they may act upon that information, target practices which need to improve and re-orientate services. Always, the first step is obtaining the relevant information.

According to Donabedian (1980), there are two main elements in the provision of optimal medical care: technical care and interpersonal communication or psychosocial care. Much research now indicates that patients with cancer are satisfied with the quality of technical care they are receiving from their doctors (Wiggers et al., 1990). The same research also shows that patients are less satisfied with psychosocial aspects of care including communication and information provision. There are even suggestions that doctors are not detecting those patients who experience high levels of psychological and emotional distress and debilitating side-effects (Ford et al., 1994; Hardman et al., 1989). A survey of patients receiving chemotherapy for their cancer revealed significant gaps in oncologists awareness of patient psychosocial outcomes. Using an interactive computer program, Newell et al. (unpublished) surveyed 196 adult patients attending the medical oncology department about their levels of side effects, anxiety, depression and perceived needs. During the study period, medical oncologists caring for these patients were asked to complete a brief deskpad checklist for each patient. The checklist asked them to rate each patient's level of side effects, anxiety, depression and perceived needs. The study found that although medical oncologists' perceptions of their patients' levels of side effects were fairly accurate, patients' levels of anxiety, depression and perceived needs were less accurately perceived: only 27% to 45% of patients being accurately classified.

This study highlights the importance of constant monitoring of provider performance with the aim to improve care provision. While continuous quality improvement and quality assurance systems have a tradition in clinical aspects of medical care (Fallowfield, 1995), they are less prevalent amongst psychosocial dimensions of care. Quality assurance activities ensure that patients are receiving best practice by providing clinicians with up-to-date and relevant information not easily obtainable. It is important though that the quality assurance is performance-specific and relevant to routine practice and not merely activities of passive uptake of information, such as journal reading or conference attendance (Curry & Putnam, 1981; Stinson & Mueller, 1980). The latter types of adult education have been found to be less successful at influencing practices and improving care (Lomas et al., 1989).

4. Cost-Effective Interventions

If the conduct of quality assurance reveals that psychosocial care is less than adequate, how are providers expected to change their practices and help patients if they are not equipped with the appropriate patient interventions? It is important that acceptable and cost-effective strategies of improving patient outcomes are made available to providers.

It is crucial that interventions designed to ease the psychosocial burden of cancer undergo a strict process of development and evaluation. The United States Preventive Services Task Force (1989) have published a system of categorising the quality of research evidence based on the type of design employed by the study. The system is widely accepted (Cochrane Collaboration, 1994; Guyatt et al., 1994). According to this system, the highest level of evidence involves the use of randomised controlled trials. In these studies subjects are randomly allocated to intervention or control conditions. The use of a control group allows the effects of the intervention to be separated from extraneous influences. The random allocation of subjects increases the likelihood that the two groups are equal in all aspects except receipt of the intervention. In other words, if the evaluation finds that the intervention improves patient outcomes, we may be confident that the results are true. If evaluation finds that the intervention produces no benefits, we may be similarly confident that the results are true. The second level of evidence is that obtained from non-randomised controlled trials or well-designed cohort, case-control and multiple time series studies. These types of studies are more open to various types of biases including selection bias, systematic biases, observer biases and recall bias (United States Preventive Services Task Force, 1989). Each of these biases compromise our confidence that the results of the evaluation are true. The third level of evidence includes that obtained from descriptive studies, reports of expert committees, opinions of respected leaders and based on clinical experience. Although the weakest type of evidence, they are commonly applied as often other types of experimental designs are not possible logistically or ethically. In addition, they hold a certain amount of face validity.

As an example of where this system of classification of evidence was applied in psychosocial cancer care, the development of guidelines for breaking bad news to patients will be outlined (Girgis & Sanson-Fisher, in press). The guidelines aimed to provide clinicians with a series of steps they may follow which help patients recall information about their diagnosis and treatment options and adjust to their diagnosis more readily. They stemmed from an acknowledgment that patients were not satisfied with the amount and type of information they were provided at diagnosis and a lack of satisfaction in doctors' interpersonal skills at this time.

The first step in developing the guidelines involved a systematic search of the literature to find accounts of randomised controlled trials which have demonstrated successful methods of breaking bad news. A MEDLINE search was undertaken for the years 1973 to 1993. A total of 302 citations were identified. The search yielded only 4 randomised controlled trials with most other articles reporting opinion, or descriptive data. One of the trials examined the effects of use of euphemisms and uncertainty in communicating with cancer patients on anxiety and emotional adjustment (Dunn et al., 1993). The remaining three examined the relative effectiveness of different strategies of communication in improving recall and satisfaction with information provided to cancer patients (Damien et al., 1991; Dunn et al., 1993; Reynolds et al., 1981).

Given the lack of randomised controlled trials, a consensus process was employed to develop the guidelines. Thus, the next step was the drafting of a list of guidelines, based on the results of the literature review. The third step involved presenting the list to a broad consensus panel (N = 28) of medical oncologists, general practitioners, surgeons, nurse consultants, social workers, clergy, human rights representatives and patients with cancer (N = 100). Each panel member was asked to rate each guideline on a Likert type scale which assessed whether they felt the item was important to use when breaking bad news or not important. Finally, the guidelines were amended based on the results of the ratings and based on more than 70% of patients rating them as either essential or desirable (Girgis & Sanson-Fisher, in press). Table 17.1 displays the resulting steps for breaking bad news.

Interestingly, when the ratings of oncologists, other health care providers and patients were compared, some discrepancies were evident. In general,

Table 17.1   Steps for breaking bad news

1.	Privacy and adequate time
2.	Assess understanding
3.	Simple and honest
4.	Patients to express feelings
5.	Broad time frame for the prognosis
6.	Arrange review
7.	Discuss treatment options
8.	Offer assistance to tell others
9.	Details of support services
10.	Document information given

patients listed items as essential much more significantly than oncologists. For example, although 92% of patients felt that having bad news broken in quiet and private places as essential, only 67% of oncologists did so. Similarly, although 71% of patients rated the arrangement of a review 24 hours later as essential, only 36% of oncologists did so. The results of this comparison highlights the difficulty in using 'opinions' or 'consensus' to form guidelines. Who's opinion do you use when trying to reach consensus? No doubt, the strongest evidence, that of randomised controlled trials, should be sought.

5. Implement System of Routine Feedback

The value of the data collection process can be significantly enhanced with its appropriate clinical application (Goldberg, 1986). In their basic form, data on the psychosocial outcomes of patients reflect issues of importance to patients and, as such, issues which should be targeted and addressed by health care providers. Thus, it appears that the provision of feedback to providers on these variables has the potential to greatly assist providers to achieve optimal quality care in two major ways. First, feedback has the potential to assist providers in identifying particular groups within their patient sample who may require increased or unique types of care. Second, feedback has the potential to assist providers in identifying treatment or supportive care areas which may require more attention or improvement. Supplying such feedback to treatment centres may also be acknowledged as a quality assurance activity.

The provision of tailored patient and provider specific feedback to providers has demonstrated considerable benefit for clinical care (Davis et al., 1992; Rogers, 1983). However, whether it changes practice may vary according to the type of feedback received (Davis et al., 1992). There are a number of potential types of feedback which may be used. Reports of overall global summaries of data received from patients across a number of treatment centres can be given to each treatment centre. This form of feedback involves the collation of data on the prevalence of each outcome, such as quality of life, from all data collection sites. These data can allow the closer examination of the predictors of various outcomes, such as low quality of life, including any treatment centre variables. In this way, some form of feedback relating to the relative differences between treatment centres may be obtained; for example, '68% of patients taking part in the survey reported receiving adequate information from their providers about their treatment regime. Some variation in the proportion of patients receiving adequate information resulted across treatment centres'. However, global feedback does not provide treatment centre specific feedback to each clinic. Consequently, this form of feedback alone, although less costly than other forms, has produced minimum provider effects in past research (Davis et al., 1992).

A form of feedback which has shown more potential than global estimates of patient outcomes is the provision of feedback which is specific to the treatment centre or clinician (Davis et al., 1992). The effectiveness of this type of feedback is accentuated by being performance-specific, and individual specific. It is even more relevant if it is provided as close to the time of surveying as possible. To increase the information potential of the feedback, comparisons may be presented of patients' actual self-reported outcomes with those which the treatment centre or clinician would wish to achieve. For example, the clinic may select a goal of: '90% of patients attending the clinic should report receiving adequate information from their providers about their treatment regime' and the actual results may be: '68% of patients attending the clinic report receiving adequate information from their provider about their treatment regime'. Similarly, the clinic may adopt a goal which has been advocated as 'best practice'. For example, in Australia, the National Health and Medical Research Council have recently released Guidelines for the Management of Women with Early Breast Cancer (NHMRC, 1995). The publication contains sections which clearly outline the type and amount of psychosocial support and information women should be receiving. These guidelines may be used as benchmarks against which to measure actual care within the format of a feedback report.

A combination of the two forms of feedback outlined above may be used to provide constructive feedback on the status of patient outcomes within individual treatment centres or clinics and in comparison with other treatment centres or clinicians. The inclusion of peer comparison in feedback reports has been an important predictor of the success of feedback at improving various clinical practices (Davis et al., 1992).

Thus, it appears that feedback is most likely to be effective at motivating clinician behaviour change if it provides performance-specific data, goals, is immediate, is clinic or clinician targeted, and includes peer comparison. Methods of providing such comprehensive feedback are often costly and cumbersome. For example, data need to be collected from large samples of patients, some data may need to be collected from clinicians, the data need to be collated, analysed and presented back to clinics in an acceptable manner, relatively quickly. An innovative method of providing feedback is through the use of interactive computer programs. Placed in clinic waiting areas, patients and providers are able to regularly complete computer surveys. The computer programs are able to quickly produce feedback reports which display the data collected from patients and clinicians against information which has been pre-programmed, such as 'best practice' goals or personal targets. Thus, the main advantage of the use of computers in providing feedback is that they carry out most of the necessary tasks quickly and cost-effectively. Another advantage of the computer is that they are acceptable to patients. Newell et al. (unpublished) asked patients receiving chemotherapy for their cancer to rate the acceptability of a 15 minute computer survey. The results showed that, despite little previous experience with computers, 97% of patients reported to find the computer 'easy to use', 98% indicated that they felt it was a 'good way for the doctor to get information', and 90% of patients said that they would be 'happy to do it at each visit'.

6. Provide Training

The main purpose of feedback is to increase the awareness of the target of inadequacies in his or her performance with the aim to motivate improvements in practices (Rogers, 1983). Although much research has shown that feedback is an important ingredient in the drive to improve the quality of health care, often feedback alone is insufficient. Clinicians may be aware of their deficiencies in counselling skills or information transfer skills, but are not equipped with the skills to change their practices. Girgis et al. (in press) found that most surveyed surgeons reported to feel 'not at all competent' at increasing patients' ability to remember what they have been told, at encouraging patients to express anxieties about their condition and at breaking bad news to patients about their diagnosis or prognosis, despite believing that these skills were important or very important in being a good surgeon. In these cases it is important that effective methods of training interactional skills are employed.

A large number of studies have now demonstrated that relatively brief training programmes can result in a considerable improvement in interactional skills. In an extensive review of the literature, Kern et al. (1989) assessed over 200 studies which had explored the impact of interactional skills training and concluded that training resulted in a positive impact. Based on the seminal work of Maguire, there is now widespread scientific support for the inclusion of a number of elements into the training of interactional skills (Maguire & Rutter, 1976; Maguire et al., 1986). Among these elements is the inclusion of a strong rationale for the adoption of desired skills (Sanson-Fisher et al., 1991). The rationale provides a basis from which the need for interactional skills, as well as strategies for interacting effectively with patients, can be established. Information on the behaviour being studied such as a definition of the problem behaviour, the prevalence, burden of illness and the potential role of medical practitioners have also been shown to be effective in interactional skills training (Sanson-Fisher et al., 1991).

Other strategies such as rehearsal, practice and feedback have been found to be effective in the teaching of interactional skills. By asking clinicians to practice the introduced skills, with real or simulated patients, significant improvements in interactional skills competence has been shown (Rutter & Maguire, 1976). Improvements in consultation skills and the collection of diagnostic information following training have also been reported for direct feedback strategies using either video, audiotapes or peers (Maguire et al., 1986). The peer feedback approach, as discussed previously, has been shown to be superior to video feedback in enhancing medical students' smoking cessation skills (Roche, 1993).

Recently, Campbell et al. (1996) trained senior medical students to better provide HIV/AIDS counselling using a training programme based on the above elements. In summary, the program included a written package, a lecture, students practising skills by making a video, peer feedback on the video, and small-group discussions. During an evaluation, the researchers measured students' performance in counselling simulated patients (using a videotape) at baseline and three months following the intervention program. They found that students receiving the programme showed significantly greater improvement in pre and post-test counselling skills over three months than did the controls (see Figure 17.3).

CONCLUSION

This paper has argued that various opportunities for ways of improving the

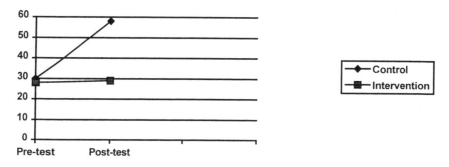

Figure 17.3 Results of a randomised controlled trial of a training program to teach medical students interactional skills: HIV/AIDS counselling.

psychosocial outcomes of patients with cancer continue to exist despite the large body of research which is published annually. First, there is a need for more rigorous and standardised measures of psychosocial outcomes. The measures will form the basis on which to base further work in this area. Second, there is a need for baseline information regarding the prevalence of various psychosocial patient outcomes. While the data on patient quality of life and satisfaction with care appears to be expanding, more thorough data are required in the areas of psychological distress and patient perceived needs. Further, data are required which provide information on those patients most in need of psychosocial intervention. Third, research indicates that oncologists are not detecting, on a regular basis, those patients who experience distress or high levels of unmet need. The implementation of quality assurance programmes will ensure that deficiencies in performance are noted and acted upon. Fourth, interventions which are designed to improve the psychosocial care and outcomes of patients should be evaluated rigorously and their cost-effectiveness determined. Fifth, perhaps as a component of quality assurance, feedback systems should also be implemented into clinics. The feedback should be quick, tailored, performance-related and incorporate peer comparison. Finally, where necessary, clinicians should be provided with the skills essential for the provision of optimal psychosocial care. To maximise the uptake and maintenance of these skills, training should include the provision of a strong rationale, demonstration of goal behaviours, opportunities for practice and feedback.

References

Aaronson, N. K., Ahmedzai, S., Bullinger, M. et al. (1991) For the EORTC Study Group on Quality of life. The EORTC core quality of life questionnaire: interim results of an international field study. In *Effect of Cancer on Quality of Life*, pp. 185–203, edited by D. Osoba. Boca Raton, Florida: CRC Press Inc.

Anastasi, A. (1976) *Psychological Testing*. New York: MacMillan.

Campbell, E., Weeks, C., Walsh, R. & Sanson-Fisher, R. (1996) Training medical students in HIV/AIDS test counselling: results of a randomized trial. *Medical Education*, **30**, 134–141.

Curry, L. & Putnam, R. W. (1981) Continuing medical education in Maritime Canada: the methods physicians use, would prefer and find most effective. *Can. Med. Assoc. J.*, **124**, 563–566.

Damien, D. & Tattersall, M. H. N. (1991) Letters to patients: improving communication in cancer care. *Lancet*, **338**, 923–926.

Davis, D., Thomson, M., Oxman, A. & Haynes, R. (1992) Evidence for the effectiveness of CME. A review of 50 randomised controlled trials. *JAMA*, **268**, 1111–1117.

Derogatis, L. R., Morrow, G. R., Fetting, J. et al. (1983) The prevalence of psychiatric disorder among cancer patients. *JAMA*, **249**, 751–757.

Donabedian, A. (1980) *The Definition of Quality and Approaches to its Assessment*. Michigan: Health Administration Press.

Dunn, S. M., Butow, P. N., Tattersall, M. H. N., Jones, Q. J., Sheldon, J. S., Taylor, J. J. & Sumich, M. D. (1993) General information tapes inhibit recall of the cancer consultation. *Journal of Clinical Oncology*, **11**, 2279–2285.

Dunn, S. M., Patterson, P. U., Butow, P. N., Smartt, H. H., McCarthy, W. H. & Tattersall, M. H. (1993) Cancer by another name: a randomised trial of the effects of euphemism and uncertainty in communicating with cancer patients. *Journal of Clinical Oncology*, **11**, 9989–996.

Fallowfield, L. J. (1988) Psychological complications of malignant disease. *Baillieres Clinical Oncology*, **2**, 461–478.

Fallowfield, L. (1995) Improving the quality of communication and quality of life in cancer care. *Cancer Forum*, **19**, 129–131.

Foot, G. G. L. (1996) *Needs Assessment in Tertiary and Secondary Oncology Practice: A Conceptual and Methodological Exposition.* (doctoral thesis). University of Newcastle.

Foot, G. & Sanson-Fisher, R. (1995) Measuring the unmet needs of people living with cancer. *Cancer Forum*, **19**, 131–135.

Ford, S., Fallowfield, L. J. & Lewis, S. (1994) Can oncologists detect distress in their outpatients and how satisfied are they with their performance during bad news consultations? *Br. J. Ca.*, **70**, 767–770.

Girgis, A. & Sanson-Fisher, R. (in press) Breaking bad news: consensus guidelines for medical practitioners. *J. Clinical Oncology.*

Girgis, A., Sanson-Fisher, R. W. & McCarthy, W. H. (in press) Communicating with patients: surgeons' perceptions of thier skills and need for training. *Aust. NZ. J. Surgery.*

Goldberg, D. (1986) Use of the General Health Questionnaire in clinical work. *BMJ*, 293, 1188–1189.

Guyatt, G. H., Sackett, D. L. & Cook, D. J. (1994) Users guide to the medical literature. II. How to use an article about therapy or prevention. *JAMA*, **271**, 59–63.

Hardman, A., Maguire, P. & Crowther, D. (1989) The recognition of psychiatric morbidity on a medical oncology ward. *J. Psychol. Res.*, **33**, 235–239.

Johnston, M. (1980) Anxiety in surgical patients. *Psychol. Med.*, **10**, 145–152.

Kern, D. E., Grayson, M., Barker, L. R., Roca, R. P., Cole, K. A., Roter, D. & Golden, A. S. (1989) Residency training in interviewing skills and the psychosocial domain of medical practice. *J. Gen. Int. Med.*, **4**, 422–431.

Linder-Pelz, S. (1982) Toward a theory of patient satisfaction. *Soc. Sci. Med.*, **16**, 577–82.

Lindley, C. (1992) Quality of life measurements in oncology. *Pharmacotherapy*, **12**, 347–352.

Lomas, J., Anderson, G., Pierre, K., Vayda, E., Enkin, M. & Hannah, W. (1989) Do practice guidelines guide practice? The effect of a consensus statement on the practice of physicians. *New Engl. J. Med.*, **321**, 1306–1311.

Maguire, P., Fairbairn, S. & Fletcher, C. (1986) Consultation skills of young doctors: I. Benefits of feedback in interviewing as students persist. *BMJ*, **292**, 1573–1578.

Maguire, P. & Rutter, D. (1976) Training medical students to communicate. In *Communication Between Doctors and Patients*, edited by A. E. Bennett. London: Oxford University Press.

Moinpour, C. M., Feigl, P., Metch, B., Hayden, K. A., Meyskens, F. L. & Crowley, J. (1989) Quality of life end points in cancer clinical trials: review and recommendations. *J. Natl. Cancer Inst.*, **81**, 485–95.

Muir, C., Waterhouse, J., Mack, T., Doll, R., Payne, P. & Davis, W. (1987) *Cancer Incidence in Five Continents* 5. Lyon: International Agency for Research on Cancer.

Newell, S., Girgis, A., Sanson-Fisher, R. & Stewart, J. Assessing the psychosocial outcomes of chemotherapy patients. Under editorial review.

Newell, S., Girgis, A., Sanson-Fisher, R. & Stewart, J. Are touchscreen computer surveys acceptable to medical oncology patients? Under editorial review.

NHMRC (1995) *Clinical Practice Guidelines for the Management of Early Breast Cancer*. Canberra: NHMRC.

Perkins, J. & Sanson-Fisher, R. Measuring the psychological outcomes of patients receiving radiotherapy. Under Editorial Review.

Reynolds, P. M., Sanson-Fisher, R. W., Poole, A. D., Harker, J. & Byrne, M. J. (1981) Cancer and communication: information-giving in an oncology clinic. *BMJ*, **282**, 1449–1551.

Roche, A. (1993) Drug and alcohol medical education: skills training for early and brief intervention. (doctoral thesis). University of Newcastle.

Rogers, E. (1983) *Diffusion of innovation*. New York: Free Press.

Rutter, D. R. & Maguire, G. P. (1976) History-taking for medical students: II. Evaluation of a training programme. *Lancet*, **ii**, 558–560.

Sanson-Fisher, R. (1993) Primary and secondary prevention of cancer: opportunities for behavioural scientists. *Intal. Rev. Health Psych.*, **2**, 117–145.

Sanson-Fisher, R. W., Redman, S., Walsh, R., Mitchell, K. R., Reid, A. L. A. & Perkins, J. (1991) Training medical practitioners in information transfer skills: the new challenge. *Medical Education*, **25**, 322–333.

Shapiro, T. (1987) How to help patients get through chemotherapy. *RN*, **March**, 58–60.

Stinson, E. R. & Mueller, D. A. (1980) Survey of health professionals information habits and needs. *JAMA*, **243**, 140–143.

United Kingdom Cochrane Centre Internet Server. *1994 Cochrane Collaboration Handbook*.

United States Preventive Services Task Force (1989) *Guide to Clinical Preventive Services: An assessment of the Effectiveness of 169 Interventions*. Baltimore: Williams & Wilkins.

Ware, J. E. & Davies, A. R. (1983) Behavioural consequences of consumer dissatisfaction with medical care. *Eval. Program Plann.*, **6**, 291–297.

Wiggers, J., Donovan, K., Redman, S. & Sanson-Fisher, R. (1990) Cancer patient satisfaction with care. *Cancer*, **1**, 610–616.

World Health Organization (1958) *The first ten years of the World Health Organization*. Geneva: World Health Organization.

Zigmund, A. S. & Snaith, R. P. (1983) The Hospital anxiety and depression scale. *Acta Psychiatr. Scand.*, **67**, 361–370.

Chapter 18

CAFFEINE AND STRESS

Jack E. James, PhD

CAFFEINE AND STRESS

Considering current population patterns of caffeine use, there is a high probability of the simultaneous occurrence of exposure to the drug and everyday life experiences, including psychosocial 'stress'. Indeed, for reasons which have yet to be explicated, caffeine consumption appears to increase during periods of increased stress (Conway, Vickers, Ward & Rahe, 1981). However, while the literature on the human use of caffeine contains frequent references to stress, there have been few attempts to gather together the disparate findings. Accordingly, this chapter draws upon several separate strands of biomedical and behavioural research to illustrate some of the main health implications of the co-occurrence of caffeine and stress.

Caffeine Consumption

European colonisation in the sixteenth and seventeenth centuries resulted in the introduction of coffee and tea to many parts of the world in which caffeine foods and beverages had been unavailable previously (James, 1991). With increased availability, global consumption increased steadily, such that caffeine is now the most widely-consumed psychoactive substance in the world (Gilbert, 1984). Caffeine use transcends most social barriers, including age, gender, geography, and culture. With more than 80% of the world's population using the drug daily, consumption trends continue to rise. Coffee is the major dietary source of caffeine. Tea is consumed more widely, but qualifies as the second major source of caffeine because it is generally lower than coffee in caffeine content. On average, tea beverages are about one half to two-thirds the caffeine concentration of coffee. Approximately 90% of dietary caffeine is consumed as coffee and tea, with the remaining 10% being consumed mostly as cola soft-drinks.

Although some prescription and nonprescription medications, chocolate, and chocolate-flavoured drinks also contain caffeine, these sources generally account for a small fraction of daily caffeine intake. In the developed countries, per capita intake varies between about 200 to 400 mg per day (approximately two to six cups of coffee or tea per day) (James, 1997b).

Pharmacology of Caffeine

Following oral ingestion, caffeine is rapidly absorbed from the gastrointestinal tract into the bloodstream (Arnaud, 1987). Approximately 90% of the caffeine contained in a cup of coffee is cleared from the stomach within 20 minutes, and peak plasma concentration is typically reached within about 40–60 minutes (Rall, 1990). Once ingested, caffeine is readily distributed throughout the entire body. Concentrations in blood are highly correlated with those found in the brain, saliva, breastmilk, semen, amniotic fluid, and fetal tissue (James, 1997b). The drug has an elimination half-life of about 5 hours in humans (Pfeifer & Notari, 1988), and when ingested in typical amounts, results in plasma concentrations that remain at pharmacologically active levels for most of the waking hours. In adults, caffeine is virtually completely transformed by the liver, with less than 2% of the ingested compound being recoverable in urine unchanged (Arnaud, 1987).

Mechanism of Action

Caffeine exerts a variety of pharmacological actions at diverse sites, both centrally and peripherally, which are generally believed to be mostly due to competitive blockade of adenosine receptors (Fredholm, 1995). The drug has a similar molecular structure to adenosine, a neuromodulator which acts upon specific cell-surface receptors distributed throughout the body. It is generally accepted that most of the effects of caffeine are due primarily to antagonism of endogenous adenosine, although some effects may also be mediated by catecholamines and possibly by the renin-angiotensin system. Some of the main actions of adenosine are summarised in Table 18.1, which

Table 18.1 Some acute biological effects of adenosine[1]

Biological system	Effect
Central nervous system	Decreased transmitter release, sedation
Cardiovascular	Dilates cerebral and coronary blood vessels
Renal	Antidiuresis
Respiratory	Bronchoconstriction
Gastrointestinal	Inhibition of acid secretion
Metabolic	Inhibition of lipolysis

[1]These effects are broadly opposite to those of caffeine.

shows that adenosine generally functions to inhibit physiological activity. By blockading adenosine receptors, caffeine has broadly stimulant effects.

Tolerance and Physical Dependence
Repeated exposure to caffeine has been reported to increase the number of adenosine receptors in the brain (Daly, Shi, Nikodijevic & Jacobson, 1994), and caffeine tolerance in humans has been reported in relation to the cardiovascular effects of the drug and its disruptive effects on sleep (Zwyghuizen-Doorenbos, Roehrs, Lipschutz, Timms & Roth, 1990). However, while repeated exposure to caffeine produces a degree of tolerance to some of its effects, *complete* tolerance usually does not occur in the context of typical habitual patterns of consumption. This is evident in the fact that, irrespective of prior history of use, the response magnitude to successive doses is generally inversely proportional to plasma caffeine (Smits, Thien & van't Laar, 1985a). Figure 18.1 shows that overnight abstinence, which characterises usual patterns of consumption, results in almost complete depletion of systemic caffeine by early morning (Lelo, Birkett, Robson & Miners, 1986; Pfeifer & Notari, 1988; Shi, Benowitz, Denaro & Sheiner, 1993). Converging evidence suggests that the pattern of diurnal depletion of systemic caffeine experienced by most consumers prevents the development of complete tolerance (James, 1997b). That is, although caffeine ingested during the day produces a progressive diminution in responsiveness to each successive dose (e.g. Goldstein, Shapiro, Hui & Yu, 1990; Lane & Manus, 1989), consumers begin each day

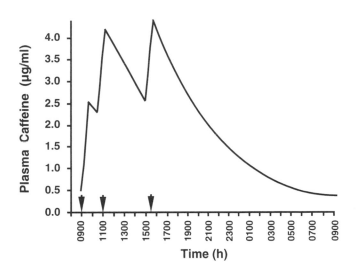

Figure 18.1 Expected 24-hour plasma caffeine concentration (μg/ml) time course associated with caffeine equivalent to 1 cup of coffee ingested three times daily. Arrows indicate when caffeine has been consumed.

largely re-sensitised because systemic caffeine levels are depleted by overnight abstinence (Smits et al., 1985a).

Chronic exposure to caffeine leads to physical dependence, with headache, sleepiness and lethargy being the most frequently-reported symptoms of caffeine withdrawal (Griffiths, Evans, Heishman, Preston, Sannerud, Wolf et al., 1990; Hughes, Higgins, Bickel, Hunt, Fenwick, Gulliver et al., 1991; Silverman, Evans, Strain & Griffiths, 1992. Abrupt cessation of as little as 100 mg (one cup of coffee) per day can produce symptoms, which may begin within about 12 to 16 hours, peak at around 24 to 48 hours, and persist for up to one week (Griffiths et al., 1990; Hughes, Oliveto, Bickel, Higgins & Badger, 1993; Hughes, Oliveto, Helzer, Higgins & Bickel, 1992). A pattern of weekend caffeine withdrawal headache has been reported in persons whose consumption of caffeine during weekends is less than during the week (Couturier, Hering & Steiner, 1992). Although symptoms specific to caffeine may be relieved by ingesting the drug, little attention has been given to the effects of caffeine withdrawal on either reactivity to, or ability to cope with, stress.

Caffeine, Stress and Cardiovascular Health

The potential for adverse effects induced by the co-occurrence of caffeine and stress may be greatest in relation to the threat of cardiovascular disease arising from elevated blood pressure. It has been shown conclusively that caffeine has the potential to elevate blood pressure (See James, 1991, 1997b for reviews). Effects peak within a range of 5–15 mm Hg systolic and 5–10 mm Hg diastolic, may last several hours, and have been observed across a wide age range, in both normotensive and hypertensive men and women. Moreover, strong evidence exists that caffeine may exacerbate some of the cardiovascular effects of stress. This was first reported by Henry and Stephens (1980) in a study in which mortality and disease incidence were monitored in mice living in large community cages. As conditions became more crowded and competitive, the incidence of cardiovascular and renal disease increased. Further increases in disease were observed when coffee was substituted for drinking water.

In the first experimental study of caffeine and stress in humans, Lane (1983) found that the pressor effects of caffeine and stress (mental arithmetic) were additive. This initial study involved participants who were virtual non-users of caffeine, and the findings were replicated in subsequent studies involving non-users (Lane & Williams, 1985) and habitual consumers (Lane & Williams, 1987). Subsequent experimentation has repeatedly confirmed the additive nature of the pressor effects of caffeine and stress (e.g. Greenberg & Shapiro, 1987; James, 1990; Lovallo, Pincomb, Sung, Passey, Sausen & Wilson, 1989), including stress encountered in the natural environment (France & Ditto, 1989, 1992; Lane, Pieper, Barefoot, Williams & Siegler, 1994; Pincomb, Lovallo, Passey, Brackett

& Wilson, 1987). These findings concerning the additive nature of the respective pressor effects of caffeine and stress have significant implications for population cardiovascular disease. For a time, concern was dampened by the belief that habitual use of caffeine leads to the development of complete hemodynamic tolerance, but this belief has been shown to be ill-founded by recent systematic investigation of the chronic pressor effects of habitual caffeine use.

Pressor Effects of Habitual Caffeine Use
It is important to note that most of what is known about the pharmacological effects of caffeine in humans has been provided by studies of the classic 'drug-challenge' type. Typically, a single, relatively large, caffeine challenge (often equivalent to 3–4 cups of coffee) is administered after an overnight fast and a period of caffeine abstinence. While this approach is suitable for elucidating acute effects, it may not be adequate for studying the effects of habitual caffeine exposure, characterised by the daily ingestion of 3–5 caffeine beverages consumed at intervals. Indeed, as mentioned above, it has long been suspected that repeated exposure to caffeine produces tolerance to the pressor effects of the drug, thereby giving rise to the suggestion that the pressor effects observed in the experimental laboratory do not generalise to the everyday conditions under which caffeine is ordinarily consumed.

However, contrary to the tolerance hypothesis, no stable differences in caffeine-induced pressor effects have been found between habitual consumers (in whom chronic caffeine tolerance may be presumed to have reached steady state), and infrequent users (in whom tolerance is unlikely to have developed) (James, 1990). More specifically, it has been shown that the magnitude of caffeine-induced pressor effects is inversely related to plasma caffeine concentration at the time the drug is ingested, irrespective of prior history of exposure (Goldstein et al., 1990; Smits, Thien, & van't Laar, 1985b). That is, in both consumers and non-consumers alike, as plasma caffeine levels rise, the pressor action of additional doses of the drug diminishes. Hence, a second caffeine challenge, given within one or two hours of the first, produces a discernible, but smaller, pressor effect than that caused by the first challenge (Goldstein et al., 1990; Lane & Manus, 1989). As plasma levels fall, the hemodynamic effects of the drug increase. In other words, the magnitude of caffeine-induced pressor effects throughout the day may be predicted to be inversely proportional to the caffeine concentration time course shown in Figure 18.1.

Of the various factors that influence plasma caffeine level, elimination half-life and time since the drug was last consumed are generally the main determinants (James, 1993, 1996). Given that the half-life of caffeine in humans is typically about 5 hours, and the fact that the drug is usually consumed in separate portions throughout the day (with fewer portions consumed later in the day followed by overnight abstinence), plasma caffeine concentration is typically highest in the late afternoon and lowest on awakening in the morning (Lelo et al., 1986). Overnight abstinence of 10–12 hours is characteristic of the consumption patterns of the majority of consumers, leading to almost complete depletion of systemic caffeine by early morning. This, in turn, renders the consumer sensitive to the hemodynamic effects of the drug when re-exposure next occurs (typically, shortly after awakening) (Shi et al., 1993; Smits et al., 1985a)

In one of the comparatively few systematic studies of the effects of habitual caffeine consumption, significant decreases in blood pressure were found in habitual consumers who changed from drinking 5 cups of regular coffee per day to an equivalent amount of decaffeinated coffee (van Dusseldorp, Smits, Thien & Katan, 1989). Similar results were obtained in a number of recent studies in which ambulatory monitoring was used to measure blood pressure level for extended periods. To date, there have been seven such studies, four of which reported persistent caffeine-induced pressor effects (Green & Suls, 1996; James, 1994a; Jeong & Dimsdale, 1990; Superko, Myll, DiRicco, Williams, Bortz & Wood, 1994) and three reported no effect (Eggertsen, Andreasson, Hedner, Karlberg & Hansson, 1993; MacDonald, Sharpe, Fowler, Lyons, Freestone, Lovell et al., 1991; Myers & Reeves, 1991). Interestingly, the seven studies are distinguishable on the basis of the length of the time epochs used to analyse results (James, 1993, 1997a). Readings were averaged across shorter time periods in the four positive studies, and longer time periods in the three negative studies. Since the hemodynamic effects of caffeine generally peak within about one hour post-ingestion, and are substantially diminished within about 3 hours (Robertson, Frölich, Carr, Watson, Hollifield, Shand et al., 1978), significant pressor effects were probably obscured in the three negative studies because blood pressure readings were averaged across inappropriately long epochs.

Figure 18.2 summarises results obtained from one study in which ambulatory blood pressure was measured for 24-hour periods in healthy normotensive men and women who were maintained on a regimen of moderate caffeine intake equivalent to 1–1.5 cups of coffee consumed 3 times daily (morning, mid-morning and mid-afternoon) (James, 1994a). When averaged across 2-hour epochs, blood pressure level correlated well with systemic caffeine levels. Blood pressure increases peaked at 6 mm Hg systolic and 5 mm Hg diastolic by late morning, while increases of 2–4 mm Hg persisted for several hours of the day. Compared to the effects of caffeine ingested after a sustained period of abstinence, habitual caffeine consumption diminished peak pressor effects by only 25%. That is, habitual use of the drug produced only *partial* (rather than complete) caffeine tolerance. In addition to confirming the presence of persistent post-ingestion increases in blood pressure, 24-hour monitoring revealed modest blood pressure *decreases* during times of the day when participants had been caffeine-abstinent for several hours (see Figure 18.2).

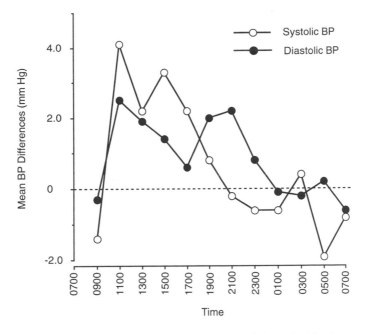

Figure 18.2 Mean differences in ambulatory systolic and diastolic blood pressure (BP) obtained during a double-blind caffeine-free regimen versus caffeine (equivalent to 1-1.5 cups of coffee) three times daily. (Adapted from results reported previously (James, 1994a).)
Difference scores were obtained by subtracting mean blood pressures obtained during the caffeine-free condition from pressures obtained at the same time of day during the caffeine condition.

Probable Population Effects of Habitual Caffeine Consumption
The various lines of evidence outlined above converge to suggest that, contrary to common belief, habitual caffeine consumers do not develop immunity to the pressor effects of the drug (James, 1997b). Although comparatively modest, the blood pressure increases reported in recent studies are large enough to be clinically significant (James, 1994a; Jeong & Dimsdale, 1990; Superko et al., 1994), especially in persons who are predisposed to cardiovascular disease. Effects of this magnitude could contribute to errors in clinical diagnosis, and undermine the benefits of anti-hypertensive medication. More importantly, since the population distribution of blood pressure in the 'normal' range has a positive and essentially linear association with cardiovascular disease (MacMahon, Peto, Cutler, Collins, Sorlie, Neaton et al., 1990), any contribution by caffeine to population blood pressure levels threatens to contribute to the overall incidence of cardiovascular mortality and morbidity. Although caffeine-induced pressor effects are not constant (but depend on when caffeine was

last consumed), current evidence indicates that habitual consumers experience elevations in blood pressure for substantial periods of every day (James, 1994a; Jeong & Dimsdale, 1990; Superko et al., 1994). Factors determining the extent of harm arising from increases in population blood pressure include the size of the change in blood pressure, the duration of exposure to the factor responsible for the change, prevalence of exposure to the putative factor, and incidence of the pathological conditions to which elevated blood pressure contributes (e.g. coronary heart disease) (Collins, Peto, MacMahon, Herbert, Fiebach, Eberlein et al., 1990).

Recently, James (1997a) has argued that consideration of these factors suggests that the widespread use of caffeine probably contributes to population cardiovascular disease. Although the size of the reduction in population blood pressure that might accompany a reduction in caffeine use is likely to be modest in absolute terms, exposure to caffeine is generally long (virtually life-long in the majority of consumers), the prevalence of exposure is very high (more than 80% in most countries), and the incidence of cardiovascular disease is high throughout the world. If caffeine consumption has the effect of elevating average population blood pressure by 2–4 mm Hg (a reasonable inference considering recent experimental data), and 80% of the population are assumed to be habitual consumers (Gilbert, 1984), extrapolation based on epidemiologic blood pressure data (MacMahon et al., 1990) suggests that population-wide cessation of caffeine use could lead to 9–14% less coronary heart disease and 17–24% less stroke. To summarise, the available evidence indicates that habitual consumers are not immune to the pressor effects of caffeine, and that caffeine-induced increases in blood pressure are additive to the pressor effects of acute psychophysiological stress (at least that produced in the laboratory). Indeed, in this respect, it may be reasonable to conceptualise caffeine as an additional (avoidable) cardiovascular stressor, capable of exacerbating the effects of everyday sources of psychological stress which may not always be so readily avoided.

Caffeine, Stress and Psychological Well-being

Considering the combined effects of caffeine and stress on cardiovascular reactivity, it seems plausible that under some circumstances the co-occurrence of caffeine and stress might exacerbate already elevated levels of central nervous system (CNS) arousal, and thereby undermine psychological well-being. The areas of psychological functioning that appear to be most pertinent to a consideration of the combined effects of caffeine and stress include psychosis, anxiety, and insomnia. In addition, the psychological implications of caffeine use in children deserves special consideration.

Psychosis
There has been considerable interest in the possible involvement of caffeine

in schizophrenia and other serious psychiatric disorders, with the most dramatic accounts being provided by several reports of alleged caffeine-induced psychosis (e.g. Stillner, Popkin & Pierce, 1978; Zaslove, Beal & McKinney, 1991). As a typical example, Druffel (1988) described a truck driver who became acutely agitated after being harassed by 'unidentified flying objects' (consisting of several white balls of light) and 'possessed' during an overnight cross-country trip. The driver had consumed the approximate equivalent of eight cups of coffee in the form of 'No-Doze' (caffeine) tablets and an unspecified number of coffee and cola drinks within a period of several hours. The anecdotal nature of this and several similar case reports casts doubt on the generality of the suggested involvement of caffeine. Nevertheless, it is interesting to note that a common feature of such case reports is the suggestion that psychotic symptoms may have been precipitated following the ingestion of an unusually large amount of caffeine at a time of intense stress. In the case of the truck driver described above, possible precipitating stressors included excessive sleep deprivation, intense time pressure, and physical exhaustion. It is conceivable that under such circumstances increased CNS activation induced by the ingestion of large amounts of caffeine may contribute to a lowering of the threshold for psychotic events.

Anxiety
Considering the CNS-stimulant properties of caffeine, there is interest in knowing whether caffeine contributes to disorders typically regarded as involving pronounced CNS activation. Particular attention has been given to problems of anxiety. Attempts have been made to examine the population relationship between caffeine consumption and anxiety by correlating self-reported caffeine use with scores on self-report inventories of anxiety (Eaton & McLeod, 1984; Hire, 1978; Lynn, 1973). This approach, however, is subject to confounding due to the fact that caffeine use is self-selected. Hence, persons who are adversely affected by the drug may avoid it (Boulenger, Uhde, Wolff & Post, 1984). Such systematic (i.e. non-random) avoidance would tend to weaken any positive association, potentially giving rise to no association or even an inverse association. Conversely, as mentioned above, caffeine consumption has been reported to increase during periods of increased stress (Conway et al., 1981). Such circumstances might be expected to contribute to a positive association between caffeine use and anxiety, because the CNS-stimulant properties of the drug would tend to exacerbate any stress-induced feelings of anxiety. Thus, theoretical considerations provide no clear prediction of the likely population association between caffeine use and anxiety. Indeed, because the relevant surveys have produced inconsistent results (Eaton & McLeod, 1984; Hire, 1978; Lynn, 1973), the association also remains unclear empirically.

Attention has been given to the relationship between caffeine and anxiety amongst psychiatric patients (e.g. Greden, Fontaine, Lubetsky &

Chamberlin, 1978; Winstead, 1976), because their use of the drug has been observed to be higher than that of the general population (Greden et al., 1978; James & Crosbie, 1987; Winstead, 1976). However, many of the findings are open to alternative interpretation, because of inadequate control of potentially important confounders, including participant expectations (heavier users in these studies may have been led to expect adverse effects) and the fact that caffeine use is positively correlated with other potentially anxiogenic factors such as cigarette smoking. Consequently, James, Crosbie and Paull (1987) attempted to control for patient expectations and usage of 'other' substances (cigarettes, alcohol, prescription and nonprescription medication) in a survey of 173 psychiatric inpatients. Although heavier caffeine users reported more somatic symptoms, no significant association was found between caffeine consumption and anxiety. In a subsequent study, James and Crosbie (1987) sought to further examine the association between caffeine and psychological well-being in the context of unusually heavy habitual use, while simultaneously controlling for concurrent substance use. Ninety-six subjects were divided into three groups of equal size, matched on age and sex, consisting of psychiatric patients, university students, and a non-psychiatric, non-student sample chosen specifically because of their habitually high caffeine intake. The results indicated that caffeine use contributed to increased anxiety only in the heavy user group, whose self-reported mean caffeine intake was at the exceptionally high level of more than 2 g (i.e. in excess of the equivalent of 20 cups of coffee) per day.

Particular attention has also been given to the anxiogenic potential of caffeine in patients with panic disorder, with several studies reporting that this group has an exaggerated sensitivity to the drug (e.g. Boulenger et al., 1984; Breier, Charney & Heninger, 1986; Charney, Heninger & Jalow, 1985; Lee, Flegel, Greden & Cameron, 1988). However, most of the findings are based on subjects' self-reports of adverse effects, and are thereby open to an alternative interpretation. Specifically, while not necessarily experiencing more intense effects, patients might be more inclined than non-patients to label the psychoactive effects of caffeine as symptoms of anxiety. Nevertheless, objective evidence of exaggerated caffeine sensitivity has been observed in the response of panic disorder patients to a novel taste test (DeMet, Stein, Tran, Chicz-DeMet, Sandahl & Nelson, 1989). Previous research had shown that the ability to taste quinine is enhanced if caffeine is present in the solution (Schiffman, Diaz & Beeker, 1986). Compared to normal controls and patients with posttraumatic stress disorder, DeMet et al. (1989), reported that panic disorder patients showed an exaggerated response to a caffeine challenge.

This finding, which has been independently replicated (Apfeldorf & Shear, 1993), has been interpreted as evidence of the involvement of adenosine as part of the causal mechanism of panic disorder. It has been suggested that panic disorder patients may have either an increased number of adenosine receptors, or that adenosine mechanisms in these persons may have a greater affinity for caffeine (Apfeldorf & Shear, 1993; DeMet et al., 1989). As such, suppression by caffeine of the adenosine receptor system is consistent with accounts of pronounced caffeine-induced anxiogenic effects reported by patients with panic disorder (Breier et al., 1986; Charney et al., 1985; Lee et al., 1988). At one level, these findings lend support to the inclusion in *DSM-IV* (1994) of 'caffeine-induced anxiety disorder', which is recommended if the clinical evidence relating to a particular case suggests that caffeine has contributed to symptoms of pronounced anxiety, panic attacks, or obsessions or compulsions. However, notwithstanding evidence that caffeine may exacerbate existing anxiety disorder, there is little objective support for the existence of a separate clinical syndrome of anxiety that is primarily caffeine induced.

Insomnia
To the extent that life stress may interfere with sleep, evidence of increased caffeine consumption during periods of heightened stress (Conway et al., 1981) should be a matter of concern, especially in view of the popular belief that caffeine is also capable of interfering with sleep. Research on caffeine and sleep can be categorised into three broad groupings, consisting of cross-sectional surveys, experimental studies involving subjective indices of sleep, and experimental studies involving objective sleep measures (see James, 1991). Of these three main approaches, cross-sectional surveys have yielded the least consistent results. While some surveys have suggested a positive correlation between caffeine consumption and sleep problems (Hicks, Hicks, Reyes & Cheers, 1983a; Hicks, Kilcourse & Sinnott, 1983b; Pantelios, Lack & James, 1989), others reported no such association (e.g. Broughton & Roberts, 1985; Lack, Miller & Turner, 1988). More consistent results have been obtained in experimental caffeine-challenge studies involving subjective sleep measures. These have generally found that caffeine is capable of delaying sleep onset and/or adversely affecting quality of sleep (e.g. Dorfman & Jarvik, 1970; Smith, Maben & Brockman, 1993). The most consistent results concerning caffeine and sleep have been provided by challenge studies conducted under sleep-laboratory conditions involving objective measurements (e.g. EEG) of sleep parameters, which leave no doubt about the potential of caffeine to disrupt sleep, especially by increasing sleep onset latency (e.g. Penetar, McCann, Thorne, Kamimori, Galinski, Sing et al., 1993; Rosenthal, Roehrs, Zwyghuizen-Doorenbos, Plath & Roth, 1991).

The anti-soporific effects of caffeine are recognised by *DSM-IV*, which contains the diagnosis of 'caffeine-induced sleep disorder'. However, epidemiologic attempts to elucidate the population distribution of caffeine-induced sleep problems have yielded inconsistent findings (Janson, Gislason, De-Backer, Plaschke, Bjornsson, Hetta et al., 1995; Shirlow & Mathers, 1985). Indeed, there is a perplexing degree of inconsistency between the strength of the laboratory findings regarding the disruptive effects of caffeine on sleep, and the paucity of evidence implicating caffeine as a factor in the etiology of sleep disorders as they exist in the general population. However, it should be noted that most of the laboratory studies conducted to date examined the acute effects of caffeine. While more needs to be learned about whether tolerance to the anti-soporific effects of caffeine develops with habitual use, current evidence suggests that partial (rather than complete) tolerance may develop with repeated use (Bonnet & Arand, 1992). More importantly, attention needs to be given to the possible influence of *pattern* of caffeine consumption on sleep problems. Whereas caffeine is typically administered immediately before bedtime in the sleep laboratory, most consumers reduce their caffeine intake during the latter part of the day. Thus, although caffeine has demonstrated potential to disrupt sleep, its actual role in either precipitating or exacerbating sleep disorders, with or without exposure to stressful life events, remains unclear.

The demonstrated ability of caffeine to delay sleep onset has led to interest in the possibility of its use in the work place as a means of maintaining wakefulness, especially when the work is monotonous and/or the workers are likely to be experiencing sleep deprivation (e.g. during shiftwork). Although caffeine is likely to promote wakefulness during periods immediately following its ingestion, little is known about delayed effects, either on sleep indices during subsequent periods of sleep or on more general indices of somatic and psychological well-being. Moreover, the frequent claim, sometimes in authoritative texts (e.g. Rall, 1990) and sometimes by representatives of commercial interests (James, 1994b), that caffeine enhances cognitive performance is ill-founded. While there are many reports of caffeine-induced improvements in performance on motor and psychomotor tasks such as tapping (e.g. rate of tapping a telegraph key), digit-symbol substitution, stimulus recognition, and vigilance tracking, there are also many reports of caffeine having no effect on the performance of such tasks (Dews, 1984; James, 1991, 1998; Stavric, 1988). With more complex cognitive tasks (e.g. prose memory, word-list recall, Stroop test), the findings variously indicate improvements, no effect, or decrements in performance following ingestion of caffeine. Even when enhanced performance is reported, the overall evidence suggests that effects are likely to be modest and unstable (James, 1994c, 1995, 1997b).

Children
Headache, irritability, inattention, tiredness, and other potential symptoms of stress are common in children. Interestingly, essentially the same symptoms are induced by caffeine withdrawal, at least, in adults. As such, it is surprising that comparatively little research has been conducted on the effects of caffeine in children, especially given that caffeine is widely consumed by children (Barone & Roberts, 1984). In one of the few available studies, Rapoport, Berg, Ismond, Zahn and Neims (1984) found that level of

habitual caffeine intake was a reliable predictor of child behaviour during experimental periods of abstinence and re-exposure to caffeine. In particular, 'high' consumers, when deprived of caffeine, had higher scores on an anxiety questionnaire and scored lower on measures of autonomic arousal. Conversely, 'low' consumers, when exposed to caffeine, were reported as being more emotional, inattentive, and restless. The findings were interpreted as indicating underlying physiological differences between high and low caffeine consuming children. It is unclear, however, whether the differences were caused by history of caffeine use, or whether pre-existing physiological differences encouraged some children to consume more caffeine beverages and others to consume less.

The suggestion that children who have had differing levels of exposure to caffeine may also show subtle physiological differences draws attention to a potentially important but neglected area of caffeine research. It is well-known that most pregnant women continue to consume caffeine during pregnancy, thereby raising questions as to whether caffeine may be responsible for congenital abnormalities. To date, the search has been primarily concerned with gross morphological abnormalities, and the general opinion is that caffeine does not contribute significantly to such defects in humans. However, the question of whether maternal use of caffeine might have more subtle effects, especially in respect of postnatal physiology and behaviour, has been largely ignored. A longitudinal study by Streissguth, Barr, Martin and Herman (1980), which was only partly concerned with caffeine, provides one of the few relevant human studies. The investigators found that alcohol is a behavioural teratogen (i.e. capable of producing congenital abnormalities) with detectable effects in children at eight months, and that nicotine also has teratogenic effects detectable in the behaviour of children at four years (Streissguth, Martin, Barr & Sandman, 1984). Caffeine was not found to be teratogenic in the earlier study, nor apparently in the later one (although no specific data were presented). However, in view of the fact that nicotine was not identified as a teratogen at eight months but was found to be teratogenic at four years, the possibility exists that maternal caffeine may have effects that are detectable in children older than four years. This possibility is all the more plausible in light of the fact that, over the past decade, strong evidence has emerged of an inverse association between caffeine and birth weight (James, 1997b). As such, important questions arise in relation to the possible effects of maternal caffeine use on fetal growth, and subsequent behavioural and psychological development in the children of caffeine-consuming mothers.

TREATMENT OF PHYSICAL DEPENDENCE

Despite growing concerns over the potential adverse effects of habitual caffeine use, very few reports exist of systematic efforts for assisting habitual consumers to reduce their caffeine consumption. Foxx and Rubinoff (1979) appear to have been the first to report the use of a systematic programme of caffeine-reduction. Using a single-subject experimental design, favourable results were reported for three subjects who received a program of behavioural intervention based on nicotine and cigarette 'fading' methods that had been developed for smokers (e.g. Foxx & Axelroth, 1983; Foxx & Brown, 1979). Foxx (1982) obtained additional follow-up data on the three subjects, and reported that the reduced intake of all three was substantially maintained for more than three years after the termination of treatment. In essence, treatment consisted of a combination of self-monitoring and a series of predetermined step-wise reductions in daily caffeine consumption in the direction of a specified terminal goal of reduced daily intake. Similar procedures were subsequently used with a single subject by Bernard et al. (1981) who reported equally favourable results. These generally promising initial findings were confirmed in a larger study by James et al. (1985) in which 27 chronic heavy caffeine consumers were monitored before and during a four-week treatment programme and at six- and 18-week follow-up.

Despite the consistently favourable results, it should be noted that the caffeine-reduction studies mentioned above relied on subject self-reports of caffeine consumption. As such, the reliability of the findings is open to question. This problem is not unique to the assessment of caffeine use. Just as bioanalytic techniques for directly quantifying levels of drug exposure have become an integral part of research into the use and effects of other substances (e.g. alcohol, nicotine), objective methods of quantification are needed to advance our understanding of the effects of caffeine. Accordingly, James et al. (1988) employed bioanalytic methods to examine the reliability of self-monitored caffeine intake and level of procedural compliance in a systematic programme of caffeine reduction. Plasma concentrations of caffeine and its primary demethylated metabolites (paraxanthine, theophylline, and theobromine) were measured in conjunction with self-reported caffeine intake during the course of a caffeine-fading regimen similar to that employed by James et al. (1985). Overall, the twelve subjects, each with a history of heavy caffeine use, provided highly reliable self-reports of caffeine intake during the course of the 18-week programme. However, while the general efficacy of the caffeine-fading procedure was also supported, there were indications that maintenance effects may not necessarily be as good as had been reported in previous studies.

Unlike the earlier studies, subjects in the James et al. (1988) study showed signs of significant relapse at twelve-weeks follow-up. It has long been known that the accuracy of self-reports is enhanced when subjects are aware that their behaviour may be independently checked. Hence, the independent measure provided by the plasma assays may have encouraged subjects to be more accurate than the subjects of previous studies in reporting follow-up caffeine intake. Although disappointing, the relapse observed by James et al. (1988) is consistent with generally reported therapy outcomes for excessive substance use. Since relapse continues to be a major problem in the management of virtually every form of substance use, it would be surprising if long-established patterns of heavy caffeine consumption showed none of the same recidivist characteristics. Although the reasons for the relapse observed by James et al. (1988) remain unclear, it would not appear to have been due to the influence of withdrawal effects, since the resumption of higher levels of consumption did not occur until many weeks after the original treatment goal had been achieved.

SUMMARY

Caffeine use far exceeds use of any other psychoactive substance and typical patterns of use mean that psychosocial stress is often experienced against a background of pharmacologically active levels of the drug. This combination of caffeine and stress has implications for both somatic health and psychological well-being. Recent findings indicate that life-long daily use of caffeine probably contributes to the development of cardiovascular disease (possibly being responsible for 10% of premature deaths from coronary heart disease and 20% from stroke), and that the cardiovascular effects of the drug are additive to those caused by psychosocial stress.

Regarding psychological function, clinical case studies indicate that the ingestion of large amounts of caffeine during a period of extreme psychological stress may contribute to the occurrence of psychotic episodes. Although there is little consistent evidence to suggest that caffeine use is capable of inducing a clinical syndrome of anxiety, the findings do suggest that caffeine may exacerbate existing anxiety disorders, particularly, panic disorder. While evidence from laboratory-based studies shows that caffeine taken before bedtime reliably increases sleep onset latency, it remains unclear to what extent (if at all) typical patterns of caffeine use contribute to sleep problems in the general population. Notwithstanding the fact that caffeine is widely consumed by children, there have been very few studies of the effects of the drug on children. It is conceivable that caffeine use may contribute to common emotional and behavioural problems in children, and that many childhood complaints, such as headache, irritability, inattention, and tiredness, may be due to caffeine withdrawal.

To date, there have been relatively few studies designed to evaluate the efficacy of intervention strategies aimed at helping people to reduce their intake of the drug. Promising initial results have been reported for treatment consisting of a combination of self-monitoring and step-wise reductions (fading) in daily intake, but further research is needed to establish the long-term maintenance of treatment effects.

Overall, the available evidence indicates that habitual caffeine use has a number of potentially adverse somatic and psychological effects, and that in some instances the drug may exacerbate the effects of psychosocial stress. In light of these findings, and the ubiquity of caffeine and stress in contemporary life, the extent and nature of combined caffeine-stress effects warrants extensive further research.

Acknowledgement

The author is indebted to Elizabeth Gregg for her helpful comments on an earlier draft of this chapter.

References

American Psychiatric Association (1994) *Diagnostic and Statistical Manual Of Mental Disorders* (4th edn). Washington, DC: American Psychiatric Association.

Apfeldorf, W. T. & Shear, M. K. (1993) Caffeine potentiation of taste in panic-disorder patients. *Biological Psychiatry*, **33**, 217–219.

Arnaud, M. J. (1987) The pharmacology of caffeine. *Progress in Drug Research*, **31**, 273–313.

Barone, J. J. & Roberts, H. (1984) *Human Consumption of Caffeine*. Berlin: Springer-Verlag.

Bernard, M. E., Dennehy, S. & Keefauver, L. W. (1981) Behavioural treatment of excessive coffee and tea drinking: A case study and partial replication. *Behavior Therapy*, **12**, 543–548.

Bonnet, M. H. & Arand, D. L. (1992) Caffeine use as a model of acute and chronic insomnia. *Sleep*, **15**, 526–536.

Boulenger, J.-P., Uhde, T. W., Wolff, E. A., III & Post, R. M. (1984) Increased sensitivity to caffeine in patients with panic disorders. *Archives of General Psychiatry*, **41**, 1067–1071.

Breier, A., Charney, D. S. & Heninger, G. R. (1986) Agoraphobia with panic attacks. Development, diagnostic stability, and course of illness. *Archives of General Psychiatry*, **43**, 1029–1036.

Brezinovt, V. (1975) Two types of insomnia: Too much waking or not enough sleep. *British Journal of Psychiatry*, **126**, 439–445.

Broughton, R. & Roberts, J. (1985) A survey of subjective sleep measures and performance in working adults. *Sleep Research*, **14**, 89.

Charney, D. S., Heninger, G. R. & Jalow, P. I. (1985) Increased anxiogenic effects of caffeine in panic disorders. *Archives of General Psychiatry*, **42**, 233–243.

Collins, R., Peto, R., MacMahon, S., Herbert, P., Fiebach, N. H., Eberlein, K. A., Godwin, J., Qizilbash, N., Taylor, J. O. & Hennekens, C. H. (1990) Blood pressure, stroke, and coronary heart disease. Part 2, short-term reductions in blood pressure: overview of randomised drug trials in their epidemiological context. *Lancet*, **335**, 827–838.

Conway, T. L., Vickers, R. R., Jr, Ward, H. W. & Rahe, R. H. (1981) Occupational stress and variation in cigarette, coffee, and alcohol consumption. *Journal of Health and Social Behaviour*, **22**, 155–165.

Couturier, E. G., Hering, R. & Steiner, T. J. (1992) Weekend attacks in migraine patients: Caused by caffeine withdrawal. *Cephalalgia*, **12**, 99–100.

Daly, J. W., Shi, D., Nikodijevic, O. & Jacobson, K. A. (1994) The role of adenosine receptors in the central action of caffeine. *Pharmacopsychoecologia*, **7**, 201–213.

DeMet, E., Stein, M. K., Tran, C., Chicz-DeMet, A., Sandahl, C. & Nelson, J. (1989) Caffeine taste test for panic disorder: Adenosine receptor supersensitivity. *Psychiatry Research*, **30**, 231–242.

Dews, P. B. (ed.) (1984) *Caffeine: Perspectives from Recent Research*. Berlin: Springer-Verlag.

Dorfman, L. J. & Jarvik, M. E. (1970) Comparative stimulant and diuretic actions of caffeine and theobromine in man. *Clinical Pharmacology and Therapeutics*, **11**, 869–872.

Druffel, A. (1988) The caffeine zone. *International UFO Reporter*, **13**, 18–22.

Eaton, W. W. & McLeod, J. (1984) Consumption of coffee or tea and symptoms of anxiety. *Journal of Public Health*, **74**, 66–68.

Eggertsen, R., Andreasson, A., Hedner, T., Karlberg, B. E. & Hansson, L. (1993) Effect of coffee on ambulatory blood pressure in patients with treated hypertension. *Journal of Internal Medicine*, **233**, 351–355.

Foxx, R. M. (1982) Behavioral treatment of caffeinism: A 40-month follow-up. *Behavior Therapist*, **5**, 23–24.

Foxx, R. M. & Axelroth, E. (1983) Nicotine fading, self-monitoring and cigarette fading to produce cigarette abstinence or controlled smoking. *Behaviour Research and Therapy*, **21**, 17–27.

Foxx, R. M. & Brown, R. A. (1979) Nicotine fading and self-monitoring for cigarette abstinence or controlled smoking. *Journal of Applied Behavior Analysis*, **2**, 111–125.

Foxx, R. M. & Rubinoff, A. (1979) Behavioral treatment of caffeinism: Reducing excessive coffee drinking. *Journal of Applied Behavior Analysis*, **12**, 344–355.

France, C. & Ditto, B. (1989) Cardiovascular responses to occupational stress and caffeine in telemarketing employees. *Psychosomatic Medicine*, **51**, 145–151.

France, C. & Ditto, B. (1992) Cardiovascular responses to the combination of caffeine and mental arithmetic, cold pressor, and static exercise stressors. *Psychophysiology*, **29**, 272–282.

Fredholm, B. B. (1984) *Cardiovascular and Renal Actions of Methylxanthines*. New York: Alan R. Liss.

Fredholm, B. B. (1995) Adenosine, adenosine receptors and the actions of caffeine [Astra Award Lecture]. *Pharmacology and Toxicology*, **76**, 93–101.

Gilbert, R. M. (1984) *Caffeine Consumption*. New York: Alan R. Liss.

Goldstein, I. B., Shapiro, D., Hui, K. K. & Yu, J. L. (1990) Blood pressure response to the 'second cup of coffee'. *Psychosomatic Medicine*, **52**, 337–345.

Greden, J. F., Fontaine, P., Lubetsky, M. & Chamberlin, K. (1978) Anxiety and depression associated with caffeinism among psychiatric inpatients. *American Journal of Psychiatry*, **135**, 963–966.

Green, P. J. & Suls, J. (1996) The effects of caffeine on ambulatory blood pressure, heart rate, and mood in coffee drinkers. *Journal of Behavioral Medicine*, **19**, 111–128.

Greenberg, W. & Shapiro, D. (1987) The effects of caffeine and stress on blood pressure in individuals with and without a family history of hypertension. *Psychophysiology*, **24**, 151–156.

Griffiths, R. R., Evans, S. M., Heishman, S. J., Preston, K. L., Sannerud, C. A., Wolf, B. & Woodson, P. P. (1990) Low-dose caffeine physical dependence in humans. *Journal of Pharmacology and Experimental Therapeutics*, **255**, 1123–1132.

Henry, J. P. & Stephens, P. M. (1980) Caffeine as an intensifier of stress-induced hormonal and pathophysiologic changes in mice. *Pharmacology, Biochemistry and Behavior*, **13**, 719–727.

Hicks, R. A., Hicks, G. J., Reyes, J. R. & Cheers, Y. (1983a) Daily caffeine use and the sleep of college students. *Bulletin of the Psychonomic Society*, **21**, 24–25.

Hicks, R. A., Kilcourse, J. & Sinnott, M. A. (1983b) Type A-B behavior and caffeine use in college students. *Psychological Reports*, **52**, 338.

Hire, J. N. (1978) Anxiety and caffeine. *Psychological Reports*, **42**, 833–834.

Hughes, J. R., Higgins, S. T., Bickel, W. K., Hunt, W. K., Fenwick, J. W., Gulliver, S. B. & Mireault, G. C. (1991) Caffeine self-administration, withdrawal, and adverse effects among coffee drinkers. *Archives of General Psychiatry*, **48**, 611–617.

Hughes, J. R., Oliveto, A. H., Bickel, W. K., Higgins, S. T. & Badger, G. J. (1993) Caffeine self-administration and withdrawal: incidence, individual differences and interrelationships. *Drug and Alcohol Dependence*, **32**, 239–246.

Hughes, J. R., Oliveto, A. H., Helzer, J. E., Higgins, S. T. & Bickel, W. K. (1992) Should caffeine abuse, dependence or withdrawal be added to DSM-IV and ICD-10? *American Journal of Psychiatry*, **149**, 33–40.

James, J. E. (1990) The influence of user status and anxious disposition on the hypertensive effects of caffeine. *International Journal of Psychophysiology*, **10**, 171–179.

James, J. E. (1991) *Caffeine and Health*. London: Academic Press.

James, J. E. (1993) Caffeine and ambulatory blood pressure. *American Journal of Hypertension*, **6**, 91–92.

James, J. E. (1994a) Chronic effects of habitual caffeine consumption on laboratory and ambulatory blood pressure levels. *Journal of Cardiovascular Research*, **1**, 159–164.

James, J. E. (1994b) Caffeine, health and commercial interests. *Addiction*, **89**, 1595–1599.

James, J. E. (1994c) Does caffeine enhance or merely restore degraded psychomotor performance. *Neuropsychobiology*, **30**, 124–125.

James, J. E. (1995) Caffeine and psychomotor performance revisited. *Neuropsychobiology*, **31**, 202–203.

James, J. E. (1997a) Is habitual caffeine use a preventable cardiovascular risk factor? *Lancet*, **349**, 279–281.

James, J. E. (1997b) *Understanding Caffeine: A Biobehavioral Analysis*. Thousand Oaks, CA: Sage Publications.

James, J. E. (1998) Acute and chronic effects of caffeine on performance, mood, headache, and sleep. *Neuropsychobiology*, **38**, 32–41.

James, J. E. & Crosbie, J. (1987) Somatic and psychological health implications of heavy caffeine use. *British Journal of Addiction*, **82**, 503–509.

James, J. E., Crosbie, J. & Paull, I. (1987) Symptomatology of habitual caffeine use amongst psychiatric patients. *Australian Journal of Psychology*, **39**, 139–149.

James, J. E., Paull, I., Cameron-Traub, E., Miners, J. O., Lelo, A. & Birkett, D. J. (1988) Biochemical validation of self-reported caffeine consumption during caffeine fading. *Journal of Behavioral Medicine*, **11**, 15–30.

James, J. E., Stirling, K. P. & Hampton, B. A. M. (1985) Caffeine fading: Behavioral treatment of caffeine abuse. *Behavior Therapy*, **16**, 15–27.

Janson, C., Gislason, T., De-Backer, W., Plaschke, P., Bjornsson, E., Hetta, J., Kristbjarnason, H., Vermeire, P. & Boman, G. (1995) Prevalence of sleep disturbances among young adults in three European countries. *Sleep*, **18**, 589–597.

Jeong, D. & Dimsdale, J. E. (1990) The effects of caffeine on blood pressure in the work environment. *American Journal of Hypertension*, **3**, 749–753.

Lack, L., Miller, W. & Turner, D. (1988) A survey of sleeping difficulties in an Australian population. *Community Health Studies*, **XII**, 200–207.

Lane, J. D. (1983) Caffeine and cardiovascular responses to stress. *Psychosomatic Medicine*, **45**, 447–451.

Lane, J. D. & Manus, D. C. (1989) Persistent cardiovascular effects with repeated caffeine administration. *Psychosomatic Medicine*, **51**, 373–380.

Lane, J. D., Pieper, C. F., Barefoot, J. C., Williams, R. B. J. & Siegler, I. C. (1994) Caffeine and cholesterol: interactions with hostility. *Psychosomatic Medicine*, **56**, 260–266.

Lane, J. D. & Williams, R. B., Jr. (1985) Caffeine affects cardiovascular responses to stress. *Psychophysiology*, **22**, 648–655.

Lane, J. D. & Williams, R. B. (1987) Cardiovascular effects of caffeine and stress in regular coffee drinkers. *Psychophysiology*, **24**, 157–164.

Lee, M. A., Flegel, P., Greden, J. F. & Cameron, O. G. (1988) Anxiogenic effects of caffeine on panic and depressed patients. *American Journal of Psychiatry*, **145**, 632–635.

Lelo, A., Birkett, D. J., Robson, R. A. & Miners, J. O. (1986) Comparative pharmacokinetics of caffeine and its primary demethylated metabolites paraxanthine, theobromine and theophylline in man. *British Journal of Clinical Pharmacology*, **22**, 177–182.

Lovallo, W. R., Pincomb, G. A., Sung, B. H., Passey, R. B., Sausen, K. P. & Wilson, M. F. (1989) Caffeine may potentiate adrenocortical stress responses in hypertension-prone men. *Hypertension*, **14**, 170–176.

Lynn, R. (1973) National differences in anxiety and the consumption of caffeine. *British Journal of Social and Clinical Psychology*, **12**, 92–93.

MacDonald, T. M., Sharpe, K., Fowler, G., Lyons, D., Freestone, S., Lovell, H. G., Webster, J. & Petrie, J. C. (1991) Caffeine restriction: Effect of mild hypertension. *British Medical Journal*, **303**, 1235–1238.

MacMahon, S., Peto, R., Cutler, J., Collins, R., Sorlie, P., Neaton, J., Abbott, R., Godwin, J., Dyer, A. & Stamler, J. (1990) Blood pressure, stroke, and coronary heart disease. Part 1, prolonged differences in blood pressure: prospective observational studies corrected for the regression dilution bias. *Lancet*, **335**, 765–774.

Myers, M. G. & Reeves, R. A. (1991) The effect of caffeine on daytime ambulatory blood pressure. *American Journal of Hypertension*, **4**, 427–431.

Pantelios, G., Lack, L. & James, J. E. (1989) Caffeine consumption and sleep. *Sleep Research*, **18**, 65.

Penetar, D., McCann, U., Thorne, D., Kamimori, G., Galinski, C., Sing, H., Thomas, M. & Belenky, G. (1993) Caffeine reversal of sleep deprivation effects on alertness and mood. *Psychopharmacology*, **112**, 359–365.

Pfeifer, R. W. & Notari, R. E. (1988) Predicting caffeine plasma concentrations resulting from consumption of food or beverages: A simple method and its origin. *Drug Intelligence and Clinical Pharmacy*, **22**, 953–959.

Pincomb, G. A., Lovallo, W. R., Passey, R. B., Brackett, D. J. & Wilson, M. F. (1987) Caffeine enhances the physiological response to occupational stress in medical students. *Health Psychology*, **6**, 101–112.

Rapoport, J. L., Berg, C. J., Ismond, D. R., Zahn, T. P. & Neims, A. (1984) Behavioral effects of caffeine in children. Relationship between dietary choice and effects of caffeine challenge. *Archives of General Psychiatry*, **41**, 1073–1079.

Robertson, D., Frölich, J. C., Carr, R. K., Watson, J. T., Hollifield, J. W., Shand, D. G. & Oates, J. A. (1978) Effects of caffeine on plasma renin activity, catecholamines and blood pressure. *New England Journal of Medicine*, **298**, 181–186.

Rosenthal, L., Roehrs, T., Zwyghuizen-Doorenbos, A., Plath, D. & Roth, T. (1991) Alerting effects of caffeine after normal and restricted sleep. *Neuropsychopharmacology*, **4**, 103–108.

Schiffman, S. S., Diaz, C. & Beeker, T. G. (1986) Caffeine intensifies taste of certain sweeteners: Role of adenosine receptor. *Pharmacology, Biochemistry and Behavior*, **24**, 429–432.

Schiffman, S. S. & Warwick, Z. S. (1989) *Use of Flavor-amplified Foods to Improve Nutritional Status in Elderly Persons*. New York: The New York Academy of Sciences.

Shi, J., Benowitz, N. L., Denaro, C. P. & Sheiner, L. B. (1993) Pharmacokinetic-pharmacodynamic modeling of caffeine: tolerance to pressor effects. *Clinical Pharmacology and Therapeutics*, **53**, 6–14.

Shirlow, M. J. & Mathers, C. D. (1985) A study of caffeine consumption and symptoms: Indigestion, palpitations, headache and insomnia. *International Journal of Epidemiology*, **14**, 239–248.

Silverman, K., Evans, S. M., Strain, E. C. & Griffiths, R. R. (1992) Withdrawal syndrome after the double-blind cessation of caffeine consumption. *New England Journal of Medicine*, **327**, 1109–1114.

Smith, A. P., Maben, A. L. & Brockman, P. (1993) The effects of caffeine and evening meals on sleep and performance, mood and cardiovascular functioning the following day. *Journal of Psychopharmacology*, **7**, 203–206.

Smits, P., Thien, T. & van't Laar, A. (1985a) The cardiovascular effects of regular and decaffeinated coffee. *British Journal of Clinical Pharmacology*, **19**, 852–854.

Smits, P., Thien, T. & van't Laar, A. (1985b) Circulatory effects of coffee in relation to the pharmacokinetics of caffeine. *American Journal of Cardiology*, **56**, 958–963.

Somani, S. M. & Gupta, P. (1988) Caffeine: A new look at an age-old drug. *International Journal of Clinical Pharmacology, Therapy and Toxicology*, **26**, 521–533.

Stavric, B. (1988) Methylxanthines: Toxicity to humans. 2. Caffeine. *Food and Chemical Toxicology*, **26**, 645–662.

Stillner, V., Popkin, M. K. & Pierce, C. M. (1978) Caffeine-induced delirium during prolonged competitive stress. *American Journal of Psychiatry*, **135**, 855–856.

Streissguth, A. P., Barr, H. M., Martin, D. C. & Herman, C. S. (1980) Effects of maternal alcohol, nicotine, and caffeine use during pregnancy on infant mental and motor development at eight months. *Alcoholism: Clinical and Experimental Research*, **4**, 152–164.

Streissguth, A. P., Martin, D. C., Barr, H. M. & Sandman, B. M. (1984) Intrauterine alcohol and nicotine exposure: Attention and reaction time in 4-year old children. *Developmental Psychology*, **20**, 533–541.

Superko, H. R., Myll, J., DiRicco, C., Williams, P. T., Bortz, W. M. & Wood, P. D. (1994) Effects of cessation of caffeinated-coffee consumption on ambulatory and resting blood pressure in men. *American Journal of Cardiology*, **73**, 780–784.

van Dusseldorp, M., Smits, P., Thien, T. & Katan, M. B. (1989) Effect of decaffeinated versus regular coffee on blood pressure. A 12-week, double-blind trial. *Hypertension*, **14**, 563–569.

Watt, A. H., Bayer, A., Routledge, P. A. & Swift, C. G. (1989) Adenosine-induced respiratory and heart rate changes in young and elderly adults. *British Journal of Clinical Pharmacology*, **27**, 265–267.

Winstead, D. K. (1976) Coffee consumption among psychiatric inpatients. American *Journal of Psychiatry*, **133**, 1447–1450.

Zaslove, M. O., Beal, M. & McKinney, R. E. (1991) Changes in behaviors of inpatients after a ban on the sale of cafeinated drinks. *Hospital and Community Psychiatry*, **42**, 84–85.

Chapter 19

IMPLEMENTATION OF RELAXATION THERAPY WITHIN A CARDIAC REHABILITATION SETTING

Jan van Dixhoorn, MD, PhD

STATUS OF RELAXATION INSTRUCTION WITHIN CARDIAC REHABILITATION

Relaxation instruction is rarely an explicit part of a cardiac rehabilitation program. Although its effectiveness has been demonstrated in a number of studies and clinical feasibility has been reported by several authors, relaxation instruction did not reach the status of a treatment modality in its own right as it did for other health problems. The seven world congresses on cardiac rehabilitation that have been held so far never addressed the issue adequately. Interest in psychophysiological self-regulation techniques is very limited within the field of cardiology. Cardiac rehabilitation centers on exercise training and patient education. Relaxation practice is not uncommon, but it is usually included as one component of an exercise or educational program. The available time for instruction as well as its quality and depth will probably be at a superficial level in that situation. Thus, the contribution of instruction in relaxation and in skills for dealing with stress to the recovery of cardiac patients has a potential that remains largely unrealised.

By contrast, within the area of psychophysiological self-regulation, the application of relaxation to a wide range of health problems is being documented and updated, but to the exclusion of cardiac rehabilitation. In two major textbooks on relaxation and stress management cardiac rehabilitation is not mentioned as a potential area of application (Lehrer & Woolfolk, 1993; Lichstein, 1988). The journal 'Biofeedback & Self-Regulation' contains almost no papers with cardiac patients as subjects, with the exception of papers dealing with heart rate feedback.

This situation is unsatisfactory but also interesting. It is particularly interesting since cardiovascular health has been a common outcome measure in studies on the effect of stress on health. Cardiovascular risk factors that play an intermediate role are common endpoints, but the actual occurrence of illness and cardiac death have been used as well. The last few years have seen an increasing number of reports on the effect of stress and stress management on the prognosis of cardiac patients, that is, *after* the illness has occurred (Linden et al., 1996; Williams & Chesney, 1993). This will hopefully stimulate interest and further study. Nevertheless, the worlds of stress research and stress management on the one hand, and of clinical cardiological care and rehabilitation on the other hand, seem to do their best *not* to meet.

STUDIES OF RELAXATION INSTRUCTION

Clinical Reports

In the United States, Fardy (1986), Sime (1980), and Hackett and Cassem (1982) recommended the use of relaxation, especially as an aid to the regular exercise program. Fardy wrote: 'Incorporating relaxation techniques at the end of cool-down is an innovation that can further enhance the quality of the exercise session' and referred to a 1978 manual of cardiac rehabilitation. He continues: 'Too often, persons maintain their hectic pace throughout the day and try to squeeze the exercise session into an already busy schedule. It is questionable whether those who approach exercise in that manner derive full benefit from it. Relaxation exercises may ensure at least brief respite from the frantic activity of the day' (Fardy, 1986, p. 428). The technique that he recommends involves concentration, deep breathing, and learning to contract and relax peripheral muscles. Sime (1980) considers patients recovering from myocardial infarction excellent candidates for long-term behavioral therapy, such as progressive relaxation. In particular he considers it appropriate to include relaxation training during each session the patient attended for exercise training, for several reasons: 'Exercise therapy generally requires participation three to five times a week for six months. This frequency and time would also be sufficient to accomplish fairly effective training in progressive relaxation'. Although programs nowadays take much less time, they do provide an occasion for regular practice. Furthermore, he argues that exercise may produce some acute reduction in muscle tension, thus facilitating the relaxation process. Patients develop awareness of tension levels more easily when overall somatic tension is lower at the outset. Sime had the opportunity to do a pilot study. 'Sensory awareness relaxation training was utilized at the outset followed immediately by group progressive relaxation training. The patients were lying in a supine position on soft gymnasium mats with a 15 inch cushion under the lower legs to relieve strain upon the lower back. Training sessions were 20 minutes in duration, three times a week for a period of six months. Initially, many of the patients thought the program was ridiculous, but within 1 to 5 sessions the majority had experienced a very pleasant relaxation response. As a result the relaxation session became the highlight of the program and it appears to be a permanent aspect of the total program'. His experience of the initial resistance is quite typical as well as the growing enthusiasm when the contribution of relaxation becomes clear.

Uncontrolled Studies

Luthe (1972) summarized the results of the early studies of autogenic training with cardiac patients, which were all uncontrolled clinical reports. For instance, Polzien saw a reduction of asymptomatic ST depression (silent ischaemia) in 28 out of 35 patients. Kenter treated 42 patients with angina pectoris and found marked improvement in 34 of them. He observed that small groups (4–5) were best and that outdoor patients had better results than hospitalized patients. Luthe was convinced of the utility of autogenic training: 'a well trained person has better possibilities of adjusting favourably to ischemic conditions in case they should develop' and he adds: 'The American Heart Association and other organisations interested in the prevention of heart disease appear to be blissfully unaware of one of the most effective approaches in their own field' (Luthe, 1972, p. 445).

Davidson et al. (1979) studied the acute effect of relaxation in six patients who had metallic markers implanted during cardiac surgery. The relaxation procedure consisted of muscle tension and relaxation, deep slow breathing, relaxed posture and peaceful thoughts. They were asked to practise at home for a week. The results during a 10 minute relaxation period indicated a decrease in sympathetic tone, evidenced by a decrease in norepinephrine and myocardial contractility.

Benson et al. (1975) studied the effect of the relaxation response on 11 patients with stable ischaemic heart disease and premature ventricular contractions (PVC). Holter ECG recording for 48 hours and an exercise test were done before instruction and after a period of four weeks home practice. The results indicated an average decrease of PVC during sleeping hours that was statistically significant and a substantial overall decrease (> 50%) in 5 patients. During stress testing arrhythmia decreased in four patients.

These results indicate, firstly, that substantial clinical benefit may indeed occur, and secondly, that adequately controlled studies are called for to validate the belief in relaxation benefit.

Controlled Studies

A summary of controlled studies is given in Table 19.1. They were selected on the basis that relaxation instruction was an intervention in its own right. Almost all these studies investigated the additional value of relaxation

Table 19.1 Controlled studies of relaxation

Author, Year	Design	Intervention	Patients	Improvement	Follow-up
Kavanagh, Shepard et al., 1970	C E random	exercise, n = 22, weekly sessions hypnotherapy, n = 9, weekly sessions; 1 year	AMI	both groups effetive in cardiorespiratory improvement, ST-segment	post
Polackova, et al., 1982	C E matched	usual care, n = 48 + autogenic training n = 131, one individual and 36 group sessions, twice weekly	AMI	6 out 11 psychological scales, heart rate	post
Krampen & Ohm, 1984	C E quasi	usual rehabilitation, n = 59, + relaxation, n = 46, 6 weekly group sessions, 1½ hour, muscle relaxation + four autogenic formulas	AMI	general state of health, ergometry, wellbeing	post
Ohm, 1987	C E quasi	usual rehabilitation, n = 186 + relaxation, n = 234, 6 weekly group sessions, 1½ hour, muscle relaxation + four autogenic formulas	AMI CABG AP	general and cardiovascular state of health, sense of self-awareness and self-control return to work	post 6 months
Bohachick, 1984	C E random	exercise rehabilitation, n = 19 + progressive relaxation, n = 18, 3 weeks, 3 times per week	CAR-DIAC	diastolic blood pressure, anxiety, depression, somatisation	post
Cunningham, 1980	C E1 E2 ?	usual care, n = 15 + exercise rehabilitation, n = 15 + relaxation tape, n = 15	AMI CABG	no differences between groups in depression scores or locus of control	post

Table 19.1 Continued

Author, Year	Design	Intervention	Patients	Improvement	Follow-up
Munro, et al., 1988	C E quasi	exercise rehabilitation and patient education, n=30 + relaxation, n=27, one individual session, tape, home practice	AMI	diastolic blood pressure	post and 3 months
Langosch, et al., 1982	C E random	usual rehabilitation, n=30 + relaxation, n=28, 8 group sessions in 2 weeks, muscle relaxation, breath observation, two autogenic formulas	AMI	cardiac complaints	post
				relaxation practice	6 months
Winterfeld, et al., 1991	C E random	drug, n=14 + "attentive relaxation", n=20, home practice, 2 months. twice daily	CABG	heart rate, systolic blood pressure, peripheral blood circulation	post
van Dixhoorn, et al., 1987, 1989, 1990	C E random	exercise rehabilitation, n=80 + relaxation, n=7e, 6 individual sessions, muscle relaxation, "breath relaxation"	AMI	training benefit, ST-depression, wellbeing	post
				respiration rate, return to work, heart rate, relaxation practice	3 months
				respiration rate, cardiac recurrences	2–5 years

Table 19.1 *Continued.*

Author, Year	Design	Intervention	Patients	Improvement	Follow-up
Nelson, Baehr, et al., 1994	C E quasi	patient education, n=20, 8 daily group sessions relaxation, n=20, 8 daily group sessions, muscle relaxation and stress coping skills	AMI	arrhythmias, overall cardiac status, ability to work	6 months
Turner, Linden, et al., 1995	C E random	exercise rehabilitation, n=15 + relaxation, n=30, 8 weekly group sessions, autogenic training	AMI CABG	blood pressure reactivity, perceived health status, serum lipid levels	post
Trzciennieckal-Green, Steptoe, 1996	C E random	usual care, n=50 + relaxation, n=50, 10 weekly group sessions in autogenic training	AMI CABG	anxiety, depression, wellbeing, daily activity	6 months

C=control treatment, E=Experimental treatment, quasi=quasi-experimental design, AMI=Acute Myocardial Infarction, CABG=Coronary Artery Bypass Grafting, AP=Angina Pectoris training to usual care and in particular to exercise rehabilitation, except in the studies of Kavanagh et al. (1970) and Nelson et al. (1994), where two treatments were compared. Relaxation instruction demonstrates typically the value of skills training and practice. In the one study that failed to show effect (Cunningham, 1980) the intervention consisted solely of the distribution of a relaxation tape, without any supervised practice. This indicates that relaxation training has a specific value in learning to deal with stress, beyond and additional to the effects of patient information and improving fitness, which are equally designed to improve coping with the stress of the illness.

Apparently, the earliest relevant controlled study was done by Kavanagh, Shepard, Pandit, & Doney (1970), at a time when the value and safety of exercise training was still under investigation. They randomly assigned 31 myocardial infarction patients to either exercise (n = 22) or hypnotherapy (n = 9). Over a period of one year, attendance was high, 84% in the weekly exercise group and 72% in the weekly hypnotherapy meeting. With time, even the most sceptical patients developed an enthusiastic attitude towards hypnotherapy. Contrary to the authors' expectation, no one requested transfer to exercise and even the slowest patient learned the technique within five sessions. In both groups, resting heart rate decreased after one year and mean aerobic power increased by 20–25%. A surprise finding was a decrease in ST-depression. Thus, both therapies were effective in improving cardiorespiratory fitness. The authors suggest that hypnotherapy has a role in the early treatment of patients following myocardial infarction, particularly if they cannot or will not participate in an adequate exercise program. In later studies Kavanagh and Shepard (1974) further investigated this strategy, and then left the subject of relaxation, because the psychiatrist who taught the hypnotherapy classes changed his job (personal communication).

In the study by Nelson et al. (1994), 20 myocardial infarction patients followed a structured educational program and 20 patients followed the stress management program. Both programs took place during hospitalization, in eight group sessions for 2–6 patients, after an introductory individual session, conducted by the same therapist. Stress management focussed heavily on skills training, starting with four sessions in progressive relaxation, whereby muscle movement substituted for actual tension of muscle groups to facilitate awareness and relaxation. Then followed training in relaxation by recall and respiratory control. When a sufficient sense of relaxation was obtained, skill in application of relaxation in a variety of settings was trained. Patients practised twice daily. At a six month follow-up after hospital discharge, the cardiac status was significantly more often stable in the stress management group than in the educational program group, they reported fewer episodes of arrhythmias, less chest pain, and were less often unable to work for cardiac reasons. Recommendations to practise relaxation and watch for stress had been given to the educational program group as well (an entire session was devoted to it), but the practice of skills had not been rehearsed. However, a much higher proportion of patients in the experimental group remembered such advice, they more often were aware of stress, practised relaxation and handled stress more actively. The authors conclude that actual rehearsing and practising of skills is important for acquiring a sense of control that may protect for the untoward effects of stress.

The study of van Dixhoorn et al. reported post-treatment effects, as well as at three months follow-up and 2–3 years later. They randomly assigned 156 myocardial infarction patients to either exercise plus six sessions of individual relaxation and breathing instruction or exercise rehabilitation only. The experimental group turned out to have higher well-being (van Dixhoorn et al., 1990b), less training failure and less silent ischemia at post-treatment (van Dixhoorn et al., 1989), lower resting heart rate and more frequent return to work at follow-up (van Dixhoorn, 1994), lower respiration rates at post treatment and at follow-up, and even 2–3 years later (van Dixhoorn & Duivenvoorden, 1989). Moreover, the patients experienced fewer cardiac events (van Dixhoorn et al., 1987). In a recent report, the patients were followed up for five years. They turned out to have fewer coronary surgeries. The occurrence of cardiac events and rehospitalizations was reduced by 30% (van Dixhoorn, 1997a).

The usual format of the intervention consisted of 6 to 10 group sessions. Exceptions included the study of Polackova et al. (1982) who provided 36 sessions during four months, the study of Kavanagh et al. (1970) who provided weekly sessions during one year, and the studies of Cunningham (1980) and of Munro et al. (1988) who offered little training but relied heavily on home practice with the aid of a tape. Another exception is the study by van Dixhoorn and Duivenvoorden (1989) where patients were taught solely on an individual basis, because that allowed the use of biofeedback and manual techniques as a guide for practice. According to Sime (1980), a thorough training in self-regulation techniques like progressive relaxation requires several months of supervised training as well as home practice. This extensive form of training is rarely offered, probably because of budget, time and personnel constraints. Six to 10 sessions may be a minimal but is not an optimal number.

Another issue is the selection of patients. Most studies enroll all of the patients within a clinical setting that fulfills the inclusion criteria, with the exception of the studies of Polackova et al. (1982) and of Trzcienniecka-Green and Steptoe (1996) who recruited patients willing and motivated to learn stress management. In the latter study, all patients had followed regular rehabilitation (including relaxation instruction) and still had sufficient problems to motivate them to sign up for the special relaxation classes. This is a sensible policy since it increases the likelihood of a positive effect, but it does not demonstrate that relaxation is effective for all cardiac patients. Langosch et al. (1982) reported that only 60% of the regular rehabilitation patients were willing to join the relaxation and stress management classes, which were offered as additional to the usual rehabilitation program. He argues that in view of the fact that post-infarction patients are generally somewhat unwary of psychotherapy, this may be a realistic quota. The other studies however do not indicate large percentages of refusals. Both Sime (1980) and Kavanagh et al. (1970) wrote that patients may be resistant initially, but became enthusiastic once they gained the experience of relaxation.

In order to include all patients who enter a rehabilitation program, it seems important to introduce relaxation as a normal part of the program on the one hand, and to offer adequate opportunity to experience the actual procedures and effects on the other hand. The quasi-experimental design that some studies used was partly due to this. Krampen and Ohm for instance offered the two conditions of their study on alternate months in order to avoid contagion and to present the relaxation classes as a normal part of the program (Krampen & Ohm, 1984). Random assignment would have made that difficult in their setting. It could not be used in a subsequent study by Ohm, which would otherwise have been the single largest clinical trial of relaxation therapy for cardiac patients (Ohm, 1987).

Most studies recruited myocardial infarction patients. Winterfeld studied only patients after cardiac surgery (Winterfeld et al., 1991), whereas three studies had mixed populations, both MI and CABG patients, and in one study mention was only made of 'cardiac' patients (Bohachick, 1982). There was no indication that either diagnostic category had better outcomes or needed a different approach.

It is striking that the outcome variables which show differences between experimental and control or comparison groups were both physiological-medical and social-psychological. Thus, Krampen and Ohm rightfully conclude that a short course in relaxation can be effective and that its effect goes beyond teaching relaxation skills: it concerns general effectiveness of rehabilitation (Krampen & Ohm, 1984). The effects are not only psychological. Training in psychophysiological self-regulation is able to improve the medical and physiological condition of cardiac patients in a substantial and meaningful way. This may be seen as a further argument that stress has indeed a deleterious effect on already ill patients, that it is clinically worthwhile and relevant to help patients deal with it adequately and that physiological parameters should be included in evaluations of relaxation therapy (Turner et al., 1995).

Important tests of clinical relevance are the longterm outcome and the effect on cardiac morbidity and mortality. Unfortunately, most studies are limited to pre-post assessment and only a few extend the follow-up to six months. This is a short period to assess mortality and morbidity, although more cardiac events occur in the first year after hospital discharge. The longterm effect of cardiac rehabilitation, however, only appears when pooled results of several studies are examined over a period of some years

(Lau et al., 1992). The addition of relaxation instruction is apparently very cost-effective, and would remain cost-effective when treatment is given on an individual basis or for a long time period. It deserves serious consideration, therefore, to extend the follow-up period in future studies to at least a year and preferably longer, and to include measures of morbidity and medical costs.

STUDIES OF PSYCHOSOCIAL INTERVENTIONS IN CARDIAC PATIENTS

Relaxation instruction is often a component of psychosocial interventions. The effectiveness of such programs may count as an argument that supports the inclusion of relaxation in cardiac rehabilitation. However, relaxation instruction may not receive proper attention when it functions as one component of a complex treatment package. It may be given as a standardized instruction, without adequate training and rehearsal of skills, without discussion of relaxation experiences and transfer to cope with stressors in daily life. Moreover, the demonstration of the effect of a complex treatment does not allow any conclusion as to the respective roles of the ingredients. Much of the observed benefit may not be specifically linked to the content of the program, but may be attributable to nonspecific factors like emotional support, establishment of hope and a sense of control (Linden et al., 1996).

Meta-analysis of the cumulative effects in the long term of 12 psychosocial intervention studies have been carried out by Linden et al. (1996). They showed that these programs were effective in reducing cardiac mortality as well as morbidity. Cardiac all-cause mortality was reduced by roughly 51% within two years and nonfatal cardiac events by roughly 46%. The authors concluded that these findings suggest that psychosocial interventions deserve routine inclusion within cardiac rehabilitation programs. However, they add that the interventions vary greatly in length and intensity. Many of them are complex and consist of several treatment modalities including relaxation instruction (Friedman, et al., 1986; Ornish et al., 1990) and/or are delivered over a long period of time, of one year or more (Frasure-Smith & Prince, 1989; Friedman et al., 1986; Ornish et al., 1990). Thus, routine provision of the same lengthy and complex intervention to all patients may not be cost-efficient. More work is therefore urgently needed to identify which patient is likely to benefit most from which kind of treatment and to identify effective components.

In most of the studies, the control or comparison group received usual cardiological care, and did not participate in cardiac rehabilitation. Cardiac rehabilitation centers primarily on exercise training, although its purpose is not only to improve physical fitness, but also quality of life and psychological functioning, and to modify risk factors and improve prognosis. Meta-analysis has demonstrated that cardiac rehabilitation reduces the risk of death by approximately 20%, which is equivalent to the effect of beta-blockers and anti-coagulants (Lau et al., 1992). The *additional* effect of the psychosocial programs, additional to an exercise-based program, is not yet established.

Nonspecific factors probably play an important role in both exercise-based cardiac rehabilitation and psychosocial programs. It is not clear which components of the rehabilitation programs are effective, in particular whether improving physical fitness is an essential intermediate process or whether exercise serves more as an acceptable setting for behavioral and psychological changes (Fletcher et al., 1988). If both types of program share non-specific factors as a basis for their effect, the choice for the format and setting of an intervention depends partly on the feasibility and acceptability within the target population.

Probably the only way to decide upon the relative contribution of specific and non-specific factors is in an experimental design, where the combination of two treatments is compared to a single treatment. In eight of the controlled studies of relaxation reviewed above, the study design met this requirement. All of them found that relaxation instruction had an additional effect. This can be taken as an argument that relaxation instruction does have a specific contribution and should be viewed as a treatment in its own right that will improve the recovery process of cardiac patients.

IMPLEMENTATION OF RELAXATION[1]

Choice of Format

In order to reach as many patients as possible, an exercise rehabilitation setting is preferred over a psychology based program, because it seems more acceptable, both within cardiology and among cardiac patients, ie, generally, cardiac patients prefer a somatic and exercise based approach in comparison to a purely psychological approach. Cardiac rehabilitation is supposed to be comprehensive and multidisciplinary, and a psychosocial program should be part of it. It would be very costly to deliver the complete program to all patients. It needs to be understood, therefore, that exercise training does not have to be given in full to all patients.

An exercise-based program is a good starting point, but the staff need to

---

[1] The views and recommendations in this section regarding implementation are partly derived from the studies reviewed, but mainly from the personal experience of the author in teaching relaxation to cardiac patients for over 20 years, and in teaching a national course in relaxation instruction for cardiac rehabilitation staff for more than 10 years, organised by the Dutch Heart Foundation.

tailor the program to the needs of the patient and should not be afraid to stop or limit the exercise component. A major drawback of the usual exercise-based rehabilitation program is that, once patients enter the training, they simply want to and have to complete it. This would leave insufficient room for other treatments that might benefit the patient more.

A challenge for rehabilitation staff is to become flexible and follow the recovery process of the patient, rather than having the patient rigidly follow the program. This means having several treatment modalities available, offering the patient introductions in them, letting the decision of how to start be guided by preferences and specific rehabilitation goals of the patient, but observing the needs for behavioral treatments like relaxation and preparing the patient for them.

Table 19.2 outlines the implementation of a relaxation program for cardiac patients. It is recommended that the program start with a short training period, for instance 8–10 sessions, and that this be seen as a screening period to observe the patients' behaviour, needs and training response, rather than a complete training program. The training parameters can be used to *evaluate the adaptive capacity* of the patient. An increased workload and a decreased heart rate at a given workload indicate a positive training effect, which is usually attributed to the effect of the program. It can also be viewed as a sign of an already present healthy adaptive capacity. Initial training success is an indicator of sufficient physical adaptability that will enable patients to improve, even without further supervised training. Thus, they can be encouraged to practice sports, become physically more active and to return for evaluation. Supervised training can be stopped for them, unless continued participation would serve other rehabilitation goals (Fletcher et al., 1988).

Table 19.2 Implementation of relaxation therapy for cardiac patients

Choose the common setting of an exercise-based rehabilitation program.	Limit the exercise component.
Initial physical training is a screening period, observe adaptive capacity and need for other treatments.	Initial training success is a reason to stop supervised exercise. Lack of initial training success is a reason to search limiting factors.
Offer introductions in relaxation at the outset.	Provide optional separate sessions for relaxation, in groups or individual. Integrate relaxation instruction within the exercise sessions.
Evaluate repeatedly the rehabilitation goals and the means to achieve them.	Start behavioral treatments when they are indicated and the patient is open for them.

This strategy would limit the time spent on exercise sessions and yield more time for other treatments. The absence of initial training success can be taken as an indicator of factors that limit or obstruct normal physical adaptability. Cardiac factors (complications, heart failure, infarction size) appear to be only moderatly responsible for the outcome of training, but functional capacity as well as psychosocial factors are predictive (Fioretti et al., 1987; Hammond et al., 1985; van Dixhoorn et al., 1990a, Heldal et al., 1996). Depression reduces functional improvement after training (Milani et al., 1993). Thus, the absence of a training effect may not be a failure of the training, but a reason to search for and treat factors that limit the patients' adaptability. These may be found in psychosocial and behavioral treatments and in relaxation therapy. The observations in initial training provide a basis for further behavioral treatments. Because the preferential active coping style, exemplified by exercise, turned out to have been an insufficient solution in these patients, they become more motivated for the behavioral approach than at the start of rehabilitation.

It is recommended that relaxation classes be offered to all patients from the very outset of rehabilitation. Patients need the opportunity to experience and understand what relaxation is really about, and be able to overcome some of the common prejudices and misconceptions. It is important that relaxation is presented on the one hand as a clearly defined approach on its own, and on the other hand as a normal procedure and normal part of the program. After the introduction, patients should have the opportunity for continuing relaxation classes or individual instruction.

When relaxation is offered as a part of an exercise session, it will enhance the benefit of exercise, but at first it is difficult for the patient to distinguish between the two kinds of approaches. The staff know the difference and may explain it well, but when they are offered within the same context the patient may take them as one thing. For instance, we found that patients who participated in two group sessions for relaxation instruction at the start of rehabilitation often misunderstood the question 'Do you practice relaxation?', when it was posed at the end of the program. Among those who said they practised, 40% mentioned bicycling, walking or other physical activities as their form of relaxation. By contrast, patients who had participated in additional individual sessions did not misunderstand the question. They answered appropriately and had continued to practise what they had learned at the beginning. Thus, the opportunity to reach all patients is easily missed when relaxation does not stand apart as a treatment in itself. When we want the patient to understand and practise relaxation, we should present it in a clearly identifiable form that the patient will recognize.

Contribution of Relaxation to Rehabilitation Goals

A state of low tension (relaxation) is only one of the means by which relaxation contributes to rehabilitation. The clinician needs to observe the actual response of the individual patient to the instruction and possibly adapt the instruction to support the process that is most meaningful for the individual patient. Relaxation contributes to various rehabilitation goals in a variety of ways.

It supports the goal to improve physical fitness and functional capacity, because it facilitates the restorative processes that are the basis of a physical training effect. Training consists of increasing workloads beyond the level that is habitual to the individual. This strong stimulus causes damage to the body, which is repaired in the resting period after training. Repair is more than restoring the previous state; it results in a 'supercompensation', to anticipate future transgressions of the habitual level of workload. Thus, the body becomes stronger. The ability to repair and anticipate constitutes the adaptive capacity. It is weakenend by stress and strengthened by adequate rest. The state of relaxation promotes the trophotropic activities in the body that are necessary for repair and thus contribute to a physical training effect.

This explanation is a form of cognitive restructuring (Smith, 1988) that teaches the cardiac patient a healthy respect for rest and relaxation, and makes relaxation meaningful and useful, instead of a waste of time. The explanation fits in with the purpose of exercise rehabilitation, but expands it to emphasize the need for a balance of rest and effort. This concept translates easily to the process of return to work and recovery of social activities and emphasizes the need for regular breaks in the working day.

Becoming aware of one's physical limits and recognizing the moment to stop work or activity is just as important as increasing work capacity. Relaxation instruction that addresses sensory awareness is helpful to learn to differentiate the various bodily signals that indicate when strain is too high and when rest is required. This awareness supports the patients' sense of control, because they are often afraid to exert themselves too much without knowing it.

The close encounter with death leaves a shaken sense of security and a basic mistrust in the body which heals slowly. Exercise training is effective psychologically because it helps the patient to confront and overcome fear of effort. Relaxation is also effective because it provides a direct experience of inner tranquillity, safety and security. Moreover, physical complaints often arise at moments of rest, when the patient stops being busy. Those complaints are avoided but not solved by becoming physically active. They can be addressed directly by familiarizing oneself with the state of being non-active, the physical sensations that may come along and may feel unpleasant.

Physical complaints that resemble cardiac complaints may be easily attributed to the heart and cause the patient to ask for medical help. Relaxation instruction helps to monitor such signs more neutrally and differentiate those with a cardiac origin from those who have a functional origin, for instance arising from musculoskeletal strain, hyperventilation or nervous preoccupation. The reduced number of medical consultations and cardiac surgeries after relaxation instruction that was found in one study (van Dixhoorn, 1997) could be due to such improved coping with physical symptoms.

The influence of emotions and mood on physical function is often unrecognized by cardiac patients. During the recovery process they are more vulnerable and may experience these influences more concretely and acutely, but interpret them as a strange phenomenon or a sign of illness. Reporting their experiences after relaxation instruction helps them learn to verbalize and understand sensations that they previously tended to ignore. This process of increasing psychosomatic integration may result in an increased awareness of conflicts. Thus, they may not only feel better after relaxation but also feel the presence of difficulties more acutely. We found that at one year follow-up of relaxation therapy patients reported retrospectively more often that they had had a difficult time after infarction and that they had changed. These increased realistic perceptions probably stimulate healthy behavior.

Rules in Relaxation Instruction

Relaxation instruction can be taught by any of the disciplines within cardiac rehabilitation. The professional background is of less importance than the degree of expertise in teaching relaxation. It is recommended that staff develop their experience and widen the scope of instruction modalities. Moreover, a reformulation of the procedures for relaxation instruction is recommended when it is implemented on a large scale to reach all cardiac patients. These rules are now the basis for relaxation instruction as formulated in the Guidelines for Cardiac Rehabilitation in The Netherlands.

Table 19.3 Rules in instructing relaxation

Alternate active and passive attentional states.	Leave experience open: no expectation, norms or judgment.
Provide phrases for self-instruction (what and how to do) rather than phrases for self-suggestion (what to feel and how to be).	Provide means for eliciting a perceptible change in somatic tonus.
Provide different modalities of relaxation instruction and adapt modality to response of patient.	Do not tell how to breathe provide means whereby breathing can become easier.
Differentiate and discuss sensory experiences, emotional response and cognitive interpretation.	Seek cooperation of patient in exploring individual possibilities for self-regulation.

The basic principle to alternate active (tensing) and passive (relaxing) phases during the instruction is essential. It underlies the methods of such instructors of relaxation as Jacobson, Feldenkrais, Alexander, and Mitchell and teaches the patient to monitor one's body passively. Usually patients remember the active part of the instruction and the point has to be made repeatedly and strongly that the main purpose is to notice differences after the active part has been relaxed. The patient has to compare his or her state during and after the active part. This is further emphasized by the clinician by leaving the outcome of the instruction open. The patient will pay closer attention to the changes within himself when the clinician does not indicate in any way what is expected, what is good or proper. This non-judgmental attitude is acceptable when the clinician offers clear instructions on what to do that have a high likelihood of eliciting perceptible changes in somatic tension. When instructions for the active part can be trusted to elicit a change in tension, the clinician does not have to describe what the patient could feel. The clinician does not have to become suggestive, but can simply inquire into the experiences of the patient.

This approach models respect for individual experience and helps patients pay more attention to their own inner experiences. The purpose is not primarily to reduce tension, but to become more familiar with the responses of one's own living body. The cardiac patient has survived a life-threatening illness, the trust in the automatic functioning of the body has been shaken and the relationship between the living body and the conscious self needs to be redefined. Clearly perceptible somatic changes are the tools for growing body awareness and restoration of trust in spontaneous, natural processes.

The clinician needs to observe the response of the patient and adapt the instruction to that response. Most importantly, the clinician needs a variety of modalities of instruction. There are instructions for active concentration, and passively attending; instructions to contract and release a muscle group, to make small or large repetitive movements, to shift one's balance in standing or sitting positions; instructions to modify respiration directly, or to pace breathing by coupling body movements to breathing, or to stimulate spontaneous breathing by uncoupling body movements and breathing; instructions can be given verbally, or nonverbally by way of physical touch, which may be actively moving the body or passively monitoring the body; feedback can be given explicitly in a verbal way as on progressive relaxation, or manually or by way of biofeedback instrumentation. All of these different forms of instructions are followed up by inquiring into the patient's experience, both during and after instruction. Thus, the patient is not told how to breathe, but is given an instruction that may help to make breathing movement easier. When that occurs and when the patient detects the change, the instruction can be used for home practice. When the change does not occur or the patient does not detect it, another form of instruction is necessary, until patients confirm the effect by their own experience. The responses and experiences are discussed after the instruction, in order to teach the patient how to express differences in tension, mood and attentiveness, and to observe and accept the experiences in a neutral fashion (Kabat-Zinn, 1990). The clinician needs to differentiate the sensory experience, from the emotional response and the patient's cognitive interpretation.

The basis for implementation is to seek the cooperation of the patient, the willingness to try out the possible benefits of techniques for internal self-regulation. When the rehabilitation setting prepares the patient for this, it is an ideal situation to teach relaxation. By contrast, when the rehabilitation setting and staff are not open for the concepts and practice of relaxation, it will be very easy to discourage the patient and few would find benefit.

References

Benson, H., Alexander, S. & Feldman, C. (1975) Decreased premature ventricular contractions through the use of the relaxation response in patients with stable ischaemic heart disease. *Lancet*, 380–381.

Bohachick, P. A. (1982) Progressive relaxation training in cardiac rehabilitation: effect on physiological and psychological variables. *Dissertation Abstracts International*, **42**, 3191.

Cunningham, J. (1980) The effects of exercise and relaxation training upon psychological variables in coronary heart patients. *Dissertation Abstracts International*, **41**, 2313–2314.

Davidson, D., Winchester, M., Taylor, C., Alderman, E. & Ingels, N. (1979) Effects of relaxation therapy on cardiac performance and sympathetic activity in patients with organic heart disease. *Psychosomatic Medicine*, **41**, 303–309.

Fardy, P. (1986) Cardiac rehabilitation for the outpatient:a hospital-based program. In *Heart Disease and Rehabilitation*, edited by M. L. Pollock, D. H. Schmidt & D. T. Mason, pp. 423–435. New York: Wiley.

Fioretti, P., Simoons, M. L., Zwiers, G., Baardman, T., Brower, R. W., Kazemir, M. & Hugenholtz, P. G. (1987) Value of predischarge data for the prediction of exercise capacity after cardiac rehabilitation in patients with recent myocardial infarction. *European Heart Journal*, **8**(suppl G), 33–38.

Fletcher, B. J., Lloyd, A. & Fletcher, G. F. (1988) Outpatient rehabilitative training in patients with cardiovascular disease: Emphasis on training method. *Heart Lung*, **17**, 199–205.

Frasure-Smith, N. & Prince, R. (1989) Long-term follow-up of the ischemic heart disease life stress monitoring program. *Psychosomatic Medicine*, **51**, 485–513.

Friedman, M., Thoresen, C. E., Gill, J. J., Ulmer, D., Powell, L. H., Price, V. A., Brown, B., Thompson, L., Rabin, D. D., Breall, W. S., Bourg, E., Levy, R. & Dixon, T. (1986) Alteration of type A behavior and its effect on cardiac recurrences in post myocardial infarction patients: summary results of the recurret coronary prevention project. *American Heart Journal*, **112**, 653–665.

Hackett, T. P. & Cassem, N. H. (1982) Coping with cardiac disease. In *Comprehensive Cardiac Rehabilitation*, edited by J. J. Kellerman, pp. 212–217. Basel: Karger.

Hammond, H., Kelly, T., Froelicher, V. & Pewen, W. (1985) Use of clinical data in predicting improvement in exercise capacity after cardiac rehabilitation. *JACC*, **6**, 19–26.

Heldal, M., Siret, S., Sandvik, L. & Dale, J. (1996) Simple clinical data are useful in predicting effect of exercise training after myocardial infarction. *European Heart Journal*, **17**, 1821–1827.

Kabat-Zinn, J. (1990) Full Catastrophe Living. New York: Delacorte Press.

Kavanagh, T., Shephard, R. & Doney, H. (1974) Hypnosis and exercise- a possible combined therapy following myocardial infarction. *American Journal of Clinical Hypnosis*, **16**, 160–165.

Kavanagh, T., Shephard, R., Pandit, V. & Doney, H. (1970) Exercise and hypnotherapy in the rehabilitation of the coronary patient. *Archives Physical Medicine Rehabilitation*, **Oct.**, 578–587.

Krampen, G. & Ohm, D. (1984) Effects of relaxation training during rehabilitation of myocardial infarction patients. *International Journal of Rehabilitation Research*, **7-1**, 68–69.

Langosch, W., Seer, P., Brodner, G., Kallinke, D., Kulick, B. & Heim, F. (1982) Behavior therapy with coronary heart disease patients: results of a comparative study. *J. Psychosomatic Research*, **26**, 475–484.

Lau, J., Antman, E. M., Jimenez-Silva, J., Kupelnick, B., Mosteller, F. & Chalmers, T. C. (1992) Cumulative meta-analysis of therapeutic trials for myocardial infarction. *New England Journal of Medicine*, **327**, 248–254.

Lehrer, P. M. & Woolfolk, R. L. (1993) *Principles and Practice of Stress Management*. Guilford Press: New York.

Lichstein, K. L. (1988) *Clinical Relaxation Strategies*. New York: Wiley.

Linden, W., Stossel, C. & Maurice, J. (1996) Psychosocial interventions for patients with coronary artery disease. *Archives of Internal Medicine*, **156**, 745–752.

Luthe, W. (1972) Autogenic therapy: excerpts on applications to cardiovascular disorders and hypercholesteremia. In *Biofeedback and Self-Control*, edited by J. Stoyva, T. X. Barber, L. V. DiCaro, J. Kamiya, N. E. Miller & D. Shapiro, pp. 437–462. Chicago: Aldine-Atherton.

Milani, R. V., Littman, A. B. & Lavie, C. J. (1993) Depressive symptoms predict functional improvement following cardiac rehabilitation and exercise program. *Journal of Cardiopulmnary Rehabilitation*, **13**, 406–411.

Munro, B. H., Creamer, A. M., Haggerty, M. R. & Cooper, F. S. (1988) Effect of relaxation therapy on post-myocardial infarction patients' rehabilitation. *Nursing Research*, **37-4**, 231–235.

Nelson, D. V., Baer, P. E., Cleveland, S. E., Revel, K. F. & Montero, A. C. (1994) Six-month follow-up of stress management training versus cardiac education during hospitalization for acute myocardial infarction. *Journal of Cardiopulmonary Rehabilitation*, **14**, 384–390.

Ohm, D. (1987) *Entspannungstraining und Hypnose bei Patienten mit koronaren Herzkrankheit in der stationaren Rehabilitation*. Regensburg: Roderer Verlag.

Ornish, D., Brown, S. E., Scherwitz, L. W., Billings, J. H., Armstrong, W. T., Ports, T. A., McLanahan, S. M., Kirkeeide, R. L., Brand, R. J. & Gould, K. L. (1990) Can lifestyle changes reverse coronary heart disease? *Lancet*, **336**, 129–133.

Polackova, J., Bockova, E. & Sedivec, V. (1982) Autogenic training: application in secondary prevention of myocardial infarction. *Activa Nervosa Sup.*, **24-3**, 178–180.

Sime, W. E. (1980) Emotional stress testing and relaxation in cardiac rehabilitation. In *Stress and Tension Control*, edited by F. J. McGuigan, W. E. Sime & J. Macdonald Wallace, pp. 41–48. New York: Plenum.

Smith, J. C. (1988) Steps toward a cognitive-behavioral model of relaxation. *Biofeedback & Self-Regulation*, **13-4**, 307–329.

Trzcieniecka-Green, A. & Steptoe, A. (1996) The effects of stress management on the quality of life of patients following acute myocardial infarction or coronary bypass surgery. *European Heart Journal*, **17**, 1663–1670.

Turner, L., Linden, W., van der Wal, R. & Schamberger, W. (1995) Stress management training for patients with heart disease. *Heart Lung*, **24**, 145–153.

van Dixhoorn, J. (1997) De betekenis van adem- en ontspanningsinstuctie in de hartrevalidatie: een vijf jaar follow-up onderzoek (Relaxation therapy in cardiac rehabilitation: a five year follow-up study). *Ned T Geneeskunde (Netherlands Journal of Medicine)*, vol. in press.

van Dixhoorn, J. (1994) Significance of breathing awareness and exercise training for recovery after myocardial infartcion. In *Clinical Applied Psychophysiology*, edited by J. G. Carlson, A. R. Seifert & N. Birbaumer, (pp. 113–132). New York: Plenum Press.

van Dixhoorn, J., Duivenvoorden, H. J. & Pool, J. (1990a) Success and failure of exercise training after myocardial infarction: is the outcome predictable? *Journal of the American College of Cardiologists*, **15-5**, 974–982.

van Dixhoorn, J., Duivenvoorden, H. J., Pool, J. & Verhage, F. (1990b) Psychic effects of physical training and relaxation therapy after myocardial infarction. *Journal of Psychosomatic Research*, **34-3**, 327–337.

van Dixhoorn, J., Duivenvoorden, H. J., Staal, H. A. & Pool, J. (1989) Physical training and relaxation therapy in cardiac rehabilitation assessed through a composite criterion for training outcome. *American Heart Journal*, **118-3**, 545–552.

van Dixhoorn, J. & Duivenvoorden, H. J. (1989) Breathing awareness as a relaxation method in cardiac rehabilitation. In *Stress and Tension Control 3*, edited by W. E. Sime, F. J. McGuigan & Wallace J. Macdonald, pp. 19–36. New York: Plenum Press.

van Dixhoorn, J., Duivenvoorden, H. J., Staal, J. A., Pool, J. & Verhage, F. (1987) Cardiac events after myocardial infarction: possible effect of relaxation therapy. *European Heart Journal*, **8**, 1210–1214.

Williams, R. B. & Chesney, M. A. (1993) Psychosocial factors and prognosis in established coronary artery disease. *Journal of the American Medical Association*, **270**, 1860–1861.

Winterfeld, H., Risch, A., Siewert, H., Strangfeld, D., Kruse, J., Engelmann, U. & Warnke, H. (1991) Der Einfluss der konzentrativeen Entspannung auf Blutdruck und Haemodynamik bei hypertonen Patienten mit koronaren Herzkrankheit und aortokoronarer Venenbypassoperation (ACVB). *Z. Physioth*, **43**, 220–224.

Chapter 20

OCCUPATIONAL STRESS: Reflections on Theory and Practice

Dianna T. Kenny, PhD

INTRODUCTION

> Whether burdened by an overwhelming flurry of daily commitments or stifled
> by a sense of social isolation (or, oddly both); whether mired for hours in a
> sense of life's pointlessness or beset for days by unresolved anxiety; whether
> deprived by long work weeks from quality time with one's offspring or
> drowning in quality time with them—whatever the source of stress, we at
> times get the feeling that modern life isn't what we were designed for (Wright,
> 1995, p. 62).

Occupational stress is currently one of the most costly occupational
health issues (Cooper & Cartwright, 1994; Cooper, Luikkonen &
Cartwright, 1996; Cotton & Fisher, 1995; Karasek & Theorell, 1990; Kottage,
1992). The deleterious implications for individuals and organisations are
manifold, and can result in serious physical and psychological illness for
individuals, and major resource loss for organisations. The extent and
progression of the problem over the past 20 years have been eloquently
documented elsewhere [see Levi (this volume); & Spielberger, Reheiser,
Reheiser & Vagg (this volume)].

Occupational stress research has concentrated on aetiology (Hart
& Wearing, 1993; Toohey, 1993), measurement (Spielberger, Reheiser,
Reheiser & Vagg, 1998), and tertiary interventions. These have focused on
either enhancement of the individual's coping capacity (Murphy, 1988) or
broader organisational level changes such as increased worker participation
in decision making, job enlargement and enrichment, redesign of jobs and
working environment, and creation of a more supportive work
environment through a range of human resource management
interventions (Cooper et al., 1996; Hart & Wearing, 1995; Levi, 1990). As
effective as some of these strategies are in large scale restructuring

enterprises, many organisations are deterred from such global changes as a means of preventing and managing occupational stress. This is due to the cost and intrusion of such strategies-and the relatively small numbers of employees manifesting stress conditions which impair occupational functioning at any one time in any one work place (Cooper & Payne, 1992). There will always, therefore, be a need to cope with occupational stress on both the macro (organisational, structural, political) and micro (individual, dyadic, triadic) levels. This paper contributes to the enhancement of managing occupational stress at the micro level.

Firstly, a systemic model for understanding occupational stress is proposed. Some extant theories of occupational stress will then be reviewed, and interventions arising from these theories are assessed. Finally, an intervention for the rehabilitation of occupational stress based on the proposed model and theoretical discussion is outlined.

The Model

In a series of recent studies (Kenny, 1995a, 1995b, 1995c, 1995d, 1995e, 1995f, 1995g, 1996), Kenny explored the causes of the failure of occupational rehabilitation to effect a sustainable return to work following workplace injury. She concluded that a systemic framework provided both the most heuristic explanation for such failures and a workable model on which to base subsequent rehabilitation interventions. Accordingly, the model for understanding occupational stress proposed in this chapter is informed by systemic theories, including cybernetics, communication theory, family therapy as applied to the systems (i.e. workplaces, organisations and workers' compensation system) in which the worker is located, and current theories of occupational stress which embrace a systemic epistemology (Bowen, 1978; Cottone, 1991; Hart & Wearing, 1995; Karasek & Theorell, 1990; Kenny, 1995e).

A systemic theoretical model for tertiary rehabilitation of occupational stress (Cottone & Emener, 1990; Kenny, 1995g) is different to other models in that the focus is on neither the individual, nor the organisation, but on the system as a whole. In this model, occupational stress is understood as the system's attempt to maintain equilibrium or to restore homeostasis (Hart & Wearing, 1995; Hoffman, 1981). Occupational stress is not considered to be symptomatic of intra psychic pathology of the identified client, as in the medical model, or a result of environmental factors, as in the sociological model. In the proposed model, a circular epistemology (Hoffman, 1981; Keeney, 1987) informs the rehabilitation process by conceptualising relationships and processes within the system as the proper subject of investigation and intervention, thereby illuminating a range of intervention strategies at both the individual and organisational levels. Another important feature of a systems theory framework that differs from current approaches is the temporal location, which is focused heuristically upon the present and future, rather than on a forensic establishment of fact based upon past actions and processes.

THEORIES OF OCCUPATIONAL STRESS

Psychological Theories

The predominant paradigm for understanding the causes of occupational injury and illness is the medical model (Johnstone & Quinlan, 1993; Quinlan & Bohle, 1991). With its emphasis on individuals rather than groups, on treatment rather than prevention, and on technological intervention rather than environmental change, the medical model has been very influential in controlling both the way in which occupational injuries and illnesses have been defined and the means by which they are managed. The major criticism of the medical model has been its focus on treating sick or injured workers rather than on producing healthy working environments (Biggins, 1986). The outcome of this approach was to perpetuate the notion that workplace injuries are 'accidents' which were not preventable and to locate the blame for the injury in the individual worker or in the hazardous nature of the work (Davis & George, 1993; Ferguson, 1988; James, 1989).

The disciplines of industrial, occupational and health psychology have not lived up to their early promise because they have adopted a managerialist orientation akin to the medical model. That is, they tend to focus on the characteristics and behaviours of individual workers and avoid addressing the role that the structure of power and authority in industry play in occupational well-being (Bohle, 1993). For example, although the relationship between monotonous, deskilled and machine-paced work and environmental and organisational factors such as shiftwork, piece work, excessively high or low work demands, and poor working conditions on psychological and physiological stress responses in workers have been demonstrated (Clegg & Wall, 1990), their impact is predominantly assessed in relation to individual attitudes and behaviour, rather than in relation to the structure of workplaces and the organisation of labour (Quinlan, 1988).

Sadly, the history of psychological theories of occupational stress, and indeed occupational injury generally, has been one of finding victims to blame, and then to intervene in a linear way to alter the performance of the latest scapegoat. Proponents of these models have variously blamed the job, the equipment, the worker, and management (Cooper, 1995; Habeck, 1993; Kenny, 1995e; Quinlan, 1988; Willis, 1994). Such theories have spawned an enormous amount of research searching for the putative factors responsible for occupational stress. Personality and organisational factors have been identified as the major culprits.

Personality has always been considered a major mediator of stress reactivity. Although certain events are regarded as normatively stressful, sensitivity to stressors varies between individuals. That is, individuals with different personalities will respond similarly to physical threats, but different responses to ego threats are related to personality differences (Eysenck, 1988). Most theories of occupational functioning agree that personality makes a significant contribution to performance and well-being, while acknowledging that the relationship between personality and environmental factors is dynamic and complex. For example, Work Adjustment Theory (Rounds, Dawis & Lofquist, 1987) is founded on the notion that stable cognitive, behavioural and emotional dispositions underpin work adjustment, but that situational influences impact upon these stable dispositions for adaptation and change, in both positive and negative ways. Similarly, Headey & Wearing (1992) found that enduring personality characteristics, such as neuroticism and extraversion, determine people's daily work experiences, use of coping strategies, and levels of psychological distress and well-being. Extraversion has been positively correlated with subjective well-being (Costa & McRae, 1980), while introversion and neuroticism are associated with increased stress (Fontana & Abouserie, 1993), emotional exhaustion and depersonalisation (Piedmont, 1993).

In similar vein, Roskies, Louis-Guerin, & Fournier, (1993) concluded that 'personality can cushion as well as aggravate the impact of occupational stress' (p. 616–7); with negative personality dispositions transforming stressors into strains and strains into symptoms. Negative affectivity, for example, has been associated with interpersonal conflict (Spector & O'Connell, 1994), negative emotions (Chen & Spector, 1991), psychological distress, physical symptoms (Watson, Pennebaker & Folger, 1986), and job strain (Decker & Borgen, 1993). The relationship between role stress and role distress has been found to be moderated by a range of personality characteristics including intolerance of ambiguity, dependency, strong affiliation needs, low risk propensity (Siegall & Cummings, 1995), and high self-focused attention (Frone, Russell & Cooper, 1991). On the positive side, humour and optimism can significantly moderate the relationship between daily hassles, self-esteem maintenance, emotional exhaustion and physical illness (Fry, 1995).

Despite the enthusiasm for the view that personality characteristics are fundamental to an understanding of occupational stress, empirical support for such moderating effects has been mixed (Frone & McFarlin, 1989). Moreover, much of the research has been atheoretical or exploratory, and it is difficult to formulate interventions based on findings that a small amount of variance in the experience of occupational stress is accounted for by a particular personality characteristic. Researchers working within this framework would, of course, recommend that interventions be aimed at increasing humour, optimism and tolerance of ambiguity and decreasing negative trait affectivity, neuroticism and dependency. However, the literature is replete with evidence that personality characteristics are notoriously difficult to modify (McRae & Costa, 1994). Even if it were possible to change personality in the desired direction, it is not certain that workplace difficulties would improve without simultaneously attending to extrinsic organisational factors that may be operating. Moreover, personality traits may be fixed to some extent, but their place in the system as antecedents or consequences will depend on the nature of the interaction between individual and environmental systems, and to any changes that may occur within that system. Personality may also be defined as a function of coping style (Eysenck, 1988). Consistent with a systemic framework, coping behaviours will also be influenced by the sources of occupational stress (O'Driscoll & Cooper, 1994) and the resources and external support available for dealing with them (Hart & Wearing, 1995).

Research into the role of organisational factors in the aetiology of occupational stress has followed a similar trajectory to the one outlined above for personality. Ever lengthening lists of putative factors have been identified. In two reviews of occupational stress, Cooper (1983, 1985) summarised and categorised six groups of organisational variables, outlined below, that may cause stress in the workplace. These are:

1. Factors intrinsic to the job (e.g. heat, noise, chemical fumes, shiftwork).
2. Relationships at work (e.g. conflict with co-workers or supervisors, lack of social support).
3. Role in the organisation (e.g. role ambiguity).
4. Career development (e.g. lack of status, lack of prospects for promotion, lack of a career path, job insecurity).
5. Organisational structure and climate (e.g. lack of autonomy, lack of opportunity to participate in decision making, lack of control over the pace of work).
6. Home and work interface (e.g. conflict between domestic and work roles; lack of spousal support for remaining in the workforce).

There is, of course, a complex relationship between occupational and organisational factors and psychological characteristics. Interpersonal conflict in the workplace, increasingly recognised as a major contributor to work disability, has a complex aetiology. Dissatisfaction with life, daily stress, neuroticism and hostility were all found to be significant risk factors for interpersonal conflicts at work for both men and women (Appelberg, Romanov, Honkasalo & Kosdenvuo, 1991).

Responses arising from a psychological framework have focused on tertiary and secondary interventions. Tertiary interventions include individual counselling, stress management programs, employee assistance programs, and workplace mediation for conflict resolution (Appelberg, Romanov, Heikkila, Honkasalo & Kosdenvuo, 1996). Secondary interventions include training and education (Bohle, 1993; Mackay &

Cooper, 1987). With respect to these approaches Bohle (1993) argued that, in general,

> Interventions of this nature imply that the problem of stress lies primarily with the individual, that the responsibility for change consequently lies primarily with workers, and that organisations are only responsible for assisting individual workers to change. ... since no attempt is made to reduce or remove environmental stressors, interventions can best be seen as attempts to increase workers' tolerance of noxious and stressful organisational, task and role characteristics (p. 111).

While advancing our understanding to some degree, both personality and organisational factors research has remained wedded to the dominant medical and psychomedical paradigms outlined above. Although they highlight important putative factors that may contribute to occupational stress, these factors, considered separately, do not inform the rehabilitation process. Let us now turn to other models and approaches that may assist in this regard.

Sociological Theories

The most radical departure from the medical model has been the approach of industrial sociologists who have brought the social organisation of work as the primary determinant of occupational injury, illness, and stress into sharp focus (Berger, 1993; James, 1989; Williams & Thorpe, 1992). The medical model's notion of health and illness is rejected as reductionist, individualistic and interventionist, in which subjects are considered as unique cases, independent of cultural, social, political, and economic structures and processes. Industrial sociologists argue that power structures, the institutionalised conflicts of interest between safety and productivity, the social division of labour, the labour process, industrial relations and politics are the root causes of occupational illness and stress (McIntyre, 1998; Peterson, 1994).

Recent changes to legislation in occupational health and safety and workers' compensation have shifted the perception of occupational health from an individual and marginalised process to a process with major economic and political implications (Kenny, 1994a; 1994b; Willis, 1989). These changes have led to the revised view that occupational illness is a social process, the dimensions of which are not individualised, unique or specific. Further, sociologists argue that for every occupational illness or injury, there are physiological and ergonomic components whose effects are mediated by the social environment, specifically, the organisation of work and the sociology of medical knowledge surrounding the illness or injury (Figlio, 1982). Negotiation over the social and political meaning of occupational illnesses and their various economic and social implications occurs prior to their being awarded the status of a syndrome (Willis, 1994). The irony of such a process is that while gaining recognition that such conditions are public issues, solutions continue to be sought in the individual. With some notable exceptions (Levi, 1998), this has been the case for occupational stress.

The major contribution of sociological approaches to occupational illness is that 'occupational health and safety has increasingly become an industrial relations issue between capital and labour; ...it has increasingly come to mediate the social relations of production' (Willis, 1994, p. 138). In other words, the focus has shifted from a fatalistic acceptance that there will be casualties of the work process to a legislated requirement that employers provide a safe workplace for all employees. The cost of compensation is increasingly shaping occupational health and safety practices and procedures and hence the labour process itself (McIntyre, 1998).

Negotiating safety in reference to occupational stress is, of course, more difficult than negotiating safety with respect to the physical hazards of the workplace. Occupational stress currently occupies a similar nebulous position in the medical nomenclature that RSI (Repetitive Strain Injury) occupied in the last decade. One must demonstrate that the incidence of illness (presence of symptoms) is connected to the organisation of work, and as stress is a transactional process involving interactions between physiological, psychological, behavioural and organisational variables, demonstrating the causal nexus is not an easy matter. Moreover, the legislated requirements may in fact have worked against the resolution of issues related to occupational stress, requiring as they do the certification of a specific illness on the Workers' Compensation certificate. Legitimating the experience of occupational stress medically may militate against an organisational or transactional solution to the problem, since certification, a process achieved through political action, has individualised the problem and returned full circle to the victim blaming approach of the medical model.

Systemic Theories

In advocating a systemic/transactional approach to occupational stress, it needs to be stated that there are circumstances in which either personality is so damaged or environmental conditions are so adverse, that the relational context of one to the other is irrelevant. These special cases must be dealt with on a case by case basis requiring unique solutions, ranging from the individual to the political.

Several theories of occupational stress that utilise social systems theory have been developed (Bacharach, Bamberger & Conley, 1991; Edwards, 1992; Frone & McFarlin, 1989; Furnham & Schaeffer, 1984; Hart & Wearing, 1995); Hobfoll, 1989; Karasek, 1979; Karasek & Theorell, 1990; Lazarus & Folkman, 1984; McGrath, 1976). Space permits only a brief summary of the relevant models here, and the interested reader is referred to the many excellent reviews available for a comprehensive coverage.

Person–Environment Fit Theories
Person-Environment (P-E) Fit theories (Caplan & Harrison, 1993; Furnham & Schaeffer, 1984) were early precursors to the dynamic systemic theories described in the next section. Caplan (1987) used P-E fit theory as a method for understanding the process of adjustment between employees and their work environment. According to this framework, occupational stress is defined in terms of work characteristics that create distress for the individual due to a lack of fit between the individual's abilities and attributes and the demands of the workplace. Caplan (1987) suggested that recollections of past, present, and anticipated P-E fit might influence well-being as well as performance.

Interventions are directed at measuring fit prior to vocational placement, or measuring discrepancy in fit in the identification of occupational stress aetiology. Interactions between person (e.g. personality traits, vocational orientation, and experience) and environment variables have been found to be better predictors of strain than either person or environmental variables considered separately (Antonovsky, 1987; Caplan, Cobb & French, 1975).

However, characteristics of jobs and characteristics of workers may influence each other in dynamic reciprocal ways. Most P-E fit theories are static and failed to address the ongoing, reciprocal influences of environment and person (Kulik, Oldham & Hackman, 1987).

Demand–Control Theories
A development and expansion of job strain models, the demand-control model (Karasek, 1979) concerns the joint effects of job demands and job control on worker well-being. Demand is subdivided into work load, work hazards, physical and emotional demands and role conflict. Control relates to substantive complexity of work, administrative control, control of outcomes, skill discretion, supervision, decision authority and ideological control (Soderfeldt, et al., 1996). Based on the dimensions of demand and control, jobs have been classified into four categories. These are high strain jobs (high demand/low control); low strain jobs (low demands/high control); active jobs (high demands/high control); and passive jobs (low demands/low control) (Landsbergis, Schnall, Dietz, Friedman & Pickering, 1992). In general, psychological distress is predicted by high demand/low control combinations (Karasek & Theorell, 1990). Conversely, an increase in control is positively correlated with job satisfaction (Murphy 1988). Control has also been implicated in occupational stress arising from organisational change processes, where control is conceptualised as a stress antidote (Sutton & Kahn, 1986). The perception of control can also be linked to personality factors, such as locus of control and private self-consciousness (Frone & McFarlin, 1989; Kivimaki & Lindstrom, 1995).

Johnson and Hall (1996) have expanded the model to include a support component incorporating coworker and supervisor social support. Social support has positive effects on well-being and buffers the impact of occupational stressors on psychological distress (Karasek, Triantis & Chaudry, 1982). Low social support has been associated with greater symptomatology, and a significant interaction with demand and control has been observed for job dissatisfaction (Landsbergis, Schnall, Dietz, Friedman & Pickering, 1992).

Communication Theory
Karasek and Theorell (1990) view occupational stress as a strategic communication of distress. Toohey, (1993, 1995) has expanded this concept into a model of functional communication. In this model, dissatisfaction at the workplace may be expressed through illness behaviour (i.e. occupational stress), which is assessed as 'a safe and acceptable manner in which to communicate distress' (Toohey, 1995, p. 57). It is certainly debatable as to how expressing one's distress in this way is either safe or acceptable in a workplace context, especially given the social stigma attached to both mental illness, and to workers' compensation claims generally. However, these methods are obviously more acceptable than outbursts of anger, physical violence or criminal acts such as theft or destruction of property. This model is just a step away from the systemic analysis of the function of the symptom in the system in which it occurs (Hoffman, 1981; Palazzoli, et al., 1986), to which we will shortly turn our attention.

Dynamic Equilibrium Theory
A recent innovative approach to understanding occupational stress has been proposed by Hart & Wearing, 1995; Hart, Wearing & Headey, 1993c; Headey & Wearing, 1992. They challenge the prevailing Cannon (1929)–Selye (1975) view of stress which is based on an engineering model where stress is understood as the force exerted on a structure, which may then show signs of strain in response to that force. The missing part of this formulation are those characteristics which create susceptibility to strain, either through innate personality traits, behaviours, resources, or organisational factors. According to the dynamic equilibrium theory, stress is not defined as a demand, a response or a process, but as a state of disequilibrium that arises when a change occurs that affects the individual's normal levels of psychological distress and well-being. To understand the cause of this change, it is necessary to separately assess the impact of personality, organisation, coping processes and both positive and negative work experiences. People may respond with both positive and negative affect to the same environment (Diener & Emmons, 1985). Psychological well-being is therefore determined by the balance between separate positive (e.g. extraversion, salutogenic life events) and negative (e.g. neuroticism, adverse life events) factors (Bradburn, 1969), each one of which has its own unique set of causes and consequences (Hart, 1994). Hart and Wearing (1995) argue that both stable personality characteristics and the dynamic interplay between coping and daily work experiences together account for

changes in levels of psychological distress and well-being.

Although often used interchangeably in the occupational stress literature, Hart and Wearing (1995) have demonstrated that psychological distress and morale operate as separate dimensions and make independent contributions to the quality of work life. That is, positive work experiences impact upon morale, and negative work experiences impact upon psychological distress. This suggests that morale may be improved by increasing positive work experiences and that psychological distress can be reduced by decreasing negative work experiences. In addition, research with teachers and police officers has indicated that these professional groups are not stressed so much by the nature of their work, but by the organisational context in which the work occurs (Headey & Wearing, 1992). The implication of this finding is that intervention should focus on developing a supportive organisational climate that enables workers to cope more adaptively with operational work demands, rather than to direct change efforts at the nature of the work per se. A core set of organisational factors, among them staff relationships and leadership quality, is related to both psychological distress and morale. Other factors, such as excessive work demands, are negative and relate only to psychological distress, while factors such as opportunities for advancement, are positive and relate only to morale (Hart, Conn, Carter & Wearing, 1993). That is, strain occurs when excess elements (e.g. demands) may threaten one need and deficit elements (e.g. lack of communication or support) may threaten another. Careful analysis of both positive and negative organisational characteristics is therefore needed before intervening to ameliorate identified problems.

Cybernetics and Systems Theory
The ecological view of humans as living systems dependent upon a healthy relationship with the environment is one of some currency in political, public health and philosophical realms. The development of this perspective into a model for explicating the antecedent processes of occupational stress based on cybernetics and systems theory has been foreshadowed, but not yet realised (Cottone & Emener 1990; Cox, 1987; Edwards 1992; Hart & Wearing 1995; Kenny 1995e; Tate, 1992). The ecological view of occupational stress is succinctly summarised, as follows:

> Work related psychosocial stressors originate in social structures and processes, affect the human organism through psychological processes, and influence health through four types of closely interrelated mechanisms— emotional, cognitive, behavioural and physiological. Situational (e.g. social support) and individual factors (e.g. personality, coping repertoire) modify the health outcome. The work-environment-stress-health system is a dynamic one with many feedback loops ... the approach (to intervention) should be systems-oriented, interdisciplinary, problem-solving oriented, health (not disease) oriented, and participative (Levi, 1990, p. 1142).

In cybernetic theory, the concept of feedback is the pivotal process. Feedback describes a process whereby the system initiates homeostatic mechanisms based upon information received. Hoffman (1981) describes feedback loops as either deviation amplifying or deviation counteracting, whereby a system either stabilises, moving to a state of equilibrium, or destabilises, moving to a state of disequilibrium. According to a cybernetic analysis, systems or organisations may undergo first or second order change. In first order change, negative feedback is the process whereby systems maintain their organisation through deviation-counteracting mechanisms such as homeostasis, morphostasis, and self correction (Sluzki, 1985). In second order change, positive feedback loops amplify deviation (i.e. create change rather than maintain stasis).

Feedback loops are initiated when an individual identifies a discrepancy between a perceived current state that creates imbalance and discomfort, and another desired psychological and/or physiological state (Frone & McFarlin, 1989). The individual then assigns significance (importance) to the discrepancy (Carver & Scheier, 1981; Cummings & Cooper, 1979; Edwards, 1992). The importance or meaning accorded this discrepancy determines whether a feedback mechanism is initiated (Edwards 1992). In an interesting variation of this theme, Buunk and Ybema (1997) have proposed that experiencing occupational stress, or any form of uncertainty, instigates a desire for social comparison information, that is, a need to discover how other people feel about the situation. Contact with similar others may lead the individual to adapt his/her stress response to those of other group members. Such a process may account, in part, for particular patterns of occurrence of occupational stress or illness that have been identified (Willis, 1994).

Although the parallel is rarely drawn, there is a strong philosophical relationship between the concept of 'discrepancy' in systems theory, 'alienation' in Marx's theory of the pathology of social change (Marx, 1982), and Durkheim's (1952) 'anomie'. Susan Sontag (1978, cited in Willis, 1994) conceived of 'illness as metaphor' within sociological theorising at about the same time that psychologists and family therapists were embracing the notion of the symptom in the identified patient as a metaphor of family dysfunction (Bowen, 1978; Haley, 1964; Minuchin, 1978; Palazzoli, Boscolo, Cecchin & Prata, 1986). Similar analogies have been offered subsequently, for example, Willis's (1994) analysis of RSI as a metaphor for alienation. Applying these concepts to the occupational stress arena, one could argue that occupational stress arises when, through either individual or organisational change processes, a discrepancy occurs between the personal values of the worker and the values of the organisation to which s/he belongs. Because managers and supervisors are key representatives of organisational culture, it is most often within the relationship between the individual and the supervisor that the individual will experience alienation (McIntyre, 1998).

The experience of occupational stress and its concrete manifestation i.e. the lodging of a workers' compensation claim, is the functional communication of distress brought about by alienation (Karasek & Theorell, 1990). In Edward's (1992) theory, alienation may be understood in terms of thwarted desires which produce negative emotions such as anger, disillusionment, or the desire for retribution or revenge. Decreased worker morale, in dynamic equilibrium theory (Hart & Wearing, 1995), may be conceptualised as a precursor to alienation if steps are not taken to remedy the morale problem early in the cycle.

REHABILITATION OF OCCUPATIONAL STRESS

Systemic theories have not yet had a major impact on the prevention or management of occupational stress. (Edwards, 1992; Frone & McFarlin, 1989). However, the processes involved in occupational rehabilitation can be conceptualised cybernetically, in terms similar to those of systemic family therapy. Bowen (1966, 1978) was a systemic family therapist who postulated the importance of the role played by triangles in family interaction. This process, called triangulation, occurs in all social groups, as twosomes form to the exclusion of, or against a third party. Bowen proposed that a two-person system may form a three-person system under stress. For instance, tension might arise between the two and the one who feels most uncomfortable or vulnerable may 'triangle in' a third party, to relieve tension and to restore the power balance. The third party, once drawn in, may form his/her own set of alliances, thus creating shifting power balances. The action may not remain localised within the original triangle, as more and more stakeholders become involved in the ongoing struggle. Bowen associates pathology with rigidity and suggests that, although all systems create triadic patterns, these patterns will become more rigid during periods of crisis or stress. The rigidity of the response patterns set up by injury/occupational stress and the central players' initial responses to the claim follow a limited and predictable path and set up a highly restricted set of choices for the stakeholders involved.

When a worker is injured/stressed, the matter is initially dealt with in the injured worker-employer dyad. If the worker and employer deal with the matter to their mutual satisfaction, no other parties need become involved, other than in a service provision capacity. That is the employer will notify the insurer, who will organise payment, and the injured worker may contact a health professional for treatment. However, if the employer is dissatisfied with the injured worker's response to his injury (e.g. by taking too much time off work, or by remaining on shortened hours of work), he may call in the insurer, not as a service provider, but as an ally against the injured worker. The insurer will respond by disputing the claim for workers' compensation, ordering expert medical opinion and instructing the worker to attend a doctor appointed by the insurance company. The injured worker may respond by attending his own doctor, no longer only as a service provider, but also as an ally who will assist the injured worker to restore the power balance by organising medical specialist opinion which is frequently contrary to the insurance doctor's opinion. The parties may then become polarised in an apparently unresolvable dilemma. One of the reasons for this is that the issue of how best to manage the injury is replaced with the issue of stakeholder integrity, particularly that of the injured worker. The genuineness of the injury becomes the focus of stakeholder involvement, rather than searching for the best solution for the worker and his/her employer. The more parties who become involved, the poorer the communication between them and the greater the suspicion and hostility. Recourse to the legal profession with protracted legal proceedings is often the next step in this process of triangulation.

Systemic concepts such as Bowen's notion of triangulation (Bowen, 1966, 1978), and Karasek's notion of stress as a form of strategic or functional communication (Karasek & Theorell, 1990), have the capacity to provide a firm underpinning to the model of tertiary rehabilitation described in this chapter.

The proposed systemic model is particularly relevant to the analysis and case management of occupational stress. It suggests that the intervention of the rehabilitation case manager should be directed at identifying the dyadic and triadic relationships and at providing clients with a functional means of communicating their distress. It is vital that this process allows the real sources of stress to be identified. In an interesting and provocative paper, Mahony (1996), building on Goffman's (1971) distinction between 'front stage' and 'back stage' explanations of behaviour, argues that certain occupational groups present 'front stage' explanations only for the causes of their occupational stress. Front stage refers to those explanations that are most likely to have currency with prevailing social norms, management, and in the case of claims for occupational stress, the Workers' Compensation authorities. She sights the example of prison officers, whose front stage explanations for occupational stress included daily exposure to personal risk, resulting in safety fears, including fears of injury and death at the hands of violent criminals. The back stage reality, that were the underlying causes of absenteeism, sick leave and occupational stress was the inherent boredom of the job (e.g. standing in a tower on guard for eight hours) and stigmatisation by outsiders. These putative back stage factors would receive much less support from management or Workers' Compensation authorities. Therefore, workers may collude in propagating the front stage reality to the detriment of developing appropriate interventions for change. Careful analysis is required to avoid intervening on the basis of front stage interpretations of the problem. This may lead to impasses, stalemates, anger, hostility, and industrial action.

Provision of the opportunity to deal with both front stage and back stage issues, that may include, among others, medical or treatment issues, industrial and legal issues, change management problems, family problems, life cycle issues, underlying or consequent psychological or psychiatric conditions, and competence and training difficulties, is a necessary component in the rehabilitation process. If successful, this communication will free both the client and significant stakeholders from the aggregation of issues (e.g. searching for truth or blame and appointing scapegoats) that has resulted in triangulation processes (see Kenny, 1995b, 1995e) that were both precursors to the claim and impediments to successful return to work. This analysis also serves to clarify expected outcomes of the rehabilitation process, as distinct from other (e.g. industrial/legal) processes which may have a bearing on the resolution of the problems (Nowland, 1997).

Due to the complex nature of the rehabilitation process and the large number of stakeholders involved, the role of the case manager is central and pivotal (Kenny, 1995c; Weil & Karls, 1985). The adoption by the rehabilitation professional of an advocacy or adversarial role, either on behalf of the worker, or on behalf of one of the other stakeholders (usually the employer) may create a major barrier to successful rehabilitation (Kenny, 1995a, 1995f; Shrey, 1993). A systemically based intervention will resolve these errors by clarifying the role of the case manager within this system as *an advocate for the rehabilitation process*, rather than for any of the stakeholders. A systems framework emphasises the importance of professional neutrality, providing clear roles and functions based upon the professional's relationship to the system as a whole, rather than to any one component (Furlong & Young, 1996). This approach also serves to clarify expected outcomes of the rehabilitation process, as distinct from other (e.g. industrial/legal) processes which may have a bearing on the resolution of the problems.

The focus of the systemic intervention is the relationship between the injured worker and the system rather than an exploration of the individual's traits, skills and capacities in isolation. It is based on the cybernetic model outlined above which has in turn been informed by the theories and processes described in the preceding sections. In this model, developed by Nowland (1997), and enlarged upon here, the case manager should:

1) *Map the stakeholders and their inter-relationships.* Both the client and the case manager need to understand who is involved, either overtly or covertly. A field map is then constructed of the overall system of stakeholders and their relationships to one another in the system. Figure 20.1 presents a prototypical example of a field map. This map includes stakeholders who may become involved once a claim for workers' compensation is lodged. Not all clients will come into contact with all parties outlined in Figure 20.1. However, the schematic representation of the field illustrates the possible dyadic and triadic relationships that can occur in the post-injury period.

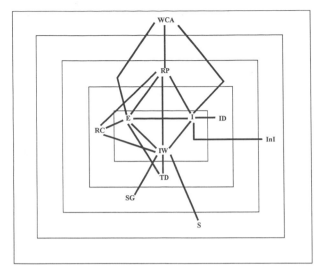

Legend.
WCA   Work Cover Authority
RP   Rehabilitation Provider
E   Employer
I   Insurer
IW   Injured Worker
TD   Treating Doctor
ID   Insurance Doctor
InI   Insurance Investigator
SG   Support Groups
S   Solicitor
RC   Rehabilitation Co-ordinator

Figure 20.1   A model of the proximal and distal stakeholders in the post-injury period and communication pathways.

2) *Identify sub-systems.* Sub-systems are identified by the commonality of their purpose and rules. Different stakeholders may belong to more than one sub-system, and through a process of identifying sub-system membership, conflicts of interest and alliances and coalitions may be clarified (i.e. Bowen's triangulation processes). The client is inevitably a member of a large number of sub-systems simultaneously (i.e. workplace, medical and rehabilitation systems, family systems and social systems). It is important to determine the relative strength and influence of each of these systems. The more intensive, committed, and socially integrated a setting, the greater is its potential impact on the outcome (Moos, 1987). In addition, the relationship of the worker to his/her work in terms of demand/control/social support may further illuminate the putative sources of stress currently experienced. It may also be possible to identify the dominant source of stress within one of the identified sub-systems.

3) *Identify the rules governing the operation of the sub-systems.* The rules governing the behaviour of the sub-systems may not be consistent with the purpose of the overall system, nor to be in the best interest of successful rehabilitation. The case manager needs to identify any homeostatic mechanisms that would operate to threaten change, and to make these rules and mechanisms explicit.

4) *Identify the issues for the client.* This step assists the client to understand the systemic causal relationship between his/her stress response and individual and systems variables. This process will highlight the initial factors as well as to identify potential barriers to resolution of the problem. A number of structured exercises can facilitate this process (Brassard

& Ritter, 1994). During this stage, it is important that the case manager obtain a clear understanding of the 'back stage' issues for the client, and to allow ample opportunity for the functional communication of distress that may constitute one of the underlying impediments to the resolution of the issues. Clarifying and separating both positive and negative work experiences may assist the client to gain some conceptual clarification of the causes of their psychological distress, as distinct from vocational dissatisfaction or morale. This step can then lead into stage 5 of the process.

5) *Apportion responsibility for management of the factors.* Different issues may need to be referred to different personnel, either within or outside the organisation. Possible sources of additional support include union representative or other employee advocate, individual counsellor, or line manager. The rehabilitation case manager co-ordinates and monitors these referrals and acts as a conduit and liaison between the client and other stakeholders.

6) *Plan and implement the rehabilitation intervention.* Once the aggregation of issues has been dealt with, the case manager can then prepare the client for return to work. During this phase, the case manager gradually relinquishes responsibility to the client and other key stakeholders in the workplace.

Systemic interventions have not previously been operationalised in this way. Predictions from the application of this model include role clarification for all stakeholders, case manager neutrality, task assignment, increased ability to manage the multivariate factors involved in a claim for occupational stress, challenging homeostatic mechanisms, and illuminating a greater range of intervention strategies through the systemic analysis of the precipitating and maintaining factors.

DIRECTIONS FOR FUTURE RESEARCH

This model for rehabilitation of occupational stress is yet to be tested empirically. Model specification and implementation would be enhanced by the following:

i) improving identification, nomenclature and classification of occupational stress claims and separating these from related factors such as morale, vocational satisfaction and attitudes towards work (Hart & Wearing, 1995).

ii) development of strategies to avoid the medicalisation, and otherwise inadequate clinical management, of occupational stress claims. Current problems are due to over-medicalisation of occupational stress (Quinlan, 1988), poor diagnostic skills in general practitioners (Kenny, 1996), poor clinical assessment practices, passive clinical management from rehabilitation providers and over-reliance on claimant self-report as the principal source of data (Cotton, 1995).

iii) an assessment of pre-program (e.g. availability of Employee Assistance Programs, grievance procedures, mediation services) and program (e.g. type of intervention, by whom, stakeholders involved, nature and frequency of contact) variables, that can be linked to successful outcomes in the management of occupational stress claims. Although there has been some recent attention to the development of stricter procedures, protocols, and role specification of the various stakeholders involved in the management of stress claims, the intervention processes that occur at the different stages of the life of the claim, and which contribute to successful/unsuccessful outcome have not, to date, been sufficiently elucidated.

References

Antonovsky, A. (1987) *Unravelling the Mystery of Health*. San Francisco: Jossey-Bass.

Appelberg, K., Romanov, K., Honkasalo, M. L. & Koskenvuo, M. (1991) Interpersonal conflicts at work and psychosocial characteristics of employees. *Social Science and Medicine*, **32**(9), 1051–1056.

Appelberg, K., Romanov, K., Heikkila, K., Honkasalo, M. L. & Koskenvuo, M. (1996) Interpersonal conflict as a predictor of work disability: A follow-up study of 15,348 Finnish employees. *Journal of Psychosomatic Research*, **40**(2), 157–167.

Bacharach, S. B., Bamberger, P. & Conley, S. (1991) Work-home conflict among nurses and engineers: Mediating the impact of role of stress on burnout and satisfaction at work. *Journal of Organisation Behavior*, **12**(1), 39–53.

Bateson, G. (1972) *Steps to an Ecology of Mind*. New York: Ballantine Books.

Berger, Y. (1993) The Hoechst dispute: A paradigm shift in occupational health and safety. In *Work and Health: The Origins, Management and Regulation of Occupational Illness*, edited by M. Quinlan, pp. 126–139. Melbourne: MacMillan Education.

Biggins, D. (1986) Focus on occupational health: What can be done? *New Doctor*, **47**, 6–10.

Bohle, P. (1993) Work psychology and the management of occupational health and safety: An historical overview. In *Work and Health: The Origins, Management and Regulation of Occupational Illness*, edited by M. Quinlan, pp. 92–115. Melbourne: MacMillan Education.

Bowen, M. (1966) The use of family theory in a clinical practice. *Clinical Psychiatry*, **7**, 345–374.

Bowen, M. (1978) Family therapy in clinical practice. New York: Aronson.

Bradburn, N. M. (1969) *The Structure of Psychological Well-being*. Chicago: Aldine.

Brassard, M. & Ritter, D. (1994) *The Memory Jogger*. MA: Methuen, Goal QPC.

Buunk, B. P. & Ybema, J. F. (1997) Social comparisons and occupational stress: The identification-contrast model. In *Health, Coping, and Well-being: Perspectives from Social Comparison Theory*, edited by B. P. Buunk & F. X. Gibbons, pp. 359–388. Mahwah, NJ: Lawrence Erlbaum Associates.

Cannon, W. B. (1929) Organisation for physiological homeostasis. *Physiological Reviews*, **9**, 399–431.

Caplan, R. D. (1987) Person-environment fit theory and organizations: Commensurate dimensions, time perspectives, and mechanisms. *Journal of Vocational Behaviour*, **31**, 248–267.

Caplan, R. D. Cobb, S. & French, J. R. (1975) Relationships of cessation of smoking with job stress, personality, and social support. *Journal of Applied Psychology*, **60**(2), 211–219.

Caplan, R. D. & Harrison, R. V. (1993) Person-environment fit theory: Some history, recent developments, and future directions. *Journal of Social Issues*, **49**(4), 253–275.

Carver, C. S. & Scheier, M. F. (1981) *Attention and Self-Regulation: A Control Theory Approach to Human Behavior*. New York: Springer-Verlag.

Chen, P. Y. & Spector, P. E. (1991) Negative affectivity as the underlying cause of correlations between stressors and strains. *Journal of Applied Psychology*, **76**(3), 398–407.

Clegg, C. & Wall, T. (1990) The relationship between simplified jobs and mental health: A replication study. *Journal of Occupational Psychology*, **63**, 289–296.

Cooper, C. L. (1983) Identifying stressors at work: Recent research developments. *Journal of Psychosomatic Research*, **27**(5), 369–376.

Cooper, C. L. (1985) The stress of work: An overview. *Aviation, Space and Environmental Medicine*, **56**(7), 627–632.

Cooper, C. L. (1995) The major types of psychological dysfunction in workplace settings. In *Psychological Health in the Workplace*, edited by P. Cotton, pp. 87–102. Victoria: The Australian Psychological Society.

Cooper, C. L. & Cartwright, S. (1994) Healthy mind, healthy organisation. *Human Relations*, **47**(4), 455–471.

Cooper, C. L., Luikkonen, P. & Cartwright, S. (1996) *Stress Prevention in the Workplace*. Dublin, Ireland: European Foundation for the Improvement of Living and Working Conditions.

Cooper, C. L. & Payne, R. L. (1992) International perspectives on research into work, well-being, and stress management. In *Stress and Well-being at Work: Assessments and Interventions for Occupational Mental Health*, edited by J. C. Quick, L. R. Murphy & J. J. Hurrell, pp. 348–368. Washington, DC, US: American Psychological Association.

Costa, P. T. & McCrae, R. R. (1980) Influence of extroversion and neuroticism on subjective well-being. *Journal of Personality and Social Psychology*, **38**, 668–678.

Cotton, P. (1995) *Psychological Health in the Workplace*. Victoria: Australian Psychological Society.

Cotton, P. & Fisher, B.(1995) Current issues and directions for the management of workplace psychological health issues. In *Psychological Health in the Workplace*, edited by P. Cotton. Victoria: Australian Psychological Society.

Cottone, R. (1991) Counselor roles according to two counseling worldviews. *Journal of Counseling and Development*, **69**, 398–401.

Cottone, R. & Emener, W. (1990) The psychomedical paradigm of vocational rehabilitation. *Rehabilitation Counselling Bulletin*, **34**(2), 91–102.

Cox, T. (1987) Stress, coping and problem solving. *Work and Stress*, **1**(1), 5–14.

Cummings, T. G. & Cooper, C. L. (1979) A cybernetic framework for studying occupational stress. *Human Relations*, **72**, 395–418.

Davis, A. & George, J. (1993) *States of Health: Health and Illness in Australia* (2nd edn.). Sydney: Harper & Row.

Decker, P. J. & Borgen, F. H. (1993) Dimensions of work appraisal: Stress, strain, coping, job satisfaction, and negative affectivity. *Journal of Counseling Psychology*, **40**(4),   470– 478.

Diener, E. & Emmons, R. A. (1985) The independence of positive and negative affect. *Journal of Personality and Social Psychology*, **47**, 1105–1117.

Durkheim, E. (1952) *Suicide: A Study in Sociology*. London: Routledge & Gegan Paul.

Edwards, J. R. (1992) A cybernetic theory of stress, coping and well being in organizations. *Academy of Management Review*, **17**(2), 238–274.

Eysenck, H. J. (1988) Personality, stress and cancer: Prediction and prophylaxis. *British Journal of Medical Psychology*, **61**, 57–75.

Ferguson, S. (1988) Occupational medicine in Australia: The past, the present and the future. *Journal of Occupational Health and Safety—Australia and New Zealand*, **4**, 481–488.

Figlio, K. (1982) How does illness mediate social relations? Workmen's compensation and medico-legal practices, 1890–1940. In *The Problem of Medical Knowledge, Examining the Social Construction of Medicine*, edited by P. Wright & A. Treacher. Edinburgh: Edinburgh University Press.

Fontana, D. & Abouserie, R. (1993) Stress levels, gender and personality factors in teachers. *British Journal of Educational Psychology*, **63**, 261–270.

Frone, M. R. & McFarlin, D. B. (1989) Chronic occupational stressors, self-focused attention, and well-being: Testing a cybernetic model of stress. *Journal of Applied Psychology*, **74**(6), 876–883.

Frone, M. R., Russell, M. & Cooper, M. L. (1991) Relationship of work and family stressors to psychological distress: the independent moderating influence of social support, mastery, active coping and self focused attention. *Journal of Social Behaviour and Personality*, **6**(7), 227–250.

Fry, P. S. (1995) Perfectionism, humour and optimism as moderators of health outcomes and determinants of coping styles of women executives. *Genetic, Social and General Psychology Monographs*, **121**(2), 211–245.

Furlong, M. & Young, J. (1996) Talking about blame. *Australian & New Zealand Journal of Family Therapy*, **17**(4), 191–200.

Furnham, A. & Schaeffer, R. (1984) Person-environment fit, job satisfaction and mental health. *Journal of Occupational Psychology*, **57**, 295–307.

Goffman, E. (1971) *The Presentation of Self in Everyday Life*. Harmondsworth: Penguin.

Habeck, R. (1993) Achieving quality and value in service to the workplace. *Bulletin of the Australian Society of Rehabilitation Counsellors*, **4**, 15–20.

Haley, J. (1964) *Strategies of Psychotherapy*. New York: Grune and Stratton.

Hart, P. M. (1994) Teacher quality of work life: Integrating work experiences, psychological distress and morale. *Journal of Occupational and Organization Psychology*, **67**, 109–132.

Hart, P. M., Conn, M., Carter, N. L. & Wearing, A. J. (1993) Development of the School Organisational Health Questionnaire: A Measure for Assessing Teacher Morale and School Organisational Climate. Paper presented at the Annual Conference of the Australian Association for Research in Education, Fremantle, Western Australia, November.

Hart, P. M. & Wearing, A. J. (1993) Problems of Instability and Change in Quality of Life Research: Implications for a Longitudinal Model of Personality, Health and Well-being. Paper presented to the First Conference of the Australian Association for Social Research, Launceston, Tasmania, January.

Hart, P. M. & Wearing, A. J. (1995) Occupational stress and well being: A systemic approach to research, policy and practice. In *Psychological Health in the Workplace*, edited by P. Cotton. Victoria: Australian Psychological Society.

Hart, P. M., Wearing, A. J. & Headey, B. (1993) Assessing police work experiences: Development of the Police Daily Hassles and Uplifts Scales. *Journal of Criminal Justice*, **21**, 553–572.

Headey, B. & Wearing, A. J. (1992) *Understanding Happiness: A Theory of Subjective Well-being*. Melbourne: Longman Cheshire.

Hobfoll, S. E. (1989) Conservation of resources: A new attempt at conceptualising stress. *The American Psychologist*, **44**, 513–524.

Hoffman, L. (1981) *Foundations of Family Therapy*. USA: Basic Books

James, C. R. (1989) *Social Sequelae of Occupational Injury and Illness*. Unpublished PhD thesis, Griffith University, Australia.

Johnson, J. V. & Hall, E. M. (1996) Dialectic between conceptual and causal inquiry in psychosocial work-environment research. *Journal of Occupational Health Psychology*, **1**(4), 362–374.

Johnstone, R. & Quinlan, M. (1993) The origins, management and regulation of occupational illness: An overview. In *Work and Health: The Origins, Management and Regulation of Occupational Illness*, edited by M. Quinlan, pp. 3–32. Melbourne: MacMillan Education.

Karasek, R. A. (1979) Job demands, job decision latitude, and mental strain: Implications for job redesign. *Administrative Science Quarterly*, **24**, 285–308.

Karasek, R. & Theorell, T. (1990) *Healthy Work: Stress, Productivity and the Reconstruction of Working Life*. New York: Basic Books.

Karasek, R. A., Triantis, K. P. & Chaudry, S. S. (1982) Coworker and supervisor support as moderators of associations between task characteristics and mental strain. *Journal of Occupational and Behavior*, **3**, 181–200.

Keeney, B. P. (1987) The construction of therapeutic realities. Special Issue: Psychotherapy with families. *Psychotherapy*, **24**(3S) 469–476.

Kenny, D. T. (1994a) Determinants of time lost from workplace injury: The impact of theinjury, the injured, the industry, the intervention and the insurer. *International Journal of Rehabilitation Research*, **17**(4) 333–342.

Kenny, D. T. (1994b) The relationship between workers' compensation and occupational rehabilitation: An historical perspective. *Journal of Occupational Health and Safety*, **10**(2), 157–164.

Kenny, D. T. (1995a) Barriers to occupational rehabilitation: An exploratory study of long-term injured workers. *Journal of Occupational Health and Safety—Australia and New Zealand*, **11**(3), 249–256.

Kenny, D. T. (1995b) Common themes, different perspectives: A systemic analysis of employer-employee experiences of occupational rehabilitation. *Rehabilitation Counseling Bulletin*, **39**(1), 53–77.

Kenny, D. T. (1995c) Failures in occupational rehabilitation: A case study analysis. *Australian Journal of Rehabilitation Counselling*, **1**(1), 33–45.

Kenny, D. T. (1995d) Case management in occupational rehabilitation: Would the real case manager please stand up? *Australian Journal of Rehabilitation Counselling*, **1**(2), 104–117.

Kenny, D. T. (1995e) Stressed organisations and organisational stressors: A systemic analysis of workplace injury. *International Journal of Stress Management*, **2**, 207–220.

Kenny, D. T. (1995f) *Occupational Rehabilitation in New South Wales*. Sydney: The University of Sydney.

Kenny, D. T. (1995g) *Barriers to Return to Work in New South Wales: Research Findings and Theoretical Considerations*. Proceedings of the National Occupational Health Conference: Brisbane, Queensland (pp. 75–78).

Kenny, D. T. (1996) The roles, functions, and effectiveness of treating Doctors in the management of occupational injury: Perceptions of key stakeholders. *The Australian Journal of Rehabilitation Counselling*, **2**(2), 86–98.

Kivimaki, M. & Lindstrom, K. (1995) Effects of private self-consciousness and control on the occupational stress-strain relationship. *Stress Medicine*, **11**(1), 7–16.

Kottage, B. E. (1992) Stress in the workplace. *Professional Safety*, **37**(August), 24–26.

Kulik, C. T., Oldman, G. R. & Hackman, J. R. (1987) Work design as an approach to person-environment fit. *Journal of Vocational Behaviour*, **31**, 278–296.

Landsbergis, P. A., Schnall, P. L., Deitz, D., Friedman, R. & Pickering, T. (1992) The patterning of psychological attributes and distress by 'Job Strain' and social support in a sample of working men. *Journal of Behavioral Medicine*, **15**(4), 379–405.

Lazarus, R. S. & Folkman, S. (1984) *Stress, Appraisal and Coping*. New York: Springer.

Levi, L. (1990) Occupational stress. Spice of life or kiss of death? *American Psychologist*, **45**(10), 1142–1145.

Levi, L. (1998) Stress management and prevention on a European community level: Options and obstacles. In *Stress and Health: Research and Clinical Applications*, edited by D. T. Kenny, J. C. Carlson, F. J. McGuigan & J. L. Sheppard. Amsterdan: Harwood Academic Publishers

Mackay, C. J. & Cooper, C. L. (1987) Occupational stress and health: Some current issues. In *International Review of Industrial and Organisational Psychology 1987*, edited by C. L. Cooper & I. T. Robertson, pp. 167–199. Chichester, UK: John Wiley and Sons.

Mahony, K. (1996) An argument for using qualitative methods to reveal the multicausality of occupational stressors in the work of Triple 0 party workers. In *Proceedings (Edited Abstracts), International Congress on Stress and Health*, edited by D. Kenny, The University of Sydney, p. 29.

Marx, K. (1982) *Capital*, Volume 1. Middlesex: Penguin.

Matheny, K. B., Aycock, D. W., Pugh, J. L., Curlette, W. L. & Silva Canella, K. A. (1986) Stress coping: A qualitative and quantitative synthesis with implication for treatment. *Counseling Psychologist*, **14**, 499–549.

McGrath, J. E. (1976) Stress and behavior in organizations. In *Handbook of Industrial and Organization Psychology*, edited by M. D. Dunnette. Chicago, IL: Rand McNally.

McIntyre, D. (1998) *The Politics and Experience of Occupational Stressors*. Unpublished PhD Dissertation. The University of Newcastle, NSW, Austrialia.

McRae, R. R. & Costa, P. T. (1994) The stability of personality: Observations and evaluations. *Current Directions in Psychological Science*, **3**(6), 173–175.

Minuchin, S. (1978) *Families and Family Therapy*. London, Great Britain: Tavistock Publications Ltd.

Moos, R. H. (1987) Person-environment congruence in work, school and health care settings. *Journal of Vocational Behavior*, **31**, 231–247.

Murphy, L. R. (1988) Workplace interventions for stress reduction and prevention. In *Causes, Coping and Consequences of Stress at Work*, edited by C. L. Cooper & R. Payne. pp. 310–309, London: Wiley.

Nowland, L. (1997) Application of a systems approach to the rehabilitation assessment of clients with an occupational stress-related injury. *The Australian Journal of Rehabilitation Counselling*, **3**(1), 9–20.

O'Driscoll, M. P. & Cooper, C. L. (1994) Coping with work-related stress: A critique of existing measures and proposal for an alternative methodology. *Journal of Occupational and Organizational Psycholog*, **67**(4), 343–354.

Palazzoli, M., Boscolo, L., Cecchin, G. & Prata, G. (1986) *Paradox and Counter Pparadox*. Palo Alto, California: Jason Aronson.

Peterson, C. L. (1994) Work factors and stress: A critical review. *International Journal of Health Services*, **24**(3), 495–519.

Piedmont, R. L. (1993) A longitudinal analysis of burnout in the health care setting: The role of personal dispositions. *Journal of Personality Assessment*, **61**(3), 457–473.

Quick, J. C., Joplin, J. R., Nelson, D. L. & Quick, J. D. (1992) Behavioural responses to anxiety: Self reliance, counterdependence, and over dependence. *Anxiety, Stress and Coping: an International Journal*, **5**(1), 41–54.

Quinlan, M. (1988) Psychological and sociological approaches to the study of occupational illness: A critical review. *The Australian and New Zealand Journal of Sociology*, **24**(2), 189–207.

Quinlan, M. & Bohle, P. (1991) *Managing Occupational Health and Safety in Australia*. Melbourne: Macmillan Australia.

Roskies, E., Louis-Guerin, C., & Fournier, C. (1993) Coping with job insecurity: How does personality make a difference? *Journal of Organisational Behaviour*, **14**(7), 617–630.

Rounds, J. B. Dawis, R. V. & Lofquist, L. H. (1987) Measurement of person environment fit and prediction of satisfaction in the theory of work adjustment. *Journal of Vocational Behavior*, **31**, 297–318.

Selye, H. (1975) *The Stress of Life* (Rev. edn). New York: McGraw Hill.

Shrey, D. (1993) Workplace-based disability management: Challenges and opportunities for joint employer rehabilitation professional initiatives. *Proceedings of the Second National Rehabilitation Conference*, pp. 27–36. Commonwealth Rehabilitation Service. Australia: Sydney

Siegall, M. & Cummings, L. L. (1995) Stress and organizational role conflict. *Genetic, Social and General Psychology Monographs*, **121**(1), 65–95.

Sluzki, C. E. (1985) A mininmal map of cybernetics. *Networker*, May–June, 26.

Soederfeldt, B., Soederfeldt, M., Muntaner, C., O'Campo, P., Warg, L. E., & Ohlson, C. G. (1996) Psychosocial work environment in human service organizations: A conceptual analysis and development of the demand-control model. *Social Science & Medicine*, **42**(9), 1217–1226.

Spielberger, C. D., Reheiser, E. C., Reheiser, J. E. & Vagg, P. R. (1998) Measuring stress in the workplace: the Job Stress. Survey in *Stress and Health: Research and Clinical Applications*, edited by D. T. Kenny, J. C. Carlson, F. J. McGuigan & J. L. Sheppard. The Netherlands: Harwood Academic Publishers.

Spector, P. E. & O'Connell, B. J. (1994) The contribution of personality traits, negative affectivity, locus of control and Type A to the subsequent reports of job stressors and job strains. *Journal of Occupational and Organizational Psychology*, **67**(1), 1–12.

Sutton, R. I. & Kahn, R. L. (1986) Prediction, understanding and control as antidotes to organizational stress. In *Handbook of Organisational Behaviour*, edited by J. W. Lorsch, pp. 272–285. Englewood Cliffs NJ: Prentice Hall.

Tate, D. G. (1992) Factors influencing injured employees return to work. *Journal of Applied Rehabilitation Counselling*, **23**(2), 17–20.

Toohey, J. (1993) *Quality of Working Life Project: A Study of Occupational Stress in Commonwealth Government Agencies*. Canberra, Australia: Comcare.

Toohey, J. (1995) Managing the stress phenomenon at work. In *Psychological Health in the Workplace*, edited by P. Cotton, pp. 51–71. Victoria: Australian Psychological Society.

Watson, D., Pennebaker, J. W. & Folger, R. (1986) Beyond negative affectivity: measuring stress and satisfaction in the workplace. *Journal of Organizational Behaviour Management*, **8**(2), 141–157.

Weil, M. & Karls, J. M. (1985) *Case Management in Human Service Practice*. California: Jossey-Bass.

Williams, C. & Thorpe, B. (1992) *Beyond Industrial Sociology: The Work of Men and Women*. Sydney: Allen and Unwin.

Willis, E. (1989) Commentary: RSI as a social process. *Community Health Studies*, **X**(2), 210–219.

Willis, E. (1994) *Illness and Social Relations*. Sydney: Allen & Unwin.

Wright, R. (1995) The evaluation of despair. *Time*, 11 September, 62–68.

Chapter 21

MEASURING STRESS IN THE WORKPLACE: The Job Stress Survey

Charles D. Spielberger, PhD Eric C. Reheiser, John E. Reheiser and Peter R. Vagg

Hazards in the workplace and their effects on health and behavior have been recognized for many years. The phrase 'mad as a hatter' came into the English language long before anyone knew that mercury in the materials used in making hats affected the central nervous system (Kahn, 1981). In the 19th century, descriptions of the 'black lung' disease of coal miners recognized a causal link between the specific characteristics of a hazardous work environment and a particular physical disorder. More recent research has shown that the emotional and physical consequences of the psychological demands of a job can also have pervasive and profound effects on the lives of workers (e.g. Kahn, 1981; Karasek & Theorell, 1990; Matteson & Ivancevich, 1982).

It is now well established that high levels of stress in the workplace adversely affect productivity and employee health and well-being (e.g. Kahn, Wolfe, Quinn, Snoek & Rosenthal, 1964; Keita & Sauter, 1992; Levi, 1981; Perrewé, 1991; Quick, Murphy & Hurrell, 1992; Ryland & Greenfeld, 1991; Sauter & Murphy, 1995). In an US nationwide study, one-third of those surveyed reported that: 'job stress is the single greatest stress in their lives' (Northwestern National Life, 1991, p. 2). The results of this study also indicated that the proportion of workers who reported 'feeling highly stressed' more than doubled from 1985 to 1990, and that workers who reported 'having multiple stress-related illnesses' increased from 13% to 25%.

Absenteeism, employee turnover, and stress-related medical problems have substantial direct costs for employers. Financial compensation of workers for stress-related problems has also increased markedly (Grippa & Durbin, 1986), as reflected most clearly in a dramatic rise in the occupational claims of employees seeking compensation for stress-induced psychological dysfunctions (Lowman, 1993). In the United States alone, according to Sauter (1992, p. 14), 'nearly 600,000 workers are disabled for reasons of psychological disorders', costing $5.5 billion in annual payments to individuals and their families.

Growing concern over the consequences of job stress for both employees and organizations is reflected in the increasing number of studies of occupational stress published in the medical and psychological literature. Figure 21.1 shows the number of publications cited in *PsycLit* over the past 20 years that included *job*, *work*, or *occupational stress* in their titles as compared with studies of *family stress*. Investigations of stress in the workplace have increased more than twenty-fold during the last two decades and continues to rise, whereas research on family stress has increased to a lesser extent and seems to have leveled off.

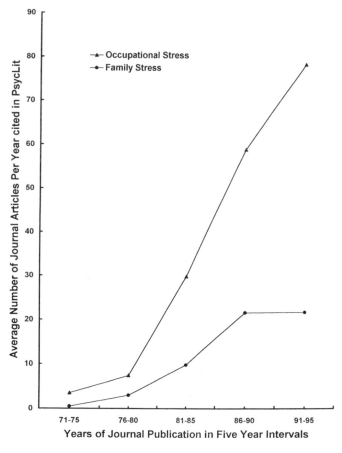

Figure 21.1   Average number of journal articles on occupational stress for each five year period, from 1971 through 1995, compared to publications on family stress for the same 25-year period

This explosive increase in research on job stress has contributed to identifying a number of major sources of stress in the workplace. However, conceptions of occupational stress have also proliferated, and definitions of this construct tend to differ from study to study (Kasl, 1978; Schuler, 1980). As noted by Schuler (1991), much of the conceptual ambiguity in definitions of occupational stress stems from the fact that some investigators have focused their attention on the specific demands or *pressures* of a particular job, whereas others are concerned primarily with the emotional, behavioral and health *consequences* of work-related stress. Because such differences in theoretical approaches to occupational stress greatly influence the procedures used to assess stress in the workplace, it is essential to understand the conceptual models that have guided the construction of job stress measures.

Jackson and Schuler (1985, p. 47) recommend that research on occupational stress focus on '... the development of good diagnostic tools for pinpointing *specific aspects about one's job* that are ambiguous or conflicting' [italics added]. In a similar vein, Murphy and Hurrell (1987) call for the construction of a generic questionnaire with a core set of questions to facilitate comparing the stress levels of various occupational groups. In developing valid psychometric questionnaires for assessing occupational stress, it is essential that the conceptual framework for constructing these measures be clearly specified (Barone, Caddy, Katell, Roselione & Hamilton 1988).

Measuring Occupational Stress

Guided by Lazarus' (1966, 1994) Transactional Process Theory of Stress and State-Trait Anxiety Theory (Spielberger, 1972, 1979), Spielberger and his colleagues (Spielberger, Grier & Pate, 1980; Spielberger, Westberry, Grier & Greenfield, 1981) constructed the *Police Stress Survey* (PSS) to evaluate the perceived severity and frequency of occurrence of stressor events encountered by law enforcement officers. In focused small-group discussions with police officers, they identified 60 specific sources of stress in police work, which were remarkably similar to those previously observed by Kroes (1976; Kroes & Gould, 1979; Kroes, Margolis & Hurrell, 1974). Findings with the PSS and normative data for Florida law enforcement officers are reported in a monograph and several brief articles (Spielberger et al., 1980, 1981; Spielberger, Grier & Greenfield, 1982).

In order to compare the stress experienced by high school teachers with that of police officers, items from the PSS were adapted to form the *Teacher Stress Survey* (TSS). Of the 60 PSS items, 39 were determined to be applicable to both teaching and police work (Grier, 1982). Each TSS item was identical to a corresponding PSS item, except that 'teacher' and 'school' were routinely substituted for 'police' and 'department'. In consultation with experienced high school teachers, 21 additional items relating to the stress experienced by teachers were generated for the TSS. It is especially interesting to note that nearly two-thirds of the PSS items, which were constructed to assess the stress experienced by law enforcement officers, were found to be equally applicable for assessing the occupational stress experienced by high school teachers (Grier, 1982).

The *Job Stress Survey* (JSS) was developed to serve as a generic measure of occupational stress. Thirty items that were included in both the PSS and the TSS surveys of occupational stress experienced by police officers and high school teachers (Spielberger & Reheiser 1994a, 1994b; Turnage & Spielberger, 1991) were selected and adapted for the JSS. In responding to the JSS, the examinee first rates the *severity* of each stressor event, on a scale from 1 to 9, and then indicates how *frequently* the stressor was encountered during the past six months. The format for responding to the JSS Severity Scale is similar to the procedure employed for rating stressful life events with the *Social Readjustment Rating Scale* (Holmes & Rahe, 1967). The perceived severity associated with each of the JSS stressor events (e.g. 'Excessive Paperwork', 'Inadequate Support by Supervisor', 'Working Overtime') is compared by the examinee to a standard stressor, 'Assignment of Disagreeable Duties'. In previous research with the PSS and TSS, this item was rated near the mid-point of the stress severity range by both police officers and teachers.

After rating the severity of the JSS stressor events, examinees are asked to report how frequently each stressor was encountered during the preceding six months by indicating, on a 10-point scale ranging from 0 to 9+, the number of days the stressor occurred. Thus, the two ratings for each of the 30 JSS items provide useful information in regard to the perceived severity of each stressor, and how often the stressor event was experienced. In rating both the perceived severity and frequency of occurrence of each stressor event, the JSS takes into account the state-trait distinction that has proved important in the assessment of anxiety (Spielberger, 1972, 1983) and other emotions, e.g. anger and depression.

Spielberger and Reheiser (1994a) factor analyzed responses to the JSS severity and frequency items for large samples of working adults employed in university, corporate and military settings. In separate analyses, two strong factors and three relatively weak factors were identified for both males and females working in these diverse settings (Spielberger & Reheiser, 1994b). However, Cattell's (1966) scree test criterion suggested that only two factors should be extracted, which were essentially the same as the two factors that were found for employees working in corporate, university, and military settings. Based on the content of the items with unique and substantial loadings, these factors were labeled Job Pressure and Lack of Organizational Support.

The main goal of the present study was to evaluate the nature and stability of the factor structure of the JSS for males and females working at higher and lower occupational levels in corporate or university settings. The two occupational levels were comprised of managerial and professional employees, and clerical and maintenance workers. Gender differences in the occupational stress experienced by employees at each of these levels were examined for the JSS Stress Index, the Perceived Severity and Frequency scales, and for the Job Pressure and Lack of Support subscales.

METHOD

Subjects

The participants in this study were 1,807 working adults employed at a large state university, or at the corporate headquarters of two large industrial companies. The factor structure of the JSS for these corporate and university employees was previously evaluated without taking occupational level into account (Spielberger & Reheiser, 1994a). In the present study, each employee was classified as either a managerial, professional, clerical or maintenance worker. University faculty and corporate engineers with college degrees were assigned to the managerial/professional group. The assignment of clerical and maintenance workers was based on the job classification of these employees in their respective work settings. In order to have a sufficient number of subjects for stable analyses of the JSS factor structure, managers and professionals were grouped together in the higher occupational level group, and clerical and maintenance workers were assigned to the lower occupational group. These groups were comprised, respectively, of 995 managers and professionals (344 females, 651 males) and 812 clerical and maintenance employees (596 females, 216 males).

Job Stress Survey

The JSS consists of 30 items that describe specific sources of stress that are commonly encountered in the workplace. Examinees first respond to each item, numbered 1–30, by rating the perceived severity of the stressor as more or less stressful than the standard stressor, 'Assignment of disagreeable duties'. The standard is assigned a score of 5, which defines the mid-point of a 9-point scale. A rating of '1' indicates very low perceived stress as compared to the standard; a rating of '9' indicates very high stress. The examinee is then instructed to report the frequency of occurrence of the same 30 stressor events, numbered 31–60, by indicating, on a 10-point scale ranging from 0 to 9+, the approximate number of days the stressor was experienced during the past six months.

JSS Severity and Frequency scores are computed by simply summing the ratings of the 30 stressor events for each scale. Severity and Frequency scores for the Job Pressure and Lack of Support subscales are obtained in a similar manner by summing the ratings for the 10 items comprising each subscale. Stress Index scores are obtained by multiplying the severity and frequency ratings for each item. The overall JSS Index score is determined by summing the Index scores for all 30 JSS items; Pressure and Lack of Support Index scores are computed in a similar manner for the 10 items comprising these subscales.

Procedure
The JSS Test forms were distributed to employees in each work setting by company or university administrators. Employees were encouraged to read the instructions carefully, and then respond to each of the JSS Severity items. After completing the Severity scale, the examinees responded to the 30 Frequency items. All participants responded individually and anonymously, and were asked to report their gender and professional classification. They were informed that their responses would be confidential, and would contribute to the development of university or company stress management programs. The rate of return was approximately 60% for the corporate employees and 70% for the university personnel.

RESULTS

Principal components factor analyses of responses to the 30 JSS Severity and Frequency items were computed separately for males and females in the two employee groups. In these analyses, one strong, one moderately strong, and three or four weak factors with eigenvalues greater than 1.00, were identified. However, for both occupational groups, Cattell's (1966) scree test criterion suggested that only two factors should be extracted. The two-factor promax solutions for males and females in both occupational level groups also provided the best simple structure, and the most meaningful interpretation of responses to the JSS Severity and Frequency items. It is interesting to note that the individual JSS items which had the strongest loadings on the Job Pressure and Lack of Support factors in the present study also had the strongest loadings on these same factors in previous research (Spielberger & Reheiser, 1994a).

The 20 JSS items that best defined the Severity and Frequency factors in the present study and in previous research were selected for further analysis in order to 'sharpen' the two factors (Vagg & Hammond, 1976). The results of separate principal components factor analyses, with promax rotations, of the responses of males and females in the two occupational groups to these 20 items are reported in Table 21.1. As may be noted, the factor structures for the Severity and Frequency items were very similar for the two occupational groups, and were remarkably stable for men and women.

Table 21.1 also shows that almost all of the Severity and Frequency items had their dominant salient loadings on the same factors for males and females in both the managerial/professional and clerical/ maintenance groups. Furthermore, in 7 of the 8 factor analyses reported in Table 21.1, the Job Pressure factor was substantially more cohesive than the Lack of Support factor, as reflected in the larger eigenvalues for the unrotated

Table 21.1 Factor loadings of JSS Severity and Frequency items on Job Pressure and Lack of Organizational Support factors for female and male managerial/professional and clerical/maintenance employees[1]

Item	JSS Severity								JSS Frequency							
	Job Pressure				Lack of Support				Job Pressure				Lack of Support			
	Manag./Profes.		Cleric./Mainten.		Manag./Profes.		Cleric./Mainten.		Manag./Profes.		Cleric./Mainten.		Manag./Profes.		Cleric./Mainten.	
	F (344)	M (651)	F (596)	M (216)	F (344)	M (651)	F (596)	M (216)	F (344)	M (651)	F (596)	M (216)	F (344)	M (651)	F (596)	M (216)
26/56	.80	.65	.78	.75					.66	.67	.66	.75				
16/46	.67	.76	.59	.74					.68	.76	.67	.71				
23/53	.64	.44	.59	.45				.31	.67	.64	.66	.66				
25/55	.62	.41	.70	.37					.63	.52	.69	.68				
11/41	.61	.70	.77	.77					.67	.57	.68	.58				
07/37	.57	.62	.57	.57					.66	.71	.63	.81				
04/34	.55	.55	.59	.59					.51	.42	.51	.56				
27/57	.53	.48	.50	.59					.48	.39	.41	(.27)				
09/39	.46	.49	.52	.50					.54	.48	.53	.46				
02/32	.40	.41	.40	.40					.58	.58	.46	.55				
06/36					.73	.74	.88	.73					.83	.78	.87	.79
13/43					.68	.65	.76	.66					.68	.64	.68	.62
03/33					.67	.55	.38	.54			(.27)		.52	.53	(.26)	.34
18/48			.31	.45	.62	.60	.31	.62					.61	.59	.45	.48
14/44					.61	.53	.66	.57					.49	.55	.53	.51
21/51					.52	.54	.72	.69					.71	.67	.79	.77
08/38					.51	.59	.61	.66					.72	.68	.63	.59
29/59					.49	.47	.47	.53					.49	.45	.51	.63
05/35			(.27)		.44	.41	.53	.56	.37	.32			.40	.41	.48	.60
19/49					.40	.42	(.28)	.48			(.28)		.32	.41	(.23)	.42
Eigenvalues: P.F.	5.56	4.43	6.80	1.69	1.78	2.07	1.53	6.51	5.40	4.95	5.96	6.39	2.40	2.22	1.74	1.56
Prom.	3.70	3.23	4.01	3.77	3.40	3.18	3.66	4.00	3.99	3.60	3.87	3.94	3.66	3.48	3.43	3.60

[1] Items are ranked in descending order of the loadings for female managerial/professional personnel on the Severity Job Pressure and Lack of Support factors.

principal factors solutions. However, for males in the clerical/maintenance group, the Lack of Support factor was larger than the Job Pressure factor.

Means, standard deviations and alpha coefficients for the 30-item JSS Stress Index, and the 10-item Job Pressure and Lack of Support Index subscales, are reported in Table 21.2. Alpha coefficients for all three JSS Index scales were .80 or higher (mdn. alpha = .85). Differences in the mean scores for the four groups were evaluated in 2×2 (Gender by Occupational Level) analyses of variance (ANOVAs). The F-values for the main and interaction effects for male and female managerial/professional and clerical/maintenance employees are also reported in Table 21.2.

No significant Gender or Occupational Level main effects, nor Gender-By-Occupational-Level interactions, were found in the analyses of the JSS Stress Index and Lack of Support Index scales. However, the main effect of Occupational Level for the JSS Pressure Index was highly significant ($p <$ .001), indicating that the managerial/professional employees experienced substantially greater stress from the pressure of their jobs than the clerical/maintenance workers. The significant Gender-by-Occupational Level interaction effect for the JSS Pressure Index was due mainly to the very low Pressure Index scores of the male clerical/maintenance workers, whose scores on this scale were significantly lower ($p < .01$) than those of the females at this occupational level.

Table 21.2   Mean, SD's and alpha coefficients for the JSS Stress Index, and the Job Pressure and Lack of Support Index subscales, for the managerial/professional and clerical/maintenance groups

JSS Index Scales:	Manag./ Profes.		Cleric./ Mainten.		Gender	Occupa level	Interact Gender/ Occupa
	F	M	F	M	F-test	F-test	F-test
ST-INDEX							
Mean	62.70	61.05	60.52	60.15	0.09	0.82	0.12
SD	31.26	29.80	36.84	39.00			
N	315	619	559	206			
Alpha	.88	.87	.91	.92			
PRESSURE							
Mean	24.29	23.50	21.65	18.05	0.54	30.20	3.93
SD	13.53	12.28	14.31	13.82		***	*
N	327	631	579	210			
Alpha	.82	.80	.85	.85			
SUPPORT							
Mean	21.18	21.13	21.80	24.07	0.15	3.79	1.90
SD	15.12	15.15	16.32	17.50			
N	326	625	564	209			
Alpha	.82	.82	.84	.85			

*** $= p < .001$, ** $= p < .01$, * $= p < .05$

Means, standard deviations, and alpha coefficients for the JSS Stress Severity Scale, and for the Pressure and Lack of Support Severity subscales, are reported in Table 21.3 for males and females in the two occupational level groups. For all three JSS scales, the alpha coefficients for the four groups were .82 or higher (mdn. = .86). In the 2 × 2 ANOVAs for the JSS Stress Severity scores, small but significant (p < .05) for Gender and Occupational Level main effects were found, for the Pressure and Lack of Support subscales. The mean Pressure Severity scores of the female managerial/professional and clerical/maintenance employees were higher than those of the males in these groups. The mean Lack of Support Severity scores for both males and females in the managerial/professional group were higher than those of the clerical/maintenance employees.

Means, standard deviations, and alpha coefficients for the JSS Stress Frequency Scale, and for the Pressure and Lack of Support Frequency subscales, are reported in Table 21.4. The alpha coefficients for the three JSS Frequency scales and subscales were all .83 or higher (mdn. = .855) for all four groups. When differences in Gender and Occupational Level were evaluated in 2 × 2 ANOVAs, the main effects of Occupational Level for the JSS Frequency Scale, and for the Pressure-Frequency Subscale, were highly significant (p < .001). These differences were due primarily to the higher Pressure Frequency scores of the managerial/professional group, as

Table 21.3 Mean, SD's and alpha coefficients for the JSS Stress Severity scale and the Job Pressure and Lack of Support Severity subscales, for managerial/professional and clerical/maintenance groups

Severity Scales:	Manag./ Profes.		Cleric./ Mainten.		Gender	Occupa. level	Interaction Gender/Occupa.
	F	M	F	M	F-test	F-test	F-test
ST-SEVERITY							
Mean	148.92	147.62	147.57	143.86	0.67	1.71	0.43
SD	33.81	30.01	39.66	38.74			
N	333	646	589	213			
Alpha	.91	.89	.93	.93			
PRESSURE							
Mean	45.74	44.98	46.30	43.48	5.28	0.22	2.12
SD	13.78	12.17	14.70	14.48	*		
N	338	648	588	214			
Alpha	.84	.82	.87	.86			
SUPPORT							
Mean	55.96	55.62	53.96	54.26	0.68	4.96	0.17
SD	14.40	13.51	16.51	15.89		*	
N	338	646	588	214			
Alpha	.84	.82	.86	.86			

*** = p < .001, ** = p < .01, * = p < .05

Table 21.4 Mean, SD's and alpha coefficients for the JSS Stress Frequency scale and the Job Pressure and Lack of Support Frequency subscales, for managerial/professional and clerical/maintenance groups.

Frequency scales:	Manag./ Profes.		Cleric./ Mainten.		Gender	Occup. level	Interaction gender/Occupa.
	F	M	F	M	F-test	F-test	F-test
ST-FREQUENCY							
Mean	113.28	112.09	103.79	101.31	0.75	13.98	0.06
SD	49.70	48.43	53.32	56.74		***	
N	327	628	571	210			
Alpha	.89	.89	.91	.92			
PRESSURE							
Mean	48.39	48.47	40.49	34.91	2.59	80.25	5.89
SD	22.40	21.61	22.44	23.25		***	*
N	334	636	585	213			
Alpha	.85	.84	.86	.87			
SUPPORT							
Mean	32.85	32.93	32.59	34.94	0.52	0.40	1.01
SD	21.69	21.06	21.60	22.93			
N	332	629	571	212			
Alpha	.84	.83	.84	.85			

*** $= p < .011$, ** $+ p < .01$, * $= p < .05$

compared to the scores of study participants in the clerical/maintenance group (See Table 21.4). The significant Gender-by-Occupational Level interaction effect for Pressure Frequency resulted from the very low scores of the males in the clerical/maintenance group, which were significantly lower than the scores of females in this group, and also substantially lower than the scores of both males and females in the managerial/professional group. No significant main or interactive effects were found for the Lack of Support Frequency subscale.

DISCUSSION AND CONCLUSIONS

The importance of developing good diagnostic tools for assessing specific sources of stress in the work place is considered to be a major priority by many occupational stress researchers (e.g. Barone et al., 1988; Jackson & Schuler, 1985). As recommended by Murphy and Hurell (1987), the *Job Stress Survey* is comprised of a generic set of core questions for assessing the perceived severity of specific stressor events and how frequently they occur in a wide range of occupations. The internal consistency of the JSS Stress Index, Severity and Frequency scales, and the Job Pressure and Lack of Support subscales, as measured by alpha coefficients, was quite high in this study for the male and female managerial/professional and clerical/maintenance groups.

In the factor analyses of the 30 JSS items, the Job Pressure and Lack of Organizational Support factors identified in the present study were remarkably stable for both male and female managerial/professional and clerical/maintenance workers. Moreover, the factor structure of the JSS for these groups was essentially the same as found in previous analyses of the JSS responses of corporate, university, and military personnel (Spielberger & Reheiser, 1994a). The results of the factor analyses of the 20 JSS items that best defined the Job Pressure and Lack of Organizational Support factors in this study were also remarkably similar for the male and female managerial/professional and clerical/maintenance workers, and highly consistent with the findings in previous JSS factor studies.

No differences were found between the managerial/professional and clerical/maintenance employees in their overall Stress Index or Lack of Support Index scores. In the comparisons of the mean scores for the JSS Pressure and Lack of Support Index subscales, the only major finding was a highly significant Occupational Level main effect of Job Pressure, indicating that, overall, the managerial/professional employees reported experiencing more stress from the various pressures of their jobs than the clerical/maintenance workers. The female clerical/maintenance workers had higher Pressure Index scores than the males at this occupational level. It should be noted however, that most of the females were secretarial and clerical workers, while the males were primarily employed in maintenance work or as grounds keepers. Thus, female clerical workers seem to experience more job pressures than male maintenance workers.

In the analyses of the scores on the JSS Stress Severity scale, no significant differences were found for Gender or Occupational Level. However, on the Lack of Support Severity scale, the managerial/ professional group had significantly higher scores than the clerical/ maintenance employees, and females at both occupational levels had higher Pressure Severity scores than the males in these groups. For the JSS Frequency scale and the Pressure Frequency subscale, the scores of the managerial/professional employees were much higher than those of the clerical/maintenance workers. Since no differences were found between the two occupational levels on Lack of Support Frequency, the overall difference in JSS Frequency scores was due primarily to the managerial/professional employees, who reported experiencing job pressures much more frequently than the clerical/maintenance workers.

Consistent with previous research, the findings of this study provide strong evidence that job pressures and lack of organizational support are major sources of stress in the workplace. These same two factors were identified in separate analyses of the severity and frequency ratings of the 30 JSS workplace stressors. Moreover, the job pressure and lack of organizational support factors that were found in this study were invariant for the males and females at both the higher and lower occupational levels. Although no differences were found in the JSS factor structure as a function of either gender or occupational level, the managerial/professional employees reported experiencing job pressures more frequently than the clerical/maintenance workers, which contributed to significant differences between these groups in their JSS Stress Frequency and Pressure Index scores.

References

Barone, D. F., Caddy, G. R., Katell, A. D., Roselione, F. B. & Hamilton, R. A. (1988) The Work Stress Inventory: Organizational stress and job risk. *Educational and Psychological Measurement*, **48**, 141–154.

Cattell, R. B. (1966) The meaning and strategic use of factor analysis. In *Handbook of Multivariate Experimental Psychology*, edited by R. B. Cattel. Skokie. IL: Rand McNally.

Grier, K. S. (1982) A comparison of job stress in law enforcement and teaching. Doctoral dissertation, University of South Florida, 1981. Dissertation abstracts International. **43**, 870B.

Grippa, A. J. and Durbin, D. (1986) Worker's compensation occupational disease claims. *National Council Compensation Insurance Digest*, **1**, 5–23.

Holmes, T. H. & Rahe, R. H. (1967) The Social Readjustment Rating Scale: A cross-cultural study of Western Europeans and Americans. *Journal of Psychosomatic Research*, **14**, 391–400.

Jackson, S. E. & Schuler, R. S. (1985) A meta-analysis and conceptual critique of research on role ambiguity and role conflict in work settings. *Organizational Behavior and Human Decision Process*, **36**, 16–78.

Kahn, R. L. (1981) *Work and Health*. New York: Wiley.

Kahn, R. L., Wolfe, D. M., Quinn, R. P., Snoek, J. D. & Rosenthal, R. A. (1964) *Organizational Stress: Studies in Role Conflict and Ambiguity*. New York: Wiley.

Karasek, R. A., Jr. & Theorell, T. (1990) *Healthy Work: Stress, Productivity and the Reconstruction of Working Life*. New York: Basic Books.

Kasl, S. V. (1978) Epidemiological contributions to the study of work stress. In *Stress at Work*, edited by C. L. Cooper & R. L. Payne, pp. 3–38. New York: Wiley.

Keita, G. P. & Sauter, S. L. (eds.) (1992) *Work and Well-being: An Agenda for the 1990's*. Washington, DC: American Psychological Foundation.

Kroes, W. H. (1976) *Society's Victim—the Policeman: An Analysis of Job Stress in Policing*. Springfield: Charles C. Thomas.

Kroes, W. H. & Gould, S. (1979) Job stress in policeman: An empirical study. *Police Stress*, **1**, 9–10.

Kroes, W. H., Margolis, B. & Hurrell, J. J., Jr. (1974) Job stress in policemen. *Journal of Police Science and Administration*, **2**, 145–155.

Lazarus, R. S. (1966) *Psychological Stress and the Coping Process*. New York: McGraw-Hill.

Lazarus, R. S. (1994) Psychological stress in the workplace. In *Occupational Stress: A Handbook*, edited by P. L. Perrwé & R. Crandall, pp. 3–14. New York: Taylor & Francis.

Levi, L. (1981) *Preventing Work Stress*. Rading, MA: Addison-Wesley.

Lowman, R. L. (1993) *Counseling and Psychotherapy of Work Dysfunctions*. Washington, DC: American Psychological Association.

Matteson, M. T. & Ivancevich, J. M. (1982) *Managing Job Stress and Health: The Intelligent Person's Guide*. New York: Free Press.

Murphy, J. R. & Hurell, J. J. (1987) *Controlling Work Stress: Effective Human Resource and Management Strategies*. San Francisco: Jossey-Bass.

Northwestern National Life (1991) *Employee Burnout: America's Newest Epidemic*. Minneapolis, MN: Northwestern National Life Insurance Company.

Perrewé, P. L. (ed.) (1991) Handbook on Job Stress [Special issue]. *Journal of Social Behavior and Personality*. Corte Madera: Select Press.

Quick, J. C., Murphy, L. R. & Hurrell, J. J., Jr. (eds) (1992) *Stress and Well-being at Work: Assessments and Interventions for Occupational Mental Health.* Washington, DC: American Psychological Association.

Ryland & Greenfeld (1991) In P. L. Perrewé (ed.). Handbook on Job Stress. [Special issue]. *Journal of Social Behavior and Personality*, 6, 39–54.

Sauter, S. L. (1992) Introduction to the NIOSH Proposed National Strategy. In *Work and Well-being: An Agenda for the 1990's*, edited by G. P. Keita & S. L. Sauter, (pp. 11–16). Washington, DC. American Psychological Association.

Sauter, S. L. & Murphy, L. R. (1995) *Organizational Risk Factors for Job Stress.* Washington D.C.: American Psychological Association.

Schuler, R. S. (1980) Definition and conceptualization of stress in organizations. *Organizational Behavior and Human Performance*, 25, 184–215.

Schuler, R. S. (1991) Foreword. In P. L. Perrewé (ed.). Handbook on job stress [Special issue] *Journal of Social Behavior and Personality*, 6(7), v–vi.

Spielberger, C. D. (1972) Anxiety as an emotional state. In *Anxiety: Current Trends in Theory and Research*, Vol. 1, edited by C. D. Spielberger (ed.), pp. 23–49. New York: Academic Press.

Spielberger, C. D. (1979) *Understanding Stress and Anxiety.* New York: Harper & Row.

Spielberger, C. D. (1983) *Manual for the State-Trait Anxiety Inventory (Form Y).* Palo Alto, CA: Consulting Psychologists Press.

Spielberger, C. D., Grier, K. S. & Greenfield, G. (1982, Spring) Major dimensions of stress in law enforcement. *Fraternal Order of Police Journal*, 10–12.

Spielberger, C. D., Grier, K. S. & Pate, J. M. (1980) The Police Stress Survey. *Florida Fraternal Order of Police Journal*, 66–67.

Spielberger, C. D. & Reheiser, E. C. (1994a) Job stress in university, corporate and military personnel. *International Journal of Stress Management*, 1, 19–31.

Spielberger, C. D. & Reheiser, E. C. (1994b) The Job Stress Survey: Measuring Gender Differences in Occupational Stress. *Journal of Social Behavior and Personality*, 9, 199–218.

Spielberger, C. D., Westberry, L. G., Grier, K. S. & Greenfield, G. (1981) *The Police Stress Survey: Sources of Stress in Law Enforcement* (Human Resources Institute Monograph Series Three, No. 6). Tampa, FL: University of South Florida, College of Social and Behavioral Sciences.

Turnage, J. J. & Spielberger, C. D. (1991) Job stress in managers, professionals and clerical workers. *Work and Stress*, 5, 165–176.

Vagg, P. R. & Hammond, S. B. (1976) The number and kind of invariant (Q) factors: A partial replication of Eysenck and Eysenck. *British Journal of Social and Clinical Psychology*, 15, 121–129.

Chapter 22

THE FRUSTRATION OF SUCCESS: Type A Behavior, Occupational Stress and Cardiovascular Disease

Don G. Byrne, PhD

INTRODUCTION

The unique excitement of Behavioural Medicine as an area of scientific and clinical inquiry is that it spans two broad domains, behaviour and biology, in such a way that the end result, if it is successful, has the potential to add to knowledge to an extent far greater than the simple sum of the two parts. In no respect is this more tangible than in the investigation of the causes of cardiovascular disease, and here the most resounding and far-reaching success, it may be argued, occurred in the late 1950s with the proposed existence of the Type A behaviour pattern (TABP). The notion of the TABP seems deceptively self-evident. However, the impact of the Type A construct on the evolution of knowledge in cardiovascular epidemiology over more than three decades now has been, and indeed remains, one of the most momentous landmarks of contemporary psychosomatic thought. There can now be no doubt that the TABP in one form or another is causally linked with risk or incidence of a variety of manifestations of CHD and the results of a multitude of studies addressing the problem from several perspectives, as summarised in Table 22.1, support this assertion.

Applying the demanding criteria for causal inference from epidemiological data outlined by Hill (1956) to extensive results arising

Table 22.1 Methodological categories of studies linking the Type A behaviour pattern to risk or incidence of coronary heart disease

1) Retrospective (cross-sectional) studies
2) Prospective (longitudinal) studies
3) Intervention (experimental) studies
4) Patho-physiological (angiographic) studies
5) Cardiovascular reactivity (psychophysiological) studies

from studies relating the TABP to CHD (see Table 22.2), it is clear that Type A behaviour, variously defined, continues to rank as a significant and prominent risk factor for major manifestations of coronary disease.

DEFINITIONS

The TABP, as noted above, has been defined in various ways by its leading commentators (Byrne, 1987a), not always totally overlapping in nature or theme, but maintaining a consistent conceptual thread across definitions. Rosenman's (1990) definition, clearly the most comprehensive in the recent literature, sets the current standard. For Rosenman, the TABP is:

> ... an action-emotion complex involving behavioral predispositions such as ambitiousness, aggressiveness, competitiveness and impatience; specific behaviors such as muscle tenseness, alertness, rapid and emphatic vocal stylistics, and accelerated pace of activities; and emotional responses such as irritation, hostility, and increased potential for anger (p. 2).

From this, it is quite clear that the TABP is neither unitary in character nor categorical in existence but is identified by a mix of predispositions, behaviours and emotional responses, and since its character is identified by a combination of attributes, its representation within a population is likely to vary widely across some empirically specified dimension. From the conceptual perspective of the psychologist these three suggested 'elements' of the TABP (predispositions, behaviours and emotional responses) suggest an organised, linear and very well recognised sequence of events.

One of the most simple, powerful and enduring theoretical models arising from psychology in the past two decades has been that linking predispositions, behaviours and emotional responses (Mandler, 1984). Contemporary views deriving largely from the influence of the cognitive theorists link predispositions with the uniquely individual ways in which we all perceive, interpret and form constructions of the complex world around us. From these interpretations and constructions flow reactions or behaviours evident to the external observer, the broad features of which are consistent with the message or theme of the predisposing interpretation.

Table 22.2   Hill's (1956) criteria for causal inference from epidemiological data

1) Strength of association
2) Consistency of association
3) Specificity of association
4) Temporality of association
5) Biological gradient of association
6) Biological probability of association
7) Efficacy of experimental intervention

Emotional responses then either follow, concomitant with or driven by the specific behaviour, or emerge from some combination of this and the immediate effects on the individual of the interpretive message. This simple yet compelling schema is firmly entrenched in, for example, both the theoretical and empirical works of Lazarus (1966), Zajonc & Markus (1984), and Beck and Emery (1985).

Knowing the structural elements of the TABP, however, tells us little of what the behaviour pattern actually is. But knowing what it is, is crucial since, without this knowledge, it is difficult if not impossible to understand how the TABP works or how it exerts its demonstrated pathogenic influence on the cardiovascular system. The simple model outlined above provides a start, but it is quite non-specific and applies far beyond the TABP and its effects upon the heart and circulation. One very specific suggestion has, however, prominently emerged in recent times. A substantial corpus of theory and evidence has linked the appearance of the TABP at any point in time with pre-existing environmental conditions which, through circumstances of challenge, precipitate or facilitate the appearance of behaviours making up the global TABP. Within this context, the occupational environment has received particular attention both for its ubiquity and its established empirical links with the TABP. Moreover, compelling arguments have been posited that though the TABP itself can not be thought of as constituting 'stress' by another name, the pathways of pathological influence linking the TABP with risk of CHD are very likely related to those psycho-physiological pathways traditionally associated with the deleterious effects of stress on the health of the human body (Byrne & Rosenman, 1990). Before drawing these arguments together into some integrated reformulation of Type A behaviour, it is therefore useful to review briefly the established associations between occupation and the TABP and between stress and the TABP.

TYPE A BEHAVIOUR AND OCCUPATION

Clearly, there is a body of evidence, albeit now somewhat historical in nature, which supports the view that at least some attributes of individual occupations, or the environments within which they are practised, relate statistically to risk of CHD. Nonetheless, the evidence is neither unequivocal nor consistent in its support for a strong or causal link. This raises the possibility that it is not occupation or the occupational environment *per se* that endows a risk for CHD but some interaction between the occupational situation and other psychological characteristics of the individual. The idea of interactive risk is presently capturing some attention in epidemiology (Byrne & Reinhart, 1989a). A major contender for consideration within this context involves the interaction between aspects of the occupation and the TABP.

Consideration of the TABP and of occupation suggests that they are not entirely unrelated notions (Byrne & Reinhart, 1989a). Descriptions of the TABP (see, for example, Friedman, 1969; Byrne, 1981; Herman, Blumenthal, Black & Chesney, 1981) indicate that such components as ambition, competitiveness, personal striving and time-urgency are distinctly occupationally oriented, and there is clear evidence for an association between the TABP and occupational status (Byrne, Rosenman, Schiller & Chesney, 1985; Chesney & Rosenman, 1980). The relationship between crudely measured occupational status and at least some measures of the TABP is well documented, with high-status occupations being associated with high scores on scales of the TABP (Byrne & Reinhart, 1989b), (though as Chesney et al. (1981) point out, this may not be so for all measures of TABP). Given the persuasive evidence of associations between the TABP and occupation, and the unique though less clear-cut associations which they each have with risk of CHD, the question arises as to whether some combination of the two may endow coronary risk to a degree greater than that attributable to either individually.

Few studies have systematically or empirically addressed the issue of the precise relationship between occupation and the TABP, and even fewer have looked at these two variables, in combination, in relation to risk or symptoms of CHD. Recent work by the present author has, however, examined both areas in some detail, and in large and representative samples of currently employed people. A brief overview of these may serve to illustrate the quite intimate relationship which exists between occupation and the TABP.

In an extensive study of Type A behaviour and the occupational environment undertaken in a large sample of senior government employees in Australia (Byrne & Reinhart, 1989a), questionnaires were used to comprehensively assess both the TABP and occupational structure. These consisted of: (a) Form C of the Jenkins Activity Survey (JAS) (Jenkins, Zyzanski & Rosenman, 1979), providing a Global Scale of the TABP together with Scales of Speed and Impatience (S), Job Involvement (J) and Hard Driving (H); and (b) Questions constructed to quantify (i) job characteristics related to the structure of the occupational organisation but beyond personal control, (ii) time commitment to the job, beyond the standard working hours, and (iii) degree of personal involvement allowed in occupational decisions (all questions were asked in a standard format and scored on four-point Likert scales). The nature of these measures and the rationale for their use are considered more fully by Byrne & Reinhart (1989a).

Table 22.3 presents distributions for JAS Scale scores for the entire first sample, together with percents of individuals in the Type A and Type B ranges of the distribution (using the arbitrary JAS Scale means of 0 as cut-off points). It also presents intercorrelations between JAS Scale scores.

There is little remarkable about these data except for the somewhat Type B nature of the sample with regard to the H Scale of the JAS. No sex differences were evident in these scales.

Table 22.3   Sample distributions of the Jenkins Activity Scale (JAS) scores

JAS Scale	Mean	SD
Global	−2.90	9.22
Speed and Impatience (S)	−1.73	9.56
Job Involvement (J)	−2.92	9.22
Hard Driving (H)	−4.38	9.15

Percent of subjects falling above or below the arbitrary mean of 0 on each of the scales.

	<0	>0
Global	60.9%	39.1%
Speed and Impatience (S)	58.6%	41.4%
Job Involvement (J)	61.1%	38.9%
Hard Driving (H)	71.4%	28.6%

Intercorrelations between JAS Scale scores, occupational level and occupational structure are shown in Table 22.4.

Occupational level correlated consistently, significantly, and in expected ways, with measures of occupational structure. The Global and J Scales of the JAS, too, correlated consistently, significantly and sometimes strongly with measures of occupational structure; the H Scales was less consistently related to occupational structure and the S Scale hardly at all.

Table 22.4   Correlations between Jenkins Activity Survey scale scores, occupational level and job characteristics

Occupational measures	Type A behavior pattern				
	Global Type A	Speed	Job Involvement	Hard Driving	Occupational Level
Occupational level	.15**	.07	.21***	.01	−
No. of people supervised	.12**	.06	.03	.06	.31***
No. of years in present position	−.09	−.08	−.17***	.01	.06
Time of arrival at work	−.08	−.07	.07	.03	−.11**
Time of leaving work	.23***	.13**	.34***	.21***	.28***
Length of training period required for present position	−.12**	−.02	−.06	−.09	.05
Perceived likelihood of promotion	.18***	.06	.20***	.16**	.02
Standard working hours per week	.32***	.19***	.26***	.24***	.33***
Excess working hours per week	.27***	.08	.32***	.29***	.17***
Feelings about overtime	.16***	.02**	.30***	.17***	.14***
Frequency of weekend work	.31***	.15**	.44***	.24***	.32***

**p < .01, ***p < .001.
Source: From Byrne & Reinhart, 1989a.

Since the TABP is known to relate to occupational level, partial correlations between these two variables were calculated while simultaneously controlling for measures of occupational structure, to investigate whether such associations were mediated through occupational structure, either imposed by the organisation or by the individual. These partial correlations are shown in Table 22.5. Analyses were only undertaken for the Global and J Scales of the JAS since the S and H Scales did not correlate with occupational level.

Associations between the TABP (Global and J Scales of the JAS) and occupational level generally held when those characteristics of occupational structure imposed by the organisation were controlled for. When aspects of the occupational structure reflecting the operation of personal initiative were controlled for, however, associations between the TABP and occupational level either substantially diminished or completely disappeared.

As expected, JAS Scale scores did correlate significantly and positively with occupational level, though only for the Global and J Scales of the instrument. JAS Scale scores, and particularly the Global, J and H Scales, also correlated broadly, significantly and positively with measures of occupational structure, both self- and organisationally imposed. Tacit acceptance of the interdependence of the TABP and occupation has existed for some time (Jenkins, 1978) and some limited empirical evidence is available to support this (Howard, Cunningham & Rechnitzer, 1977). Much

Table 22.5 Partial correlations between Jenkins Activity Survey Global Type A and Job Involvement scales and occupational level, controlling for job characteristics[a]

Job Characteristic	Global Type A Scale with occupational level (simple $r = .15**$)	Job Involvement Scale with occupational level (simple $r = .21***$)
No. of people supervised	.12**	.19***
No. of years in present position	.15**	.21***
Time of arrival at work	.14**	.20***
Time of leaving work	.09	.12*
Length of training period required for present position	.15**	.21**
Perceived likelihood of promotion	.15**	.19***
Feelings about overtime	.13**	.16**
Frequency of weekend work	.05	.07
Standard working hours per week	.05	.13**
Excess working hours per week	.11*	.14**

[a]Because only the Global Type A and Job Involvement scales of the Jenkins Activity Survey correlated significantly with occupational level, partial correlations are presented only for these scales.
$**p < .01$, $***p < .001$.
Source: From Byrne & Reinhart, 1989a.

of the evidence has, however, been restricted to demonstrated associations between the TABP and simple indices of occupational level, and a more comprehensive overview of the TABP in relation to components of the occupational setting has only recently emerged. It should be clear from even a thematic analysis of the TABP, however, that with its emphasis on striving, achievement orientation, competitiveness, time urgency and goal directed hostility, the behavior pattern is eminently suited to foster occupational achievement or at least the pursuit of it.

In this regard, then, it is not surprising that associations between the TABP and occupational level, largely undifferentiated in previous studies, appeared to be mediated by those characteristics of the occupational environment over which the individual exercised some personal control. This was particularly so for aspects of the occupation to do with discretionary time commitment to the job. Individuals manifesting Type A attributes centering on competition and achievement might well be expected to devote time in excess of that demanded by the organisation in order to ensure advancement. The finding is also consistent with evidence long known of the TABP, that such individuals strive to exert control over their environments, whether occupational or otherwise (Byrne, Reinhart & Heaven, 1989).

OCCUPATIONAL STRESS AND CORONARY HEART DISEASE

Sources of Occupational Stress

One major source derives from the nature of occupations themselves. Both differences within (Russek, 1960) and differences between (French & Caplan, 1970) occupations have been linked to stress. Occupational stress, it is claimed, may also result from the manner of remuneration (self-paid or salaried) existing in particular work situations (Magnus, Matroos & Strackel, 1983). Disparities in employment status for women may give rise to occupational stress (Haynes & Feinleib, 1980). The level of job demand (Haynes, Feinleib, Levine, Scotch & Kannel, 1978), the nature of the workload (Magnus et al., 1983), and the degree of perceived work satisfaction (Sales & House, 1971) have also been suggested to contribute significantly to stress in the workplace. Occupational stress has been related to individual employee personality and to the level of social support derived from the workplace (Haynes & Feinleib, 1980). The degree of personal control given to workers in relation to the job demands confronting them have, in the past decade, aroused considerable interest as a source of occupational stress (Karasek, Baker, Marxer, Ahlborn & Theorell, 1981).

The Relationship Between Occupational Stress and CHD

Differences within some occupational groups have been linked with the incidence of CHD. The exemplary work of Russek (1960) demonstrated that a group of middle-aged general medical practitioners had a measurably higher rate of CHD than a group of same-age specialists in dermatology. Russek (1965) further found that rates of CHD among sub-specialities within medicine, law and dentistry varied positively with the imputed level of occupational stress within each of these groups, though Friedman & Hellersten (1968) failed to replicate this finding in a study of occupational stress and its relationship to CHD in a sample of individuals employed in various sub-specialties of the legal profession.

Public versus the private sector employment for any single occupational group may also affect rates of CHD. In a longitudinal study involving samples of bank employees working in either the public or private sector, it was found that the incidence of CHD was greater in the sample of private bank employees. The authors explain this finding in terms of the much greater pressure experienced by employees in private as compared with public banking institutions (Kornitzer, Kittel, Debacker & Dramaix, 1981; Kornitzer, Tilly, Van Roux & Balthazar, 1975).

Apart from differences in rates of CHD within occupations, there is evidence that consistent differences in rates of CHD are also to be found between occupational groups. The high CHD mortality rate among merchant naval officers in Norway relative to the population average has been attributed (Mundal, Erikssen & Rodahl, 1982) to occupational stress, as was a similarly high CHD mortality rate among merchant naval officers in West Germany (Zorn, Harrington & Goethe, 1977). In a study investigating occupational differences in CHD prevalence, French & Caplan (1970) found that blue collar, trade employees and managers had a much higher incidence of CHD than engineers or scientists, and this was found to be the case irrespective of age. It was argued that these differences were due to the higher levels of occupational stress in blue collar workers and in managerial staff relative to engineers and scientists. Other studies have shown, however, that professions of roughly equal social status experience widely disparate rates of CHD (Kasl, 1978). The teaching profession, for example, was shown to have lower CHD rates as a group when compared with the total population, whereas other professional cohorts (lawyers, surgeons, and real estate agents, for example) had a much higher rate of CHD than the population as a whole. Again, different levels of occupational stress have been linked with these differences in rates of CHD across occupational groups.

In a major study of the occupational characteristics of patients who had experienced their first episode of acute myocardial infarction (MI) (Bolm-Audorff & Siegrist, 1983), it was found that blue collar occupations were significantly over-represented when compared with the incidence of MI in the total population. Stress in the workplace was posited as the likely reason for this finding. Within the white collar group, however, differences between the incidence of acute MI were also evident. For example, pilots, air traffic controllers, and managers all had higher rates of MI than members of other occupational groupings, and again, occupational stress was offered as a likely explanation.

Self-employed individuals have been found to have a much higher rate of CHD than those with employee status. More specifically, Magnus, Matroos & Strackel (1983) concluded that self-employed persons are at twice the risk of CHD than those persons not self-employed. It is worth noting that very little work has been done with female samples, though the little that is available seems to corroborate the evidence for male samples. Certain groups of working women have been found to be at higher risk than for CHD than other groups. In particular, clerical workers have been found to have higher rates of CHD than women generally (Haw, 1982; Haynes & Feinleib, 1980). The picture is more complicated for women than for men, however, because a large percentage of women do not work and the dual roles of working and caring for a family may compound the stress profile in a way not evident in male samples.

The relationship between work demands and CHD is far from clear. Whereas early research (Liljefors & Rahe, 1970) supports a positive association between work demands (in this case, number of hours worked) and the incidence of MI, later research has not, for the most part, confirmed this simple association. Although the Framingham study (Haynes, Feinleib & Kannel, 1980; Haynes, Feinleib, Levine, Scotch & Kannel, 1978) examined associations between work demands (measured by an index of work load) and CHD among a sample of older workers, it failed to establish such an association for younger age groups. Moreover, the work demand measure did not make a significant independent contribution to the prediction of the prevalence of CHD. Magnus et al. (1983) also failed to find an association between excessive working hours and time pressure and the incidence of CHD. In addition, Maschewsky (1982) found only equivocal support for the association between work demands (measured by items covering length of working hours, pressure on time, and responsibilities at work) and acute coronary events, although workers experiencing MI were shown to rate significantly higher on other work demand indices. Theorell & Rahe (1971) reported similarly equivocal patterns in their comparison of the work demands experienced by a group who had suffered an episode of MI and a group of healthy workers. The former rated significantly higher on some measures of work demands but the latter rated higher on other dimensions of this variable.

Results from cross-cultural research have even further confused the picture. In one study (Orth-Gomer, 1979), groups of Swedes and Americans who had suffered from CHD were compared with healthy samples in each country. Whereas the Swedish sample of CHD victims reported higher rates of job demand than the comparison sample, the opposite pattern emerged for the American sample. Overall, the links between work demands and the prevalence of acute coronary disorders seem tenuous at best, and are perhaps nonexistent.

One reason for the failure to find more consistent results in the study investigating the link between work demands and CHD may be the simplicity of the measures of work demand that have been employed. It has been suggested that composite measures of work load (including psychosocial as well as physical work stressors) are necessary to adequately assess the relationship between work stressors and CHD. Such composite measures have been positively associated with CHD in samples of individuals recovering from CHD (Magnus et al., 1983). In a further study employing a composite measure of workload, Theorell & Floderus-Myrhed (1977) found that frequency of occupationally demanding activities was significantly higher in those with MI than for the population as a whole.

It has been further suggested that job satisfaction (or rather dissatisfaction) is positively associated with rates of CHD (Sales & House, 1971), but this interpretation is under review (Frank & Weintraub, 1973). For the most part, no consistent association has been found between measures of job satisfaction and the incidence of CHD (Theorell & Rahe, 1971).

In a more sophisticated model, the lack of control that an individual feels at work and the excessive demands that individuals feel subjected to in the workplace have both been found to be positively related to CHD. Alfredson, Karasek & Theorell (1982) assessed whether high work demands and low opportunities for control at work were risk factors in CHD. Employing a large and representative sample of individuals engaged in a wide range of occupations in Sweden, they found that the hectic nature of work coupled with a lack of control over work practices was significantly associated with the risk of MI. Also they found that shift work (a high demand characteristic) and monotony (a low control characteristic) were significantly though independently related to the risk of MI. It must be pointed out, however, that where physical job requirements and other possible risk factors (e.g. cigarette smoking and low education level) were simultaneously taken into consideration, the relationship between shift work and CHD risk disappeared (Alfredson & Theorell, 1983). All other relationships were maintained.

In a further study, Karasek, Baker, Marxer, Ahkborn & Theorell (1981) investigated the relationship between actual job characteristics and the risk of CHD, and found it to be predicted by a combination of high job demands and low intellectual discretion. By matching the characteristics of control subjects who had died from CHD, Karasek et al. (1981) also found that the risk of CHD was significantly increased for individuals experiencing high work demands coupled with low personal freedom.

A longitudinal study by Langosch, Brodner & Borcherding (1983) investigated the association between job demand and control characteristics, on the one hand, and the severity and progression of CHD on the other. It was reported that the high work demands (including doing too many tasks at the same time) and lack of job control (uncontrollable job stress) were positively and significantly related to the severity of CHD as well as to the progression of that disease.

Siegrist (1984) assessed the influence on rates of CHD, of low levels of control and high levels of demand in the workplace. Time urgency (a high demand characteristic), feelings of hopelessness and anger, and severe sleep disturbances (low control characteristics) were found to be significantly related to rates of CHD, and these findings may thus also be taken to support the notion that high work demands and low control at work are important contributors to CHD.

One final factor may be added to this overview. Haynes & Feinleib (1980), in attempting to explain high rates of CHD in women holding clerical jobs relative to women in other occupational categories, invoked the suggestion that women in the former group experienced, *inter alia*, a significant lack of social support in the workplace. While there is little other evidence to link inadequate social support with CHD risk, it has recently been demonstrated for men (Orth-Gomer & Johnson, 1987), and in view of the persuasive arguments associating lack of social support with rates of psychological disorder (Henderson, Byrne & Duncan-Jones, 1981), the area may be well worthy of further investigation.

TYPE A BEHAVIOUR, ANXIETY AND AFFECTIVE DISTRESS

Traditional views of the TABP have expressly and consistently dissociated it from equivalence either with stress or distress (Rosenman, 1990). Indeed, Type A individuals are reported to be largely unaware of the time-urgent, job involved, competitive and hostile behaviours which often so clearly characterise them for the external observer (Rosenman, 1988), or at least the negative aspects of these behaviours (Herman, Blumenthal, Black & Chesney, 1981), and there is some evidence that they may actively suppress recognition of these behaviours and their experiential consequences (Hart, 1983). Yet the TABP is defined, *inter alia*, as an '... action-emotion complex ...' (Rosenman, 1990, p.2), and a volume of empirical evidence links possession of the behaviour pattern with the experience of affective distress manifesting in some form or other. Of course, statistical correlations imply neither equivalence nor causality (Susser, 1973). However, in the light of the now current evidence, the links between the TABP and the experience of emotional discomfort need to be recognised and examined.

While work from several sources could be cited in discussion of this, findings from various studies undertaken and reported by the present author (Byrne et al., 1985; Byrne & Reinhart, 1990; Byrne & Rosenman, 1987) bear directly on the issue and may be presented in some detail. Table 22.6 shows associations between an interview measure of the TABP, and simultaneous measures of emotional distress and discomfort (the State Anxiety or A-State Scale of the STAI (Spielberger, Gorsuch & Lushene, 1970) and the Somatisation, Interpersonal Sensitivity, Depression and Anxiety Scales of Derogatis' (1974) Hopkins Symptom Check List or SCL 90), derived from a large sample of occupationally heterogeneous Australian males.

Table 22.6   Associations between the Structured Interview measure of the TABP and measures of emotional distress and discomfort (the SCL 90)

	Structured Interview Classification				
	A1	A2	X	B	F=
Somatisation	18.20	16.30	15.99	15.78	2.61*
Interpersonal Sensitivity	13.51	13.21	12.82	11.88	2.15
Depression	19.80	18.80	18.52	16.85	3.09*
Anxiety	14.69	13.48	13.04	12.34	3.86**

*$p < 0.05$, **$p < 0.01$
Source: From Byrne & Rosenman, 1986.

Table 22.7 presents associations between self-reported Type A behaviour and this same set of measures of emotional distress and discomfort.

State anxiety (A-State) was unrelated to the TABP as established by the SI, and failed to correlate with any JAS Scale but that of H, where the association was only marginally significant. The Somatisation, Depression and Anxiety Scales of the SCL 90 were, however, significantly associated with both interview established and self-reported Type A behaviour, though in the latter case, only with the Global and S Scales of the JAS. In this latter regard, the magnitude of associations with emotional distress was noticeably greater for the S than for the Global Scale of the JAS.

These findings were largely paralleled in a completely separate sample of Australians employed in an equally diverse range of occupations (Byrne & Reinhart, 1990), where both the Global and S Scales of the JAS correlated significantly with a range of measures of both anxiety and depression, but where associations were noticeably stronger for the S than for the Global Scale. The data may be seen in Table 22.8.

Table 22.7   Associations (Pearson product-moment correlations) between a self-report measure of the TABP (the Jenkins Activity Survey) and measures of emotional distress and discomfort (the SCL 90)

	JAS Scale			
	Global	Speed & Impatience	Job Involvement	Hard Driving
Somatisation	0.15**	0.23**	−0.02	0.06
Interpersonal Sensitivity	0.17**	0.28**	−0.05	0.09
Depression	0.15**	0.25**	−0.02	0.10*
Anxiety	0.23**	0.31**	0.06	0.09

*$p < 0.05$, **$p < 0.01$
Source: From Byrne & Rosenman, 1986.

Table 22.8 Associations (Pearson product-moment correlations) between a self-report measure of the TABP (the Global and S Scales of the Jenkins Activity Survey) and measures of emotional distress and discomfort (the A-State Scale of the STAI, the Anxiety and Depression Scales of the SCL 90), and the General Health Questionnaire.

	JAS Scale	
	Global	Speed & Impatience
A-State	0.21**	0.39**
Anxiety	0.27**	0.38**
Depression	0.15**	0.35**
GHQ	0.32**	0.31**

**$p < 0.01$
Source: From Byrne & Reinhart, 1990.

In this study, however, a measure of self-reported psychiatric symptomatology, the General Health Questionnaire (GHQ) of Goldberg (1972) was also administered, and as Table 22.8 shows, the same pattern of correlations emerged. Those with the TABP, it seems, at least as it is measured by self-report, experience greater levels of emotional distress and conspicuous psychiatric symptomatology than do those in whom the behaviour pattern is relatively less apparent.

Without labouring these simple correlations beyond their real importance, two explanations come immediately to mind to account for the findings. The first of these is, quite simply, that the experiential state of 'being Type A' engenders a state of physical discomfort. When patterns of association between the TABP and emotional distress are examined, it is clear that the behavioural scales of the JAS (the Global and S Scales) rather than the attitudinal scales (the J and H Scales) show the strongest and most consistent correlations. Thus, it may well be that the speed and time pressure characteristic of the TABP, taken together with the autonomic arousal potentially activated by the behaviour pattern, are sufficiently similar subjective states to what is commonly agreed to be anxiety (at least as James (1892) conceived of anxiety), that from an experiential perspective they may be interpreted as and described in very similar terms (Byrne, 1996). Put more bluntly, behaving in Type A ways may heighten autonomic arousal to a point where continued manifestation of the behaviour pattern becomes an affectively unpleasant experience.

The second explanation, in no way exclusively dissociated from the first, rests with the link between the TABP and both exposure to and interpretation of stressful life events (Byrne, 1981; Byrne & Rosenman, 1987). It is now clear from both these and confirmatory studies (see, for example, Vingerhoets & Flohr, 1984) that those with the TABP both encounter more life events over a specified sampling period than those without the behaviour pattern, and interpret those life events as carrying greater distressing personal impact. This is not surprising. However one measure the TABP, one consistently salient feature is that it involves a set of response tendencies, perhaps in the face of environmental challenge, which bear on the establishment and organisation of lifestyles. Indeed, given the identifying behavioural characteristics of the TABP, it would be expected that Type A individuals would organise their lives differently from those without such characteristics. The nature of Type A behavioural (and indeed attitudinal) characteristics are, by definition, totally consonant with a life-style which would expose an individual to a range of occupational, social and personal stressors in excess of that accompanying a life-style organised in the absence of these characteristics. Why those with the TABP should interpret their apparent excess of external stressors as carrying greater personal impact than those without the TABP, is not nearly so clear. It is of interest, however, to note that when the presence of N is controlled for, the association between the TABP and interpretations of life event impact largely disappear, suggesting that it may be the presence of co-existing but independent attributes, and not the existence of the TABP alone, which mostly accounts for this perhaps spurious association (Byrne & Rosenman, 1987).

Thus, both interview and self-report measures of the TABP appear to be consistently associated with measures of emotional distress or discomfort, and there are at least two plausible reasons which this might be expected. Neither reason, however, argues for an equivalence between the TABP and either emotional distress or indeed 'stress' as it is defined in the contemporary literature (Byrne & Rosenman, 1990). Rather, the emotional distress which may accompany the TABP is better seen as an *epi-phenomenon*; it is distress either driven by the behavioural expression of the TABP, or arising from the time-pressured and competitive life-style which Type A individuals set up for themselves (or perhaps a combination of these).

TYPE A BEHAVIOUR AS CORONARY-PRONE BEHAVIOUR

In the light of this evidence, the TABP should not be confused with simple presence of stress or distress, whether this derives from an occupational source or whether it has its origins elsewhere. Indeed, as Rosenman has consistently emphasised over the now long history of the TABP as an explanatory construct in cardiovascular epidemiology (Rosenman, 1990), Type A behaviour is *behaviour* and not personality. The predisposition of any individual to the TABP may well exist as a set of cognitive maps filtering environmental experiences for salient cues and setting the directions and parameters of response patterns to those cues. It is those collective responses, however, objectively evident to the outside observer, which is the TABP. If that behaviour pattern is therefore to have pathophysiological significance for CHD, as the epidemiological evidence shows it clearly does, its paths of influence must be seen to arise directly through the behaviours themselves. Evidence for a differential pathogenicity of the several recognised elements of the TABP is sketchy (Matthews & Haynes, 1986) but behavioural rather than attitudinal elements are the better predictors of CHD (Byrne et al., 1985), and this is quite consistent with the view emphasising the centrality of manifest behaviours to the overall construct.

Like all other identified risk factors[2] for CHD however, the TABP reflects the fundamental epidemiological conundrum, that nowhere near all individuals clearly and indisputably characterised by the TABP ultimately fall prey to a clinical episode of CHD. The TABP in varying degrees is evident in around 40% of the adult male population in many Western developed countries (Byrne & Reinhart, 1995) and most of these individuals live a full and expected life-span apparently free of any cardiovascular disease. Moreover, a number of recent studies have failed to report persuasive and positive, causal associations between the TABP and manifestations of cardiovascular disease, including myocardial infarction (MI) (Ragland & Brand, 1988; Shekelle, Gale & Norussis, 1985) and coronary artery atherosclerosis (Bass & Wade, 1982) (nor, it should be stated, have they been explicitly negative), prompting calls for a re-evaluation of the predictive utility of the TABP in studies of cardiovascular epidemiology (see, for example, Matthews & Haynes, 1986). It has been argued that studies unsupportive of the link between the TABP and CHD have been so because of inadequate and at times inappropriate measurement of the behaviour pattern (Byrne, 1987a); even so, it is clear that studies attempting to establish simple, linear associations between Type A behaviours and CHD have not been uniformly successful.

Rosenman's (1990) definition of the TABP clearly portrays it as a collection of behaviours and not a single behavioural entity. This view is reflected by, for example, the multi-faceted structure of the JAS (Jenkins, Zyzanski & Rosenman, 1979), albeit to an arguably limited extent (Byrne et al., 1985). Correlations between the various identified elements of the TABP are typically far less than unity (Byrne & Reinhart, 1995), though of course this is to be expected if the TABP is believed to be more than a global or monolithic construct. By extrapolation therefore, as was earlier noted, possession of the TABP by any unselected individual is likely to vary both in nature and degree from that manifested by any other unselected individual in the same population. All this being so, if Type A behaviour is now to be considered as coronary-prone behaviour, it must be conceded that only parts of the total pattern may be potentially pathogenic, and even further, that this pathogenic influence may only be evident under certain circumstances. Accordingly, the time may well have come to deconstruct

---

[2] Some would argue that the term 'risk factor' implies a universality of influence, and that the term 'risk marker' should be used instead to refer to those conditions, either exogenous or endogenous to the individual, which increase the statistical risk of illness but do not infallibly predict it.

the traditional epidemiological view of the TABP as a single, coronary-prone entity, suggesting instead a somewhat re-ordered sequence of attitudinal and behavioural events which, if ultimately supported by empirical evidence, may not only reinforce the currency of the TABP as a coronary risk factor, but endow it with even greater sensitivity in predicting individual events of CHD. Let me now venture some speculations as to what this re-ordered sequence of events might be.

In reconstructing a deconstructed model of Type A behaviour to better accommodate the obvious empirical demand for a more sophisticated explanatory sequence, the first step must clearly be the identification of the most fundamental or basic component of that model (see, for example, Craik, 1948). Price (1982) proposed a cognitive model of Type A behaviour based on the principles of social learning. The behavioural manifestations of the TABP, she asserts, arise from a set of fears linked to personal beliefs developed through socialisation and then acting in the mature individual to impart 'meaning' to current and ongoing environmental experiences (Price, 1982, p. 38). The detailed substance of this elegant argument, and in particular the proposed links between beliefs and fears, may be debated; what is far more important, however, is the assertion that the TABP has its basis in belief systems established early in life and acting as cognitive maps which regulate interpretations of subsequent environmental experiences. The notion of cognitive antecedents to all manifest behaviour is, of course, fundamental to many theories of behaviour, as this paper has earlier pointed out.

While Price (1982) has suggested that three beliefs form the foundation of Type A behaviour ('the belief that one must constantly improve himself' (p. 66), 'the belief that no universal moral principle exists' (p. 68), and 'the belief that all resources are scarce' (p. 70)), Rosenman (1988) foreshadowed what appears self-evidently to be a more basic and central cognitive set to considerations of the TABP, that being competitiveness[3]. Several reasons may be advanced to put competitiveness so prominently within a reconstructed model of the TABP. First, it has evolutionary significance; it is phylogenetically old and endows survival advantage through competition for resources (Montagu, 1976), and thus it may be fundamental to the most successful members of the species. Second, it bears a close conceptual and thematic relationship to the need for exertion of control over the environment, and the empirical evidence linking the TABP with need for control is strong and abundant (Glass, 1977). Third, there is a good deal of

---

[3] While it may be said that competitiveness is itself a behaviour and not a belief, it is theoretically more correct to see it as a motivational predisposition to behaviours of many kinds (Young, 1961), including achievement oriented behaviours, acquisitive behaviours, aggressive behaviours and behaviours designed to exert control over the environment. In this sense, competitiveness is a belief or attitude which motivates manifest behaviours rather than a behaviour in and of itself.

evidence to suggest that as well as phylogenetically programmed antecedents, competitiveness is readily acquired in the young child by modelling or vicarious social learning (Bandura, 1976). Fourth and perhaps most important, there is a direct albeit implicit conceptual link between competitiveness and so many of the manifest behaviours which give the TABP its identifiable character, including achievement oriented behaviours, behaviours reflecting time urgency and the apportionment of discretionary time to activities, hard-driven, acquisitive and accumulative behaviours, and intolerant tenacity in the face of opposition. Coincidentally, measures of competitiveness with peers, derived post hoc from Structured Interview assessments of the TABP, have been shown to predict CHD in prospective studies (Matthews, Glass, Rosenman & Bortner, 1977). Moreover, various assessments and ratings of what has been explicitly labelled 'competitive-ness' have been shown to relate to dysfunctional cardiovascular reactivity, at least in male subjects (Houston, 1988). Let me then, perhaps a little incautiously, suggest competitiveness as the cognitive set (motivational predisposition if you wish) which sits at the very base of the TABP.

The view that competitiveness may underlie a broad range of behaviours collectively typifying the TABP provides one immediate pathway through which the link between the behaviour pattern and CHD may be explored. The motivational nature of competitiveness links it directly with a state of non-specific, elevated sympathetic arousal which may become chronic if competitiveness persists, and this is strongly supported by a long history of literature on the psychology of motivation (Hoyenga & Hoyenga, 1984; Young, 1961). Moreover, as has been noted earlier in this paper, the Type A behaviours arising from competitiveness may themselves drive the individual to a state of heightened sympathetic arousal simply because they push that individual to a greater pace of activity in an effort to win the competition and achieve (Byrne & Rosenman, 1987).

There are two reasons, however, why this path to a pathophysiological influence may be secondary to a more important one. First, the evidence causally linking acute and non-specific sympathetic arousal to risk or incidence of CHD is not strong (Rosenman & Ward, 1988). Second, many individuals exhibit both competitiveness and the host of manifest Type A behaviours which I am suggesting arise from it, and few of these go on to experience a clinical event of CHD. Indeed, it seems that under some circumstances and in particular environments, many individuals not only show no sign of distress or disease, but report the experience in positive terms (Byrne & Reinhart, 1989a). Environments which allow free expression to the TABP, potential for personal control and permission to pursue achievement stand out in this respect, and if one such environment is typical, this is the 'white-collar' or executive occupational environment. By contrast, the 'blue-collar' occupational environment appears structurally better suited to the frustration of competitiveness and its accompanying Type A behaviours (Byrne & Reinhart, 1989a, 1989b, 1994). Thus, just as traditional views of the TABP link the appearance of the behaviour pattern to environmental challenge (Rosenman & Chesney, 1981), the prevailing environment may also act to frustrate the complete expression of those behaviours once evoked. It is frustration, I believe, which along with competitiveness, forms the key to the pathophysiological influence of the TABP.

The notion of frustration as a psychological construct comes with a long and classic literature (Lawson, 1965; Yates, 1962). Frustration may be defined briefly as situational denial or obstruction of a well motivated behavioural response. The most immediate and short-term consequence of frustration is behavioural persistence to achieve the desired goals (Yates, 1962). In the longer term, however, two responses become clearly apparent (Lawson, 1965); the first is aggression directed towards the environmental situation (and other individuals in it), and the second is anxiety as the frustrated individual faces the prospect of failure to achieve desired goals. In so far as the early experimental evidence allows comment, there seems to be a noticeable if somewhat loose relationship between the strength of the frustrating circumstance and the intensity of the consequent aggression and anxiety (Yates, 1962). Both anxiety (Byrne & Rosenman, 1987, 1990) and aggression (Chesney & Rosenman, 1985) have, of course, been consistently seen to accompany the TABP. In the light of this proposed model, aggression (or anger/hostility, since the two notions are essentially synonymous in this context), a construct which has until recently been posited as central to the TABP (Chesney & Rosenman, 1985), must now be viewed as a response to frustrated Type A behaviours rather than an integral element of the TABP itself.

Simply stated then, the reconstructed model of the TABP proposes competitiveness to be at the foundation of manifest Type A behaviours. Whether competitiveness is conceived of as a cognitive filter regulating interpretations of environmental experiences or a motivational state, it has the capacity to trigger individual behaviours which have now been identified as the TABP. These behaviours themselves may, by their time-pressured and achievement oriented nature, drive a level of sympathetic arousal which is elevated above some arbitrary but healthy baseline (Byrne & Rosenman, 1987). They may also lead the individual into the organisation of lifestyles which promote encounters with affectively distressing life events (Byrne & Rosenman, 1987). By and large, however, manifest Type A behaviours allowed free expression within the unique environmental circumstances of any unselected individual may have little consequence other than somewhat elevated levels of sympathetic arousal and, perhaps, feelings of some subjective distress, whether acute or chronic. Manifest Type A behaviours frustrated by unique individual environments, however, will give rise both to anxiety and aggression, possibly both intense and chronic, with the neurophysiological and neuroendocrinological sequelae which are known to accompany these states. It is these accompanying changes which might provide the biological link between the TABP and CHD. The elements of this proposed model are presented in Figure 22.1 below.

There is some very early evidence on the association between frustrated Type A behaviours and CHD. The hypothesis was tested in a sample of 1113 Australian government employees, specially sampled for their breadth of occupational levels. The TABP was measured by self-report (the Jenkins Activity Survey) and coronary risk was assessed, in this study, by a diagnosis of Angina Pectoris (AP) based on responses to a standardised clinical investigation for chest pain (the Rose Chest Pain Questionnaire). The overall prevalence of Angina Pectoris (6.7%) was somewhat high for the age group, but within reasonable bounds.

Scores on the JAS Scales of the TABP, when broken down by case status (AP or not) and the data, are shown in Table 22.9. Those with AP were significantly more Type A on the Global and H Scales than those free or coronary symptoms, while the effect approached significance for the S Scale. The self-reported TABP seems, therefore, to have some independent association with presence of coronary symptoms, though as expected, not a particularly strong one.

There was no independent association of occupational level (white or blue collar) with prevalence of self-reported Angina Pectoris. There was, however, a highly significant effect when the TABP was examined in conjunction with occupational level. These data, shown in Figures 22.2 to 22.5, reveal that by far the highest prevalence of AP is to be found in those

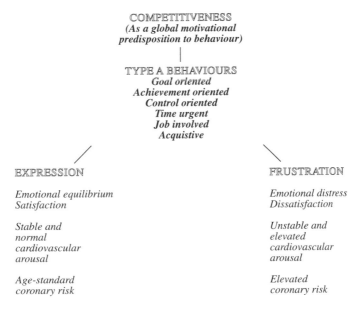

Figure 22.1 Type A Behaviour as Coronary Prone Behaviour: A Re-conceptualisation (From Byrne, 1996).

Table 22.9   Type A Behaviour (JAS Scale Scores) broken down by Self-Reported Chest Pain Status

JAS Scale/Chest Pain		Mean	SD	Cases (N=)	F
Global	Pain	−0.84	9.19	75	4.03*
	No Pain	−3.05	9.20	1038	
Speed & Impatience	Pain	0.04	8.68	75	2.74
	No Pain	−1.86	9.61	1038	
Job Involvement	Pain	−2.53	9.73	75	0.14
	No Pain	−2.94	9.19	1038	
Hard Driving	Pain	−1.67	9.48	75	7.21**
	No Pain	−4.59	9.09	1038	

*$p < 0.05$, **$p < 0.01$
Source: From Byrne & Reinhart, 1986.

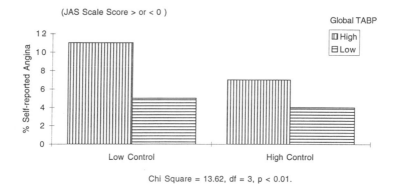

Chi Square = 13.62, df = 3, p < 0.01.

Figure 22.2   Self reported Chest Pain in Low Control (Blue Collar) and High Control (White Collar) Subjects with and without Global Type A Behaviour. (*Source*: from Byrne & Reinhart, 1989b).

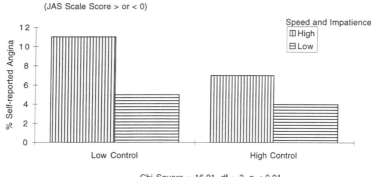

Chi Square = 16.91, df = 3, p < 0.01

Figure 22.3   Self reported Chest Pain in Low Control (Blue Collar) and High Control (White Collar) Subjects with High and Low JAS Speed and Impatience Scores (*Source*: From Byrne & Reinhart, 1989b).

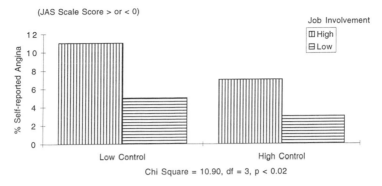

Figure 22.4   Self reported Chest Pain in Low Control (Blue Collar) and High Control (White Collar) Subjects with High and Low JAS Job-Involvement Scores (*Source*: From Byrne & Reinhart, 1989b).

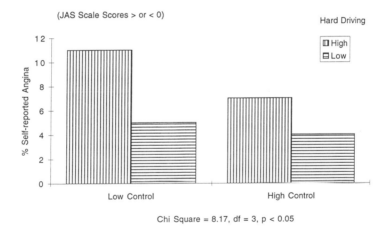

Figure 22.5   Self reported Chest Pain in Low Control (Blue Collar) and High Control (White Collar) Subjects with High and Low JAS Hard-Driving Scores (*Source*: From Byrne & Reinhart, 1989b).

who were both Type A (JAS Global, S, J and H Scales) *and* in a blue collar occupation; this effect was statistically significant.

It seems from these data, then, that at least so far as present symptoms of coronary disease (AP) are concerned, the TABP poses a far greater hazard as a coronary risk factor if found in an individual working in a blue collar occupational environment than if manifested by a white collar worker; it can not be assumed, in other words, that because the TABP is found more frequently in one occupational group (white collar workers), its toxicity as a risk factor will also be most evident in that group.

IMPLICATIONS FOR INTERVENTION IN THE WORKPLACE

Most epidemiologists would agree that the primary purpose for identifying risk factors for CHD (or indeed for any other illness) lies with enhancing the capacity of the clinician to direct intervention towards those risk factors, so reducing the probability of illness events. In examining intervention for CHD risk in the workplace there is little guiding evidence. Workplace based interventions for physical and metabolic risk factors for CHD (elevated cholesterol, cigarette smoking and the like) have met with about the same level of success as interventions directed at any unselected population and the evidence for that is well known. From the psychosocial perspective, however, the field is entirely open. There is no consistent evidence linking occupational status, however conceptualised and measured, with risk or incidence of CHD. Moreover, even if there were, any program of intervention based on enforced or recommended changes in occupational status to produce some reduction in CHD risk, the actual level of which is both unknown and undemonstrable, would be bound to failure.

Two issues arising from the literature discussed above might, however, point to where workplace based interventions could start. First, CHD risk is known to be elevated in those occupational environments characterised by high demand and low control (Alfredson, Karasek & Theorell, 1982). Second, CHD risk has been associated with occupational frustration among those individuals with the TABP (Byrne & Reinhart, 1989b) and indeed, frustration is known to be a common characteristic of many occupational environments irrespective of the behavioural characteristics of individuals occupying those environments (Byrne, 1996). Behavioural interventions to modify the TABP itself are well known and their efficacies equally well demonstrated (Byrne, 1987b). Given the potentially explosive combination of the TABP and occupational frustration, simple behavioural intervention programs for modifying the TABP could very profitably be broadly directed towards individuals or groups in the occupational setting itself. Attempts to orient such programs more specifically towards issues of occupational control would add a further level of sophistication to this. The existing literature simply do not, however, allow us to go much further than this speculation. Issues of individual motivation to change what may be (incorrectly) perceived to be occupationally advantageous behaviours (the TABP), where programs of change are applied in the work setting itself, may further confound the issue. However, given the contemporary emphasis on health promotion through workplace intervention, this will be an area attracting obvious attention in the near future.

CONCLUSIONS

The proposed reconstructed model rearranges what had traditionally been considered to constitute the TABP, departing from a global and somewhat monolithic view and suggesting, instead, a sequential process beginning with a single cognitive predisposition (competitiveness), leading to manifest and now well recognised Type A behaviours which, if frustrated in their expression, trigger both anxiety and aggression with their potentially pathogenic neuroendocrinological consequences. To the extent that a single predisposition is proposed to underlie Type A behaviours, the initiation of these behaviours transcends environmental boundaries. The traditional view of the TABP as espoused for example, by Jenkins (1978), has commonly linked the behaviour pattern at least implicitly with the occupational environment in middle-aged, middle class males, and while the reconstructed model allows the view that competitiveness as a broad cognitive predisposition regulates behavioural responses to any environment and in any individual regardless of age or gender, it allows greater specificity than has hitherto been possible as to why the occupational situation seems to consistently associated with coronary risk in the epidemiological literature. It also goes someway to explaining why, in common with all other risk factors for cardiovascular disease, the possession of the TABP does not universally predict clinical incidence of CHD. Quite simply, possession of the risk factor (in this case the TABP) is a much more powerful predictor of the clinical state if it occurs in combination with other psychosocial factors (a frustrating occupational environment in the present example) than if it occurs in isolation.

The ultimate currency of the hypothesis will rest with a demonstration of the biological link between frustrated Type A behaviours and the pathophysiology of CHD. The sequential nature of this model, together with the specificity of the nexus between manifest behaviour and frustration does, however, hold the promise of a convenient test of that hypothesis in the laboratory.

References

Alfredson, L., Karasek, R. & Theorell, T. (1982) Myocardial infarction risk and psychosocial work environment: An analysis of the male Swedish working force. *Social Science and Medicine*, **16**, 463–467.

Alfredson, L. & Theorell, T. (1983) Job characteristics of occupations and myocardial infarction risk: Effect of possible confounding factors. *Social Science and Medicine*, **17**, 1497–1503.

Bandura, A. (1976) *Social Learning Theory*. Prentice Hall: Englewood Cliffs.

Bass, C. & Wade, C. (1982) Type A behaviour: Not specifically pathogenic? *Lancet*, **2**, 1147–1150.

Beck, A. T. & Emery, G. (1985) *Anxiety Disorders and Phobias: A Cognitive Perspective*. Basic Books: New York.

Bolm-Audorff, U. & Siegrist, J. (1983) Occupational morbidity data in myocardial infarction. *Journal of Occupational Medicine*, **25**, 367–371.

Byrne, D. G. (1981) Type A behavior, life events and myocardial infarction: Independent or related risk factors? *British Journal of Medical Psychology*, **54**, 371–377.

Byrne, D. G. (1987a) Personality, life events and cardiovascular disease: Invited review. *Journal of Psychosomatic Research*, **31**, 661–671.

Byrne, D. G. (1987b) *The Behavioral Management of the Cardiac Patient*. New Jersey: Ablex Publishing Corporation.

Byrne, D. G. (1996) Type A behaviour, anxiety and neuroticism: Reconceptualising the pathophysiological paths and boundaries of coronary-prone behaviour. *Stress Medicine*, **12**, 227–238.

Byrne, D. G. & Byrne, A. E. (1990) Stress, Type A behavior and heart disease. In *Stress and Anxiety*, edited by C. D. Spielberger, I Sarason, J. Brebner & J. Strelau, pp. 233–246. Washington: Hemisphere Press.

Byrne, D. G. & Reinhart, M. I. (1989a) Work characteristics, occupational achievement and the Type A behaviour pattern. *Journal of Occupational Psychology*, **62**, 123–134.

Byrne, D. G. & Reinhart, M. I. (1989b) Occupation, Type A behaviour and self-reported angina pectoris. *Journal of Psychosomatic Research*, **33**, 609–619.

Byrne, D. G. & Reinhart, M. I. (1990) Self-reported distress, job dissatisfaction and the Type A behavior pattern in a sample of full-time employed Australians. *Work and Stress*, **4**, 155–166.

Byrne, D. G. & Reinhart, M. (1994) Type A behaviour (Jenkins Activity Scale scores), job satisfaction and risk of coronary heart disease. *Stress Medicine*, **10**, 223–231.

Byrne, D. G. & Reinhart, M. I. (1995) Type A behaviour in the Australian working population. *Australian New Zealand Journal of Psychiatry*, **29**, 270–277.

Byrne, D. G., Reinhart, M. I. & Heaven, P. C. L. (1989) Type A behaviour and the authoritarian personality. *British Journal of Medical Psychology*, **26**, 163–172.

Byrne, D. G. & Rosenman, R. H. (1986) The Type A behaviour pattern as a precursor to stressful life events: A confluence of coronary risks. *British Journal of Medical Psychology*, **59**, 75–82.

Byrne, D. G. & Rosenman, R. H. (1987) Type A behaviour and the experience of affective discomfort. *Journal of Psychosomatic Research*, **30**, 663–672.

Byrne, D. G. & Rosenman, R. H. (1990) *Anxiety and the Heart*. Washington: Hemisphere Publishing Corporation.

Byrne, D. G., Rosenman, R. H., Schiller, E. & Chesney, M. A. (1985) Consistency and variation among instruments purporting to measure the Type A behavior pattern. *Psychosomatic Medicine*, **47**, 242–261.

Chesney, M. A. & Rosenman, R. H. (1980) Type A behavior in the work setting. In *Current Concerns in Occupational Stress*, edited by C. L. Cooper & R. Payne (eds.). New York: John Wiley & Sons Ltd.

Chesney, M. A. & Rosenman, R. H. (1985) *Anger and Hostility in Cardiovascular and Behavioral Disorders*. Washington: Hemisphere Publishing Corporation.

Craik, K. J. W. (1948) *The Nature of Explanation*. Cambridge: Cambridge University Press.

Derogatis, L. R., Rickels, K., Uhlenhuth, E. H. & Covi, L. (1974) The Hopkins Symptom Check List (HSCL): A measure of primary symptom dimensions. In *Psychological Measurements in Psychopharmacology*, edited by P. Pichot , pp. 79–110. Karger: Basel.

Frank, F. D. & Weintraub, J. (1973) Job satisfaction and mortality from coronary heart disease: Critique of some of the research. *Journal of Chronic Diseases*, **36**, 351–354.

French, J. R. P. & Caplan, R. D. (1970) Psychosocial factors in coronary heart disease. *Industrial Medicine and Surgery*, **39**, 31–45.

Friedman, E. H. & Hellerstein, H. K. (1968) Occupational stress, law school hierarchy, and coronary artery disease in Cleveland attorneys. *Psychosomatic Medicine*, **30**, 72–86.

Friedman, M. (1969) *Pathogenesis of Coronary Artery Disease*. New York: McGraw-Hill.

Glass, D. C. (1977) *Behavior Patterns, Stress and Coronary Disease*. Hillsdale: Lawrence Erlbaum.

Goldberg, D. P. (1972) *The Detection of Psychiatric Illness by Questionnaire*. London: Oxford University Press.

Hart, K. E. (1983) Physical symptom reporting and health perception among Type A and B college males. *Journal of Human Stress*, **9**, 17–22.

Haw, M. A. (1982) Women, work and stress: A review and agenda for the future. *Journal of Health and Social Behavior*, **23**, 132–144.

Haynes, S. G. & Feinleib, M. (1980) Women, work and coronary heart disease: Prospective findings from the Framingham heart study. *American Journal of Public Health*, **70**, 133–141.

Haynes, S., Feinleib, M. & Kannel, W. (1980) The relationship of psychosocial factors to coronary heart disease in the Framingham study: III. Eight year incidence of CHD. *American Journal of Epidemiology*, **111**, 37–58.

Haynes, S. G., Feinleib, M., Levine, S., Scotch, N. & Kannel, W. B. (1978) The relationship at psychosocial factors to coronary heart disease: II. Prevalence of coronary heart disease. *American Journal of Epidemiology*, **107**, 384–402.

Henderson, A. S., Byrne, D. G. & Duncan-Jones, P. (1981) *Neurosis and the Social Environment*. Sydney, Academic Press.

Herman, S., Blumenthal, J. A., Black, G. M. & Chesney, M. A. (1981) Self-ratings of Type A (coronary prone) adults: Do Type A's know they are Type A's. *Psychosomatic Medicine*, **43**, 405–413.

Hill, A. B. (1956) The environment and disease: Association or causation. *Proceedings of the Royal Society of Medicine*, **58**, 295–300.

Houston, B. K. (1988) Cardiovascular and neuroendocrine reactivity, global Type A and components of Type A behavior. In *Type A Behavior Pattern: Research, Theory and Intervention*, edited by B. K. Houston and C. R. Snyder, pp. 212–253. New York: Wiley.

Howard, J. H., Cunningham, D. A. & Rechnitzer, P. A. (1977) Work patterns associated with Type A behavior: A managerial population. *Human Relations*, **30**, 825–836.

Hoyenga, K. B. & Hoyenga, K. T. (1984) *Motivational Explanations of Behavior: Evolutionary, Physiological and Cognitive Ideas*. Monterey: Brooks Cole.

James, W. (1892) *Textbook of Psychology*. London: Macmillan & Co.

Jenkins, C. D. (1978). A comparative review of the interview and questionnaire methods in the assessment of the coronary prone behavior pattern. In *Coronary Prone Behavior*, edited by T. M. Dembroski, S. M. Weiss, J. L. Shields, S. G. Haynes & M. Feinleib, pp. 71–86. New York: Springer Verlag.

Jenkins, C. D., Zyzanski, S. J. & Rosenman, R. H. (1979) *Manual of the Jenkins Activity Survey*. Palo Alto: Consulting Psychologists Press.

Karasek, R., Baker, D., Marxer, F., Ahlborn, A. & Theorell, T. (1981) Job decision latitude, job demands and cardiovascular disease: A prospective study of Swedish men. *American Journal of Public Health*, **71**, 694–705.

Kasl, S. V. (1978) Epidemiological contribution to the study of work stress. In *Stress at Work*, edited by C. Cooper & R. Payne, pp. 1–48. New York: Wiley.

Kornitzer, M., Kittel, F., Debacker, G. & Dramaix, M. (1981) The Belgian heart disease prevention project: Type A behavior pattern and the prevalence of coronary heart disease. *Psychosomatic Medicine*, **43**, 133–145.

Kornitzer, M., Thilly, C. H., Van Roux, A. & Balthazar, R. (1975) Incidence of ischemic heart disease in two cohorts of Belgian clerks. *British Journal of Preventive and Social Medicine*, **29**, 91–97.

Langosch, W., Brodner, G. & Bocherding, H. (1983) Psychological and vocational long-term outcomes of cardiac rehabilitation with post-infarction patients under the age of forty. *Psychotherapy and Psychosomatics*, **40**, 115–128.

Lawson, R. (1965) *Frustration: The Development of a Scientific Concept*. New York: Macmillan.

Lazarus, R. S. (1966) *Psychological Stress and the Coping Process*. McGraw Hill, New York.

Liljefors, I. & Rahe, R. H. (1970) An identical twin study of psychosocial factors in coronary heart disease in Sweden. *Psychosomatic Medicine*, **32**, 523–542.

Magnus, K., Matroos, A. W. & Strackel, J. (1983) The self-employed and the self-driven: Two coronary prone sub-populations from the Zeist study. *American Journal of Epidemiology*, **118**, 799–805.

Mandler, G. (1984) *Mind and Body: Psychology of Emotion and Stress*. New York: W. W. Norton.

Maschewsky, W. (1982) The relation between stress and myocardial infarction: A general analysis. *Social Science and Medicine*, **16**, 455–462.

Matthews, K. A., Glass, D. C., Rosenman, R. H. & Bortner, R. W. (1977) Competitive drive, pattern A and coronary heart disease: A further analysis of some data from the Western Collaborative Group Study. *Journal of Chronic Diseases*, **30**, 489–498.

Matthews, K. A. & Haynes, S. G. (1986) Type A behavior and coronary disease risk: Update and critical evaluation. *American Journal of Epidemiology*, **123**, 923–960.

Montagu, A. (1976) *The Nature of Human Aggression*. New York: Oxford University Press.

Mundal., R., Erikssen, J. & Rodahl, K. (1982) Latent ischemic heart disease in sea captains. *Scandinavian Journal of Work Environment and Health*, **8**, 178–184.

Orth-Gomer, K. (1979) Ischemic heart disease and psychological stress in Stockholm and New York. *Journal of Psychosomatic Research*, **23**, 165–173.

Orth-Gomer, K. & Johnson, J. V. (1987) Social network interaction and mortality: A six year follow-up study of a random sample of the Swedish population. *Journal of Chronic Diseases*, **40**, 949–957.

Price, V. A. (1982) *Type A Behavior Pattern: A Model For Research and Practice*. New York: Academic Press.

Ragland, D. R. & Brand, R. J. (1988) Type A behavior and mortality from coronary heart disease. *New England Journal of Medicine*, **318**, 65–69.

Rosenman, R. H. (1988) The impact of certain emotions in cardiovascular disorders. In *Individual Differences, Stress and Health Psychology*, edited by M. P. Janisse, pp. 2–25. New York: Springer-Verlag.

Rosenman, R. H. (1990) Type A behavior pattern: A personal overview. *Journal of Social Behavior and Personality*, **5**, 1–24.

Rosenman, R. H. & Chesney, M. A. (1981) The relationship of Type A behavior pattern to coronary heart disease. *Activitas Nervosa Superieur*, **22**, 1 45.

Rosenman, R. H. & Ward, M. M. (1988) The changing concept of cardiovascular reactivity. *Stress Medicine*, **4**, 241–251.

Russek, H. I. (1960) Emotional stress and coronary heart disease in American physicians. *American Journal of Medical Sciences*, **240**, 711–721.

Russek, H. I. (1965) Stress, tobacco and coronary disease in North American professional groups. *Journal of the American Medical Association*, **192**, 89–94.

Sales, S. M. & House, J. (1971) Job dissatisfaction as a possible risk factor in coronary heart disease. *Journal of Chronic Diseases*, **23**, 861–873.

Shekelle, R. B., Gale, M. & Norussis, M. (1985) Type A score (Jenkins Activity Survey) and risk of recurrent coronary heart disease in the Aspirin Myocardial Infarction Study. *American Journal of Cardiology*, **56**, 221–225.

Siegrist, J. (1984) Threat to social status and cardiovascular risk. *Psychotherapy and Psychosomatics*, **42**, 90–96.

Spielberger, C. D., Gorsuch, R. L. & Lushene, R. (1970) *State Trait Anxiety Inventory*. Consulting Psychologists Press: Palo Alto.

Susser, M. (1973) *Causal Thinking in the Health Sciences*. New York: Oxford University Press.

Theorell, T. & Floderus-Myrhed, B. (1977) 'Workload' and risk of myocardial infarction—a prospective psychosocial analysis. *International Journal of Epidemiology*, **6**, 17–21.

Theorell, T. & Rahe, R. H. (1971) Psychosocial factors and myocardial infarction: I. An in-patient study in Sweden. *Journal of Psychosomatic Research*, **15**, 25–31.

Vingerhoets, A. J. J. M. & Flohr, P. J. M. (1984) Type A behaviour and self reports of coping preferences. *British Journal of Medical Psychology*, **47**, 15–21.

Yates, A. J. (1962) *Frustration and Conflict*. New York: John Wiley and Sons.

Young, P. T. (1961) *Motivation and Emotion: A Survey of the Determinants of Human and Animal Activity*. John Wiley and Sons, New York.

Zajonc, R. B. & Markus, H. (1984) Affect and cognition: The hard interface. In *Emotions, Cognition and Behavior*, edited by C. E. Izard, J. Kagan & R. B. Zajonc, pp. 73–102.Cambridge: Cambridge University Press.

Zorn, E. W., Harrington, J. M. & Goethe, H. (1977) Ischemic heart disease and work stress in West German sea pilots. *Journal of Occupational Medicine*, **19**, 762–765.

Chapter 23

STRESS IN ACADEME: Some Recent Research Findings

Anthony H. Winefield, PhD

INTRODUCTION

University teaching has traditionally been regarded as a low stress occupation. Although not highly paid, academics have been envied because of the fact that they enjoyed tenure*, light work loads, flexibility, 'perks' such as overseas trips for study and/or conference purposes, and the freedom to pursue their own research interests.

Most theoretical perspectives would support such a view. Karasek (1979), for example, has proposed a theory of occupational stress (the demands-control theory) according to which jobs that combine high levels of demand with low levels of autonomy, control, or decision latitude should be the most stressful. In the past, academic jobs would clearly not have fallen in this category.

Another influential theory of occupational stress is the person-environment fit model proposed by French, Caplan and Harrison (1984). This theory sees stress as arising from a misfit (either objective or subjective) between the requirements of the job and the needs or aspirations of the individual. Again, given that most academics in the past have chosen a university career precisely because they found the work congenial (most academics have experienced both teaching and research before embarking on an academic career), such misfits would be rare.

According to both of these theories if academic work has become stressful, it must be because the nature of the work has changed. There are good reasons to believe that it has. During the past fifteen years most of the advantages associated with academic work have been eroded in many countries. Academic salaries have fallen in real terms in countries such as

---

* Since writing this in mid-1996 many Australian academics in 'tenured' positions have been made redundant.

the US, the UK, Australia and New Zealand. Increasing numbers of academic positions are now untenured; work loads have increased; and academics are under increased pressures to attract external funds for their research and to 'publish or perish'. Universities and academic Departments are being subjected to external 'quality' audits which scrutinise their research output in terms of both quantity and quality as well as teaching. Future funding support is determined by the outcomes of such audits. As Shirley Fisher (1994) says in relation to British universities in her recent book 'Stress in Academic Life':

> The demands on academics have risen rapidly over the last ten years ... there has been a steady erosion of job control. All the signs are that this will continue (p. 61).

Dr Fisher's prophetic ability has been confirmed by the recent savage cuts to higher education funding in Australia announced in the latest budget.

Not surprisingly occupational stress researchers around the world have become increasingly interested in the effects of these deteriorating employ-ment conditions and increased work pressures arising from increased bureacratic interference. I will review some recent studies carried out in the US, the UK, New Zealand and Australia which have addressed the problem of academic stress. The research questions addressed are as follows:

1. What are the perceived sources of academic stress?
2. What professional/personal characteristics are associated with academic stress?
3. Has academic stress increased in recent years?
4. How does the level of strain compare with those found in other occupational groups?
5. Are there differences in levels of academic stress between different countries?

PERCEIVED SOURCES OF ACADEMIC STRESS

Gmelch and his colleagues at Washington State University (Gmelch et al. 1984; 1986) carried out a large national survey in the United States in which they randomly sampled 40 public and 40 private universities from all 184 doctoral-granting institutions. The sample was stratified on the basis of type of discipline (the eight distinguished by Biglan, 1973), and academic rank (assistant, associate and full professor). The number of respondents was 1,221, a response rate of 67%. Factor analysis of a 45-item scale, the Faculty Stress Index, resulted in 5 factors: 1. Reward and recognition; 2. Time constraints; 3. Departmental influence; 4. Professional identity; and 5. Student interaction.

Gmelch et al. (1984) also identified the ten most serious sources of stress (of the 45 described in the FSI). These situations were those classified as the most serious sources of stress by at least a third of their respondents.

More recently, Hind & Doyle (1996) in the UK have confirmed the findings reported by Gmelch et al. (1984). First, there was remarkable agreement about the most serious sources of stress as shown in Table 23.1. Second, factor analysis of the 45-item Faculty Stress Indicator resulted in the same five factors as those described by Gmelch et al.

Another recent study from the UK identified 'inadequate resources', 'having too much work to do' and 'a feeling that the organization does not care about its staff' as the three most frequently cited sources of stress among university staff (Daniels & Guppy, 1994).

Similar results to those reported from the US and the UK were found in a recent survey carried out in New Zealand by Boyd and Wylie (1994). Their study was based on responses from more than 500 academic staff and more than 600 support staff. They identified 39 potential sources of stress of which the ten most frequently rated as 'always' or 'often' stressful are shown in Table 23.2.

Although the situations are described in somewhat different terms, it is fairly clear that the sorts of things found to be most stressful by academics are fairly similar in the different countries. Similar findings have been found in Australian universities by Dua (1994), Sharpley (1994) and by Jarrett & Winefield (1995).

One discrepant finding has been reported recently by Blix, Cruise, Mitchell & Blix (1994) in a survey carried out on 158 tenure-track teachers sampled from the California State University system. They found that their

Table 23.1   Ten situations identified as most serious sources of stress by Gmelch et al. (1984) in US universities and by Hind & Doyle (1996) in UK universities.

Situation	% indicating serious source of stress (Gmelch et al., 1984)	% indicating serious source of stress (Hind & Doyle 1996)
1 Excessively high self expectations	53%	39%
2 Securing financial support for research	50%	50%
3 Inadequate time to keep up to date	49%	56%
4 Inadequate salary	41%	47%
5 Preparing manuscripts for publication	40%	–
6 Excessively heavy workload	40%	56%
7 Job demands interfere with personal life	35%	40%
8 Unsatisfactory career advancement	34%	–
9 Frequent interruptions	33%	37%
10 Meetings that take too much time	33%	44%
11 Conflict between personal and departmental goals	–	43%
12 Inadequate time for teaching preparation	–	42%

Table 23.2   Ten situations identified as most serious sources of stress by Boyd & Wylie (1994) in NZ universities.

	Situation	% indicating serious source of stress (Hind & Doyle 1996)
1	Overall level of workload	55%
2	Deadlines/demands	50%
3	Interruptions to work	48%
4	Staffing levels for area	35%
5	University climate/morale	34%
6	Support staff time	34%
7	Level of research funding	34%
8	Method of research funding	33%
9	Lack of recognition for work	32%
10	Student numbers/class sizes	30%

participants reported higher stress scores in research-related activities unlike the participants in the study by Gmelch et al. (1984) where teaching was perceived as most stressful. This difference could be due to the different populations sampled in the two studies, to increased pressures/ reduced resources to carry out research occurring over the ten year period between the studies, or to both.

WHAT PROFESSIONAL/PERSONAL CHARACTERISTICS ARE ASSOCIATED WITH ACADEMIC STRESS?

Gmelch and his colleagues (1986) analysed each of the five factors mentioned earlier (see Table 23.3) according to professional and personal characteristics. Except for a few minor differences, there was remarkable agreement across disciplines. Not surprisingly, they found that untenured academics perceived greater stress on all five factors than tenured staff and that perceived stress declined with increased rank. Also, there were statistically significant differences between assistant and associate professors on 1. Reward and recognition; 4. Professional identity; and 5.

Table 23.3   Five Dimensions (Factors) of Faculty Stress (Gmelch et al., 1986) and items with highest factor loading.

	Factor	Items with highest loading
1	Reward and recognition	Insufficient reward for service (.74)
2	Time constraints	Feeling that I have too heavy a work load (.67)
3	Departmental influence	Resolving differences with my chair (.81)
4	Professional/identity	Preparing a manuscript for publication (.62)
5	Student interaction	Evaluating the performance of students (.62)

Student interaction (but not on 2 and 3) and statistically significant difference between associate and full professors on all five factors.

Differences between disciplines emerged on only two factors: 1. Reward and recognition and 5. Student interaction. With respect to reward and recognition, the 'soft, pure, nonlife' disciplines (e.g. history) were most stressed and with respect to student interaction, the 'soft, pure, life' displines (e.g. psychology) and the 'hard, applied, nonlife' displines (e.g. engineering) were most stressed.

Other demographic variables studied were age and sex. With respect to age, there was a decline in reported stress on only two of the five factors: time constraints and professional identity. With respect to sex, again there were differences only with respect to time constraints and professional identity. In each case women were significantly more stressed than men. This finding has been confirmed in studies by Blix et al. (1994) in the US, by Boyd & Wylie (1994) in New Zealand, and by Sharpley (1994) in Australia. On the other hand studies by the Association of University Teachers (1990) and by Abouserie (1996) in the UK, and by Jarrett & Winefield (1995) in Australia have reported no sex difference.

Abouserie (1996) found that stress was highest in more junior members of the academic staff, as did Jarrett & Winefield (1995). Finally, Richard & Krieshok (1989) in the US reported that all faculty members experienced similar role stressors, regardless of sex or rank.

HAS ACADEMIC STRESS INCREASED IN RECENT YEARS?

One of the problems inherent in much research on occupational stress is the fact that the measures of environmental stress frequently depend on self-report measures, as do measures of psychological strain, or distress. Spector & Brannick (1995) and others have called this the problem of common method variance. In the case of academic work, there is at least one objective measure of environmental stress: the student to staff ratio. Several reports have drawn attention to the deteriorating (i.e. increasing) student to staff ratios in universities in the UK, Australia and New Zealand during recent years. The increased workload implied by this is reflected in complaints by academics of insufficient time to perform their work adequately and are illustrated by the concerns expressed in the studies by Gmelch et al. (1984); Hind & Doyle (1996)—shown in Table 23.1—and by Boyd & Wylie (1994).

HOW DOES THE LEVEL OF STRAIN COMPARE WITH THOSE FOUND IN OTHER OCCUPATIONAL GROUPS?

Some studies have compared stress levels in academic and university support staff. Others have used measures that have also been widely used in studies of other occupational groups. Studies that have surveyed both academic and general staff have generally shown higher stress levels in the academic staff (Blix et al., 1994; Boyd & Wylie, 1994; Jarrett & Winefield, 1995). Sharpley (1994) on the other hand, found no overall difference. (The finding by Blix et al. was surprising because the academic staff showed significantly higher levels of person-environment fit than the administrative staff).

A possible explanation for higher stress levels in academic than in administrative university staff derives from the public nature of most aspects of academic work: undergraduate teaching, postgraduate supervision, and research. Poor performance in any of these areas is readily exposed to external scrutiny. For example, undergraduate lectures can be attended by colleagues, and lecturers are routinely subjected to student evaluations of their teaching. Student evaluations of teaching are expected to be included in 'teaching portfolios' that are taken into account by tenure and promotions committees. In the case of postgraduate supervision, poor performance is hard to conceal. Academics who fail to attract postgraduate students, or whose postgraduate students drop out, or whose theses are failed by examiners, are clearly poor performers. Finally, poor research performance is easily identified. Academics who never publish, who never attract external funding for their research, and whose publications (if any) are never cited are clearly not performing satisfactorily. There can be few occupations in which performance is so open to public scrutiny.

Jarrett & Winefield (1995) used the 12-item version of Goldberg's General Health Questionnaire as a measure of strain which has been recommended by Banks et al. (1980) as an indicator of mental ill—health in occupational studies. We found that a sample of academics from an Australian university scored more highly than other occupational groups, including engineering employees, prison officers, teachers, and transport workers. Moreover Bradley & Eachus (1995) found in a recent study of a UK higher education institution using the Occupational Stress Indicator (Cooper et al., 1988) that a sample of 306 scored significantly higher than estimated population norms (based on $N = 8038$) on the following four sources of stress: Factors intrinsic to the job; Relationships with other people; Career and achievement; and Organizational structure and climate.

ARE THERE DIFFERENCES IN LEVELS OF ACADEMIC STRESS BETWEEN COUNTRIES?

Hind & Doyle (1996) surveyed 600 academic psychologists from 85 randomly selected institutions of higher education. Overall, the levels of stress reported in the UK study were significantly higher than those from the US. This finding does not, of course, imply that UK academics experience greater job stress than their US counterparts, given that the UK data were collected more than ten years later than those from the US and the identified sources of stress will have become greater during this period.

Data collected by Jarrett & Winefield (1995) suggest that levels of academic stress in Australia may be even higher than in the UK. Jarrett & Winefield sampled all staff at an Australian university and obtained a response rate of 65% among academic staff (N = 448) and 77% of general staff (N = 1513). One of the main outcome measures used was the GHQ-12 (Goldberg, 1972). This measure was also used in two recent UK studies of academic stress. For example, Wilkinson and Joseph (1995) also used the GHQ-12 and reported a mean score of 2.15 (using binary scoring (SD = 2.98) in a sample of 105 academic staff members form the University of Essex). They pointed out that this was 'slightly higher than the widely used cut-off point of two taken to indicate risk of psychiatric disturbance' (p. 6). By contrast, the overall mean in the Jarrett & Winefield (1995) Australian university sample of 1961 was 2.44. Among the 743 members of the academic staff it was even higher, 2.84 (SD = 3.42), which is significantly higher than the mean reported by Wilkinson and Joseph (1995), t (846) = 1.97, $p < .05$.

Daniels and Guppy (1992) also used the GHQ-12 (with Likert scoring) and obtained a mean of 11.30 (SD = 4.70) on a sample of 221 academic and support staff from a British university. Again, this was significantly lower than the mean obtained in the Jarrett & Winefield sample (N = 1961) of 12.2 (SD = 5.9), t (2180) = 2.20, $p < .05$.

SUMMARY AND CONCLUSIONS

It needs to be acknowledged that some of the studies cited in this brief review have been based on low response rates (well below 50%). Such low response rates could compromise the external validity of the findings because of the danger of positive bias (i.e. the most stressed individuals might have been those most likely to participate). Nonetheless, there is overwhelming evidence that academic work is becoming increasingly stressful in many countries. Recent studies reported from the US, the UK, Australia and New Zealand have all shown high levels of stress associated with increased work loads and reduced rewards. Student to staff ratios, an objective measure of workload, have increased in most of these countries over the past 15 years as have subjective reports of increased pressure.

Moreover, the increasing tendency for academic performance to be subjected to external evaluation via quality audits, the outcomes of which determine future funding levels, have exacerbated the situation. Academics are particularly vulnerable to such pressures because every aspect of their performance—undergraduate teaching, postgraduate supervision, and research—is open to public scrutiny. Increased work loads have made it difficult or impossible for academics to maintain standards of excellence in all three areas, thereby forcing them either to choose to concentrate on one or two areas at the expense of the third or else to work excessively long hours and thereby risk exhaustion—physical, intellectual and emotional. In either case, the overall quality of their work is likely to suffer, as well as their physical and psychological well-being. The following conclusions are drawn:

1. The combination of increased workloads arising from continued funding cuts, along with external pressures from external performance audits, has resulted in a widespread perception of insufficient time (and resources) to perform at a high level.
2. The perceived sources of stress are similar across disciplines, although untenured academics and female academics seem to be most vulnerable.
3. There is persuasive evidence that academic stress has increased over the past fifteen years.
4. Academic stress levels are high by comparison with other occupational groups.
5. There is evidence that levels of academic stress are higher in the UK than in the US, and higher in Australia than in the UK.

Unless steps are taken to redress the situation, the following consequences seem inevitable: (a) academic staff will become increasingly vulnerable to 'burnout' (emotional exhaustion, depersonalisation, and reduced personal accomplishment); (b) the quality of teaching and research carried out in our universities will decline; (c) academic careers will become increasingly unattractive to the most able young people; (d) the standards of the universities will decline; (e) the intellectual life of the country will suffer.

IMPLICATIONS AND RECOMMENDATIONS

This final section considers factors that might help to reduce occupational stress in university academics. First, as Cooper (1997) pointed out recently, although there have been numerous cross-sectional studies reported in the literature documenting the psychological and physical damage associated with high levels of occupational stress, there is an urgent need for more longitudinal research. Only longitudinal research can monitor the effects on individuals of changes in the workplace. This is equally true for changes for the worse as well as changes for the better. Repeated observations of the same individuals over time can document the long-term effects of occupational stress, as well as enable investigators to evaluate the effectiveness of interventions designed to reduce stress.

Second, a possibility implied by the Person-Environment Fit theory is that academic stress may decrease with time, as different sorts of people enter the profession. For example, if being an academic in the future is going to require the exercise of entrepreneurial skills (which it has not in the past), individuals who possess such skills are more likely to be attracted to the profession and consequently experience less of a misfit than the previous generation of academics.

Third, in accordance with Demand-Control theory, interventions might be considered that reduce the demands/pressures associated with academic work and/or increase (or restore) autonomy or decision latitude. For example, the workloads of academics might be reduced by providing more research and/or teaching assistance or by introducing computer-assisted instruction.

Fourth, universities might organise stress management courses for academic staff members so that they develop effective and appropriate strategies for managing stress.

Unless some interventions are considered there seems to be a real danger that the pressures under which many academics currently operate will have serious implications for their productivity as well as their job satisfaction and psychological and physical health.

References

Abouserie, R. (1996) Stress, coping strategies and job satisfaction in university academic staff. *Educational Psychology*, **16**, 49–56.

Association of University Teachers (1990) *Goodwill under Stress: Morale in UK Universities*. England: The Association of University Teachers.

Banks, M. H., Clegg, C. W., Jackson, P. R., Kemp, N. J., Stafford, E. M. & Wall, T. D. (1980) The use of the General Health Questionnaire as an indicator of mental health in occupational studies. *Journal of Occupational Psychology*, **53**, 187–194.

Biglan, A. (1973) The characteristics of subject matter in different academic areas. *Journal of Applied Psychology*, **57**, 195–203.

Blix, A. G., Cruise, R. J., Mitchell, B. M. & Blix, G. G. (1994) Occupational stress among university teachers. *Educational Research*, **36**, 157–169.

Boyd, S. & Wylie, C. (1994) Workload and stress in New Zealand universities. New Zealand Council for Educational Research and the Association of University Staff of New Zealand.

Bradley, J. & Eachus, P. (1995) Occupational stress within a U.K. Higher Education Institution. *International Journal of Stress Management*, **2**, 145–158.

Cooper, C. L. (1997) The changing nature of work: Future stressors and their implications. Paper given at Fifth European Congress of Psychology, Dublin.

Cooper, C. L., Sloan, S. J. & Williams, S. (1988) *Occupational Stress Indicator: Management Guide*. Windsor, UK: NFER-Nelson.

Daniels, K. & Guppy, A. (1992) Control, information-seeking preferences, occupational stressors and psychological well-being. *Work and Stress*, **6**, 347–353.

Daniels, K. & Guppy, A. (1994) An exploratory study of stress in a British University. *Higher Education Quarterly*, **48**, 135–144.

Dua, J. K. (1994) Job stressors and their effects on physical health, emotional health, and job satisfaction in a university. *Journal of Educational Administration*, **32**, 59–78.

Fisher, S. (1994) *Stress in Academic Life: The Mental Assembly Line*. Buckingham: Open University Press.

French, J. R. P. Jr., Caplan, R. D. & van Harrison, R. (1984) *The Mechanisms of Job Stress and Strain*. New York: Wiley.

Gmelch, W. H., Lovrich, N. P. & Wilke, P. K. (1984) Sources of stress in academe: A national perspective. *Research in Higher Education*, **20**, 477–490.

Gmelch, W. H., Wilke, P. K. & Lovrich, N. P. (1986) Dimensions of stress among university faculty: Factor-analytic results from a national study. *Research in Higher Education*, **24**, 266–286.

Goldberg, D. P. (1972) *The Detection of Psychiatric Illness by Questionnaire*. London: Oxford University Press.

Hind, P. & Doyle, C. (1996) A cross cultural comparison of perceived occupational stress in academics in higher education. Paper given at XXVI International Congress of Psychology: Montreal.

Jarrett, R. J. & Winefield, A. H. (1995) Report on climate survey. University of Adelaide (Unpublished report).

Karasek, R. A. (1979) Job demands, job decision latitude, and mental strain: Implications for job redesign. *Administrative Science Quarterly*, **24**, 285–308.

Richard, G. V. & Krieshok, T. S. (1989) Occupational stress, strain and coping strategies in university faculty. *Journal of Vocational Behaviour*, **34**, 117–132.

Sharpley, C. F. (1994) Report of a survey of stress and health at Monash University. Melbourne: Centre for Stress Management and Research, Faculty of Education, Monash University.

Spector, P. E. & Brannick, M. T. (1995) The nature and effects of method variance in organizational research. In *International Review of Industrial and Organizational Psychology*, edited by C. L. Cooper & I. T. Robinson, Vol. 10, Chapter 8, pp. 249–274. London: Wiley.

Wilkinson, J. & Joseph, S. (1995) Burnout in university teaching staff. *The Occupational Psychologist*, **27**, 4–7.

INDEX